Lara Briden is a naturopathic doctor with more than twenty years experience in women's health. She runs a busy hormone clinic in Sydney, Australia where she treats women with PCOS, PMS, endometriosis, and many other period problems.

Follow Lara's Hormone Blog at www.larabriden.com

Twitter, Instagram, and Facebook: @LaraBriden

PERIOD REPAIR MANUAL

second edition

> NATURAL TREATMENT FOR BETTER
> HORMONES AND BETTER PERIODS

LARA BRIDEN ND

GREENPEAK
PUBLISHING

DISCLAIMER

The information contained in this book is intended to help readers make informed decisions about their health. It is not a substitute for medical treatment by a professional healthcare provider. If you have a medical problem or need medical advice, please see your doctor.

The names and details of some individuals have been changed.

Revised second edition July 2018
Second edition September 2017
First edition January 2015

For further information visit the author's website at
http://www.larabriden.com

to my patients

CONTENTS

FOREWORD

By Jerilynn C. Prior MD, Endocrinology Professor

Having worked as a clinician and scientist of women's reproductive and bone health for over forty years, I am convinced that women's self-knowledge is empowering and healing. Let me explain why I say that.

Years ago I conducted a randomized, blinded one-year therapy study that restored half of the participants who had abnormal menstrual cycles or ovulation to perfect cycles. At baseline, these 61 normal-weight, otherwise healthy women in their twenties and thirties had absent or far-apart periods or regular cycles without egg release or with repeated short times from egg release to the next period related, not to disease, but to combinations of very personal stressors. Their recovery couldn't be accounted for by the cyclic progesterone or calcium supplementation or placebo we gave during this trial, or to weight gain, or less exercise. Therefore, these women's perfectly normal menstrual cycles and ovulation, by the end of the study, were likely due to learning more about themselves in the supportive environment of a participatory, scientific study.

Self-knowledge means awareness. For example, I know I am more critical of myself than some and more ambitious than others. Self-knowledge also means "body literacy," as my educator-reporter friend Laura Wershler terms it. This body literacy allows me to appreciate, based on solid personal evidence, that my luteal phase will be short if I hike the Chilkoot trail for seven days, climbing from sea level up into the alpine, carrying a pack with a companion who is not simpatico. It also means knowing that this same combination of emotional, exertional and nutritional stressors when I was a decade younger would have made my period go away. This book will help you attain such empowering body literacy.

My first thought upon seeing the title and before reading the book, was that it would treat women's reproductive system as a rigid, inflexible machine that requires fixing by a greasy-handed, muscle-bound mechanic. I was concerned, because an engine-related concept doesn't fit with my understanding of how integrative, adaptable and self-healing our reproductive system is —if given a chance. My second thought was that this book would be full of orders to do this or avoid that inexplicable thing.

I was wrong. On reading this latest edition, I find that naturopathic physician, Lara Briden, shows great respect for the complexity and integrative powers of women's reproductive system. Furthermore, she takes an amazingly physiological and scientific approach to most aspects of women's menstrual cycles and their variations. She usually does a good job of explaining mysterious things and provides many and up-to-date medical journal references. I especially like that she identifies where the data are few, and where medical doctors and naturopaths are likely to disagree. Even better, she prepares women to speak with their physicians from a position of self-awareness, careful observation, and record-keeping, while feeling strong as self-advocates.

For women everywhere, this book is an appealing, personable and empowering introduction to understanding our body ourselves.

Jerilynn C. Prior, professor of endocrinology at the University of British Columbia, founder and scientific director of the Centre for Menstrual Cycle and Ovulation Research (www.cemcor.ca), director of the British Columbia Centre of the Canadian Multicentre Osteoporosis Study (www.camos.org) and author of the award-winning educational fiction book *Estrogen's Storm Season—stories of perimenopause* (second edition, 2017).

Introduction

Welcome to the second edition of *Period Repair Manual*. I'm excited to bring you new and updated information about how to have better hormones and better periods.

With this book, I'm even more passionate about period health than I was three years ago with the first edition. Why? Because the book is now part of a collective revolution in women's health. Mine is just one voice in a growing chorus of women's voices who are speaking up about periods and are reclaiming hormones and periods as an essential, integrated part of human health.

Women's health is not a niche topic. It is general health for half the humans on earth.

For too long, women's hormones have been thrown in the "too-hard basket" and managed with birth control. Now, I invite you to think differently about your hormones. I invite you to see them as a *force for good* that benefits every aspect of your mood and metabolism and physiology.

This book is my message to you that you are lucky to be in a female body and have female hormones. It's my assurance that your body is not complicated or mysterious or unruly. Quite the opposite. Your woman's body is strong and vital and wise, and with the right support, it knows exactly how to be healthy and have periods.

How to Use This Book

The first half of the book is all about understanding your period. What should your period be like? What can go wrong? Why do we have periods at all? In this section, I also make the case against hormonal birth control and survey alternative methods of birth control.

The second half is the treatment section. It begins with a chapter called General Maintenance, which lays the groundwork for the detailed treatment chapters that make up the rest of the book.

Please start by reading the book cover to cover because there are important topics nestled within each chapter. For example, Chapter 3 explains the Physical Signs of Ovulation, which will come in handy when we look at ovulation and progesterone later in the book. Chapter 5 describes estrogen metabolism or detoxification, and Chapter 6 is where you'll first learn about insulin resistance. Understanding those key concepts will help you to understand almost any period problem.

Special boxes

Throughout the book, you'll see definitions, tips, patient stories, and special topics.

---

 definition

Definition boxes provide simple explanations for any technical words. You can also find them in the Glossary.

(*tip*) **Tips are extra bits** of information you may find helpful.

Lara: Naturopathic doctor and period revolutionary

Patient stories are fictionalized stories based on my real patients with names and some details changed.

The final chapter is the Advanced Troubleshooting chapter, where I dive into some of the trickier health issues such as environmental toxins, digestive health, and thyroid disease. The final chapter is also where you'll find the crucial section How to Talk to Your Doctor. It provides a list of questions and statements to help you communicate with your doctor and bring you both to a better understanding of your particular health situation.

As you read, you will encounter references to different sections of the book. That will allow you to go back and piece together the different parts of your unique period story. For example, you may be struggling to get your period back after stopping birth control. I explore that problem in special sections in Chapters 2, 7, and 11. The Table of Contents and Index will help you navigate to the right sections.

Are the Recommendations Evidence-Based?

Whenever possible, I have provided a reference to a scientific study. That amounts to more than 350 studies to back up many of the recommendations.

When I have not provided a reference, it's because there was not yet published research available on that topic at the time of writing. This is the case for some of the herbal medicines and also for a couple of the special topics, such as *histamine intolerance*. Of course, I hope that scientists will one day test those treatments, but in the meantime, I want you to have the benefit of them. If that means being ahead of the curve of scientific inquiry, then so be it. One of my earliest naturopathic teachers put it this way: "If you wait for the research to catch up, then you could be waiting for a very long time."

All the recommendations are based on results I've seen with my thousands of patients over the last twenty years. And almost all of the recommendations are simple and safe to try. However, I do recommend you speak with your doctor or pharmacist about possible interactions with any existing medical condition or medication, or if you are pregnant or breastfeeding. Always cross-check the labels or packaging of any supplements for precautions and dosing instructions.

What's New in the Second Edition?

The best thing about releasing the first edition of *Period Repair Manual* was all the thoughtful feedback I received. So many questions and suggestions of how to make it better. Using that feedback, I expanded and revised the entire book, including the sections on fertility awareness method, natural progesterone, PCOS, and endometriosis.

I also gathered some of the latest research in nutrition and women's health.

What's new?

- insights from Jerilynn C. Prior MD, Endocrinology Professor
- more than 300 additional references
- expanded sections on PCOS and endometriosis
- a chapter on perimenopause and the menopause transition
- patient stories
- special topics such as *Histamine Intolerance* and *How to Choose a Probiotic*
- suggested brands of supplements.

And just a word about the suggested brands. They're listed in the Resources section, and they're to provide you with a starting place. They are by no means the only acceptable brands, as there are plenty of other good products out there. Please buy the supplement that is available to you and is not too expensive. I have not been paid to mention any product or brand name.

My Education and Background

I started my professional life as a biologist at the University of Calgary. There, I studied zoology, botany, and ecology, and worked summers collecting data on the plants and animals of the Canadian wilderness. I even published a scientific paper on the foraging behavior of male and female bats.

I was planning to pursue an academic career in biology, when one day, I saw an ad in the university newspaper, and my life took a different direction.

The ad was for the Canadian College of Naturopathic Medicine, and I was intrigued. I cut it out of the paper and taped it to my dresser mirror. "What is naturopathic medicine?" I wondered. Until that point, medicine was not something I had seriously considered because I had not been interested in working within conventional medicine.

When I began to look into naturopathic medicine, I discovered that its core philosophy is that the body can often heal itself. That resonated with everything I'd learned about the natural world in my biology studies. I understood the natural world to be a pragmatic and regenerative system. Of course, the human body had to follow the same principles, because the human body is part of the natural world.

I dropped my plans for an academic career and applied to the naturopathic college. Once accepted, I drove my little old Volkswagen three thousand kilometers east across Canada to Toronto and embarked on four more years of study.

There are currently seven accredited colleges of naturopathic medicine in North America: two in Canada and five in the United States. The first two years of naturopathic college are similar to conventional medical programs. The final two years provide hundreds of hours of training in nutritional and herbal medicine, as well as clinical training in an outpatient clinic. Graduates of accredited naturopathic colleges must complete a postdoctoral licensing exam (NPLEX).

I qualified as a naturopathic doctor in 1997 (under my maiden name, Lara Grinevitch), and promptly set up general practice in the small rural town where I'd grown up—Pincher Creek, Alberta, Canada. The 1990s were an interesting time to be a natural doctor. Even basic things like probiotics were strange to the other doctors. "Good bacteria?" said one doctor. "How ridiculous!"

It was also a particularly interesting—and somewhat scary—time for women's health. Women were faced with high-dose birth control pills, conventional hormone "replacement" therapy, and routine hysterectomies. I simply had to find better solutions for those women.

As I worked with my patients, I discovered that natural treatments yielded even better results than I had been taught to expect. I discovered that for most women, natural medicine is a viable alternative to synthetic hormones and surgery.

One condition I treated in those early years was polycystic ovary syndrome (PCOS). Back then, the conventional treatment was a surgical procedure called ovarian drilling. My approach was completely different. I had been taught that PCOS was related to an underlying problem with blood sugar and insulin, so I prescribed diet and supplements to lower insulin. A "diet solution" for PCOS was greeted with skepticism by the local doctors but I persevered and saw great results. Of course, we now know that blood sugar and insulin *are* major factors in PCOS, as we'll see in Chapter 7.

More than two decades later, I've had the opportunity to treat many, many kinds of period problems. I run a busy naturopathic practice in Sydney, Australia, where I treat women for PCOS, endometriosis, insulin resistance, thyroid disease, and many other issues.

And to my thousands of patients over the years, I just want to say thank you!

I dedicate this book to you.

Lara Briden

PART ONE

➤———————→

Understanding Your Period

Nothing in life is to be feared,
it is only to be understood.

Now is the time to understand more,
so that we may fear less.

~ *Marie Curie* ~

Chapter 1

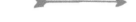

PERIOD REVOLUTION

$\int$ OMETHING BIG is happening in period health. If you've picked up this book, then you're part of the movement.

Periods are coming out into the open. They are no longer something to be endured, concealed, or regulated with hormonal birth control. As we'll see in the coming chapters, the pill has outlived its usefulness. There are better options for birth control. There are far better solutions for period problems.

More and more women are saying *No* to the pill, and *Yes*, to their own natural monthly cycles.

Period apps are part of the change. Most of my patients use them. I use one myself. When I asked my teenage stepdaughter if she uses a period app, she said "Of course," as if I'd asked a silly question.

Period apps are smartphone applications that allow you to track data about your monthly cycle. You can track your period start date. You can track signs and symptoms such as spotting, breast tenderness, and mood. You can even receive an alert when your period is likely to start! Of course, you could do the same thing with old-fashioned pen and paper, but a period app is easier and *friendlier* somehow. Your phone is right there in your bag. It's often in your hand.

By inviting our periods into our day-to-day lives, these apps make periods seem less threatening. They make periods seem *normal*, which of course they are, and always have been.

What's happening with *your* period? Does it come every month? Does it come at all? Is it heavy or painful or difficult in some way? Maybe you've just come off the pill, or are thinking about coming off the pill?

No matter your age or your situation, it's time to get to know your period. There is no better time to do so.

Your Period Is Trying to Tell You Something

Your period is not just your period. It is an expression of your underlying health. When you are healthy, your menstrual cycle will arrive smoothly, regularly, and without symptoms. When you are unhealthy in some way, your cycle will tell the story.

I invite you to think of your period as your monthly report card. Every month, it can offer a helpful account of what is happening with your health in general. That information is incredibly valuable. How better to know what you need to do—and what you need to change?

The American College of Obstetricians and Gynecologists (ACOG) agrees. In December 2015, together with the American Academy of Pediatrics, they quietly issued a groundbreaking statement called "Menstruation in Girls and Adolescents: Using the Menstrual Cycle as a Vital Sign."[1]

In it, they state:

> "Identification of abnormal menstrual patterns in adolescence may improve early identification of potential health concerns for adulthood. It is important for clinicians to have an

understanding of the menstrual patterns of adolescent girls, the ability to differentiate between normal and abnormal menstruation, and the skill to know how to evaluate the adolescent girl patient. By including an evaluation of the menstrual cycle as an additional vital sign, clinicians reinforce its importance in assessing overall health status for patients and caretakers."

I nearly cried when I read that statement. Finally!

The ACOG says doctors should always ask patients about menstruation and should advise girls to chart their cycles. By doing so, doctors will demonstrate to patients that menstruation is an important reflection of their overall health.

The ACOG is correct, of course. Menstruation is a reflection of overall health, or what they are calling a *vital sign*.

Throughout my twenty years of working with patients, I have relied on information about menstruation to help me assess health and determine the correct treatment plan. That's why I always ask my patients about their periods—even if they have come to me for something else.

Consider my patient Meagan.

Meagan: How is your period?

Meagan was 26 when she came for help with psoriasis, an immune disorder which causes dry, scaly skin patches. Her psoriasis affected her scalp and elbows and seemed to get worse with stress. Meagan said she'd inherited it from her father.

I asked Meagan a few more questions. When had it started? (When she was 13.) Did she have any allergies? (No.) Did she have any digestive problems? (No.)

Then I asked, "How is your period?"

"What do you mean?"

"Does it come every month? Do you have any pain or spotting between periods?"

Meagan said her period was fine because she took the pill.

"That's not a period," I said. "I mean, what was your period like back when you weren't on the pill?"

Meagan's period had not started until she was 16 and then it was light and irregular. Her doctor had done some blood tests and said that everything was normal. She'd recommended Meagan take the pill.

"There had to be a reason for your irregular periods," I explained. "And it could be the same underlying issue that's contributing to your psoriasis."

I ordered some extra blood tests, and all was normal except for a borderline iron deficiency, which had also come up in some of Meagan's previous tests.

A picture was starting to emerge. Meagan had a group of symptoms which suggested to me a possible sensitivity to wheat: 1) psoriasis, 2) iron deficiency, and 3) irregular periods. I explained to Meagan that the psoriasis could be, in part, an inflammatory reaction to wheat or gluten.[2] And that the same inflammatory reaction from gluten could also be contributing to both the iron deficiency and the irregular periods.[3]

Fortunately, Meagan tested negative for the most severe clinical form of gluten sensitivity: celiac disease. But I perceived that she likely had a milder form of gluten sensitivity—one that was affecting her skin and her periods. I asked her to avoid gluten for six months.

A month into treatment, Meagan stopped the pill to see if her new diet would give her regular periods. I warned her that it could take some time.

For the first two months, not much happened. Meagan's psoriasis stayed about the same, and she did not get a period.

"Recovering from gluten can take several months," I said.

Finally, after three months, her skin started to improve. After six months, she got her first period and went on to have regular periods.

The right treatment for Meagan's general health was also the right treatment for her periods. It is always like this: fix your health, and you will fix your period.

Why Hormonal Birth Control Is Not the Answer

Your doctor may not care very much about your monthly report card. She's not thinking about which subtle underlying issue is the cause of your period problems because the solution is always the same: take the pill.

The pill is a combined oral contraceptive, which is one of the types of hormonal birth control that suppress ovulation.

---

hormonal birth control

Hormonal birth control is the general term for all tablets, patches, and injections that deliver steroid drugs to suppress ovarian function. The combined pill (estrogen plus a progestin) is the most popular type.

Why does your doctor love the pill so much? Because it is a handy catch-all solution. Missing periods? Take the pill. Period pain? Take the pill. Polycystic ovary syndrome or endometriosis? Take the pill.

Then, when you want to become pregnant, you can take a fertility drug.

Conventional medical prescribing for period problems tends to look like this:

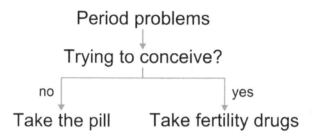

image 1 - conventional prescribing for period problems

The pill can be a predictable band-aid solution, I'll grant you. It suppresses skin oils, so it clears up pimples. It overrides hormones, so it erases pesky report card symptoms—but only as long as you keep taking it. Stopping the pill can be tricky, as we'll see in the next chapter.

Finally, the pill forces you to have a bleed, which is reassuring for both you and your doctor. But there's a problem: *a pill bleed is not a real period.*

A real period is a finale in a series of hormonal events which includes ovulation and the making of progesterone, as I'll discuss below. A real period happens approximately every 28 days because that's how long it takes your ovaries to complete the process. A real period is about the healthy functioning of your ovaries.

A pill bleed does not proceed from ovulation. Instead, it is a withdrawal bleed from the drugs that stimulate your uterine lining but *shut down your ovaries.* A pill bleed is about the dosing of a drug.

Wait a minute. Did I just say that hormonal birth control works by shutting down your ovaries and switching off your hormones? Yes. On the pill, you have no sex hormones of your own. Instead, you have steroid drugs given to you as a kind of "hormone replacement"—not unlike the hormone replacement that is given to women in menopause.

Hormone replacement might be okay if the steroid drugs were as good as your own hormones, but they're not. The steroid drugs in hormonal birth control *are not the same* as your own estrogen and progesterone, and as we'll see in the next chapter, that can pose a big problem for health.

 The pill does not regulate hormones. It switches them off entirely.

This book is your opportunity to depart from "pill medicine" and to do things differently.

Natural period repair is different from pill medicine because it's gentle and without side effects. It's also a fundamentally different approach in that it works by supporting your ovaries, not suppressing them. Natural period repair honors your period as the vital sign the ACOG says it is.

The best thing about natural period repair is that when it works, it works forever. Your period will stay healthy for as long as you remain healthy. In that way, it's a far more powerful and permanent solution than the pill could ever be.

Be a Detective

So where do you start? What is the right treatment for your health and your periods? Is it as simple as avoiding gluten, as Meagan found? Or is it something completely different?

To find your best treatment, you must first learn to interpret your period clues. This book is your step-by-step guide to doing that. First, we will look at how your period should be. Then, we will look at some of the things that can go wrong, and why. As we go, please start asking yourself questions, and start thinking about some possible answers. For example:

Does your period come at least every 35 days? If not, then you might have PCOS, which we'll discuss in Chapter 7. Or you might have a problem with your thyroid. PCOS and thyroid disease are just two of the many reasons for irregular periods.

Is your period painful? If so, then you might endometriosis, which we'll discuss in Chapter 9. Or you might need to think about inflammatory foods or take a zinc supplement.

Do you experience premenstrual breast pain? Breast pain is so common that you probably do not consider it a sign of anything at all. Mild breast pain can be a normal sign of ovulation, but more severe breast pain can mean you don't have enough iodine in your diet.

Those are fairly obvious questions. But here's the most important question of all:

Do you ovulate?

When it comes to period health, it's all about ovulation.

Ovulation is the release of an egg from your ovary. You probably understand that ovulation is essential for making a baby, but why does it matter so much for period health? Ovulation matters because it's how you progress through all the menstrual cycle phases to your menstrual flow or period.

Ovulation is also how you make progesterone, which is an amazing hormone, to say the least.

---

progesterone

Progesterone is one of several steroid hormones made by the ovary. It's essential for pregnancy but has many other beneficial functions.

Progesterone is a steroid reproductive hormone produced by a temporary gland in your ovary after ovulation. It's beneficial for mood, metabolism, and bones. It's also highly beneficial for your period. In fact, you could say, that when it comes to period health, it's all about progesterone.

We'll learn more about progesterone in the coming chapters, but suffice to say at this point, you almost certainly want more progesterone than you have right now.

Special Topic: How Do You Know If You Ovulate and Make Progesterone?

Signs of *possible* ovulation include fertile mucus and a regular cycle. Evidence of *definite* ovulation includes a rise in basal body temperature and an increase in progesterone as measured by a mid-luteal phase blood test. A period itself is not evidence of ovulation because it is possible to have an anovulatory cycle. For more information, please see the Physical Signs of Ovulation section in Chapter 3 and Progesterone Testing in Chapter 5.

---

anovulatory cycle

An anovulatory cycle is a menstrual cycle in which ovulation did not occur, and progesterone was not made.

Interpreting your period clues is something you can do on your own, to some extent. After all, you know your own body better than anyone. At some stage, however, you may need to ask your doctor or healthcare provider for help. I want your conversation with your doctor to be as productive as possible—and not just result in another prescription for the pill. Toward that goal, I have included a section called How to Talk to Your Doctor. You might find that your doctor is a lot more helpful than you'd expected—if you just know what to ask.

One final point: don't put off natural period repair. The longer you leave it, the more entrenched your period problems will become.

Hormonal patterns can be thought of as "hormonal rivers" in your body. In this analogy, your hormones flow down the gullies and trenches carved by the hormones that came before.

The best examples of "hormonal rivers" in action are the beginning of periods when you are a teenager and then the end of periods as you approach menopause. Let's look at these two times of hormonal change and adaptation.

The Beginning of Periods

When you first started having periods, estrogen was new to your body and hormone receptors.

> *hormone receptor*
>
> A hormone receptor is a docking station for hormones such as estrogen or progesterone. They exist in every type of cell and transmit hormonal messages deep into the cell.

At that young age, you react strongly to estrogen because your receptors are still quite sensitive. In the hormonal river analogy, estrogen has not yet had a chance to carve out its "river." At the same young age, you are probably not yet ovulating or making the progesterone you need to counterbalance estrogen. The result may be the heavy periods of the early teen years.

With time, you react less strongly to estrogen because your hormone receptors become less sensitive. You ideally start to ovulate and make progesterone. The result is a natural lightening of your periods.

It takes time for hormones to carve out their "rivers," and that's why it takes time to establish a healthy menstrual cycle. According to Dr Jerilynn C. Prior, a Canadian endocrinologist with expertise in reproductive hormones, it can take up to twelve years to develop a mature menstrual cycle with healthy regular ovulation and an optimal level of progesterone.[4]

Twelve years to mature your menstrual cycle.

So, what happens if you take hormonal birth control as a teen and hit the pause button on that maturation process? You will probably need some time to get things going again, and you may not see regular periods right away when you first stop birth control. That's what happened to my patient Christine.

Christine: One year to get periods

Christine had never thought much about her periods until she lost them at 29 when she came off the pill. Or rather, she perceived that she lost them. In fact, she had not had a real period since before she started the pill at 14.

Back then, her periods were irregular. This is often the case at 14, but that's not how her doctor saw it. He prescribed the pill to "regulate" Christine's periods and said it would also give her nice skin, which it did.

Christine had been on the pill for fifteen years when she decided to take a break. She wasn't ready for a baby but thought she might try for one in a few years, and she wanted to see what was happening with her fertility. She stopped the pill, but much to her dismay, she saw no sign of a period.

A few months went by, and then her doctor detected "polycystic ovaries" on a pelvic ultrasound exam. He said she might have a condition called PCOS, which was very frightening for Christine. She tried to stay calm and look for answers online and there she found some of the blog posts I'd written about the condition.

"I was so relieved by the way you speak about PCOS," Christine told me when she came in for her first appointment. "You make it sound like it is sometimes reversible."

"PCOS can be reversible," I said. "And also, we don't even yet know if you have the condition."

I ordered some blood tests for Christine and, fortunately, they were all normal. I said that she probably did not have PCOS but that we would not know for sure until she had been off the pill for longer. As we'll see in Chapter 7, PCOS is a complex hormonal condition that cannot be diagnosed by ultrasound alone. It's fairly common to have polycystic ovaries after the pill. It just meant that Christine had not ovulated that month. It did not mean she would never ovulate again.

By the time I started working with Christine, it had been five months since she stopped the pill and I thought it could be a few more until she got a period. I explained that she was in a phase of post-pill amenorrhea or "stalled menstruation," which can happen to women who start the pill at a very young age.

I thought Christine just needed time and would be okay in the long run. I was glad she didn't want a baby right away because then she might have been rushed into fertility treatment—something she probably did not need.

I suggested Christine take the herbal medicine *Vitex agnus-castus*, which promotes communication between the pituitary and ovaries. Christine took one Vitex tablet per day for three months and then had a period.

---

amenorrhea

Amenorrhea simply means no menstruation or no periods.

---

polycystic ovary syndrome (PCOS)

A common hormonal condition characterized by excess male hormones in women, covered in Chapter 7.

Getting Ready for the End of Periods

Your hormonal rivers determine how well you mature into a regular ovulatory menstrual pattern. They also determine how smoothly you transition to the end of your periods, or menopause.

If you're in your twenties or thirties, you may not be thinking much about the end of periods, but it's coming sooner than you think. The normal age for menopause is anywhere from 45 to 55. The normal age for perimenopause is up to twelve years before that, so as young as 35!

---

perimenopause

Perimenopause means "around menopause," and refers to the hormonal changes (such as increased estrogen and decreased progesterone) that occur during the two to twelve years before menopause. The final part of perimenopause is called the menopause transition.

---

menopause

Menopause is the cessation of menstruation. It's the life phase that begins one year after your last period.[5]

During perimenopause, your cycles could still be regular, but you could start to experience symptoms such as hot flashes, heavy periods, and insomnia. For more information, I invite you to read Chapter 10, which is all about the end of periods and the challenging time of perimenopause. You probably want to read Chapter 10 even if you think it doesn't yet apply to you. It's a helpful preview of what lies ahead, and will give you ways to cope when the time comes.

Going Forward

How are *your* hormonal rivers? Are your estrogen and progesterone flowing nicely? Or are your hormones not quite where you'd like them to be?

Your hormones now will determine your hormones of the future.

If you take hormonal birth control, now is the time to stop. You simply cannot go any further with your period health until you do. The pill distorts your hormonal rivers and masks your monthly report card.

And, as we'll see in the next chapter, the pill has more potential side effects than you may realize.

Chapter 2

➤———————➤

BREAKING UP WITH HORMONAL BIRTH CONTROL

We're in a strange time for women's health. It's a time when we think it's fine and normal to routinely give a drug to switch off the hormones of millions of women and girls.

What are we doing? Why should we have to shut down a woman's entire hormonal system just to accomplish the simple job of preventing pregnancy? Fertility is an expression of health, not a disease to be treated with a drug.

Imagine if hormonal birth control were proposed today for the first time. Quite likely, many women, doctors, and scientists would be appalled. But that's seeing it from a modern perspective which values women and women's hormones. The pill is far from modern. It's a relic from the 1950s when people had different ideas about things. For example, they thought the synthetic pesticide DDT was fine and normal. They thought smoking was fine and normal. And of course, they thought contraception should be illegal.

The invention of the pill helped to put an end to some of that antiquated thinking and gained women the legal right to birth control. That's something we can all celebrate.

But now it's 2018. We've progressed in so many other ways. Smartphones. Self-driving cars. Why are we still using such an outdated method of contraception?

If you think about it, fifty years of hormonal birth control shows a startling lack of imagination.

Not the Only Birth Control

It's not unusual for me to have a conversation with a patient that goes something like this:

Me: What do you do for birth control?

Patient: I don't use birth control. I use condoms.

In other words, for my patient, "birth control" is synonymous with the pill or other hormonal birth control. She thinks that if she's not using hormonal birth control, then she is not using anything at all. And bizarrely, her doctor, who should know better, may have the same idea.

I'm here to tell you that you have other birth control options. In the next chapter, we'll take a fresh look at condoms, diaphragms, intrauterine devices (IUDs), and fertility awareness methods. Contrary to what you may have been told, those methods are a reliable and perfectly reasonable choice. That's true even if you're a young woman who has not yet had children.

Pill Bleeds Are Not Periods

What if you take birth control for a reason other than contraception? For example, what if you take it to control symptoms or to "regulate" your period? If you do, you're not alone. Of all the women who take the pill, one in three takes it to regulate her period.

Hormonal birth control can certainly suppress symptoms, but let's be clear: it cannot give you a period.

As we saw in the first chapter, pill bleeds are not periods. They do not equate, in any sense, to the cycling of your own hormones.

Pill bleeds are pharmaceutically induced bleeds that are arbitrarily coordinated into a 28-day pattern to reassure you that your body is doing something natural. Having the occasional pill bleed is necessary to prevent breakthrough bleeding, but it doesn't have to be monthly. A pill bleed could just as easily be every 56 days or every 83 days, or any number of days you'd like.

There is no medical reason to bleed monthly on hormonal birth control. So, why do it? It all started in the 1950s when the pill was invented. It was invented as contraception, but contraception was not yet legal, so instead, the pill was prescribed to ostensibly "treat female disorders" and to "regulate menstruation."[6] "Regulate" was a quaint euphemism which just meant to get your period and to be "not pregnant" (wink-wink).

In other words, the whole "normalize periods" thing started as a cover story. That would be fine, except that six decades later the legacy of that story persists. Many doctors continue to prescribe birth control to "normalize" periods and "regulate" hormones, as though the pill's steroids are somehow equal to, or better than, your own hormones. The fact is, nothing could be further from the truth.

Pill steroids are *not* better than your hormones. They're not even real hormones.

Pill Drugs Are Not Hormones

Your ovarian hormones are estradiol and progesterone. They have many benefits—not just for reproduction, but also for mood, bones, thyroid, muscles, and metabolism. They're *human hormones* that are essential for human physiology.

In contrast, the steroid drugs in hormonal birth control are ethinylestradiol, drospirenone, levonorgestrel, and others. Technically, those drugs are hormones if a hormone is broadly defined as a chemical messenger. But they are *not* human hormones, and they are not part of normal human physiology. They are better described as *pseudo-hormones*.

 There's no progesterone in hormonal birth control.

One of the most common steroid drugs is levonorgestrel, which is used in many oral contraceptives and implants, as well as the Mirena® IUD, and the morning-after pill.

Levonorgestrel is a progestin, which means it's *kind of similar* to progesterone. For example, levonorgestrel is similar to progesterone in the way it suppresses ovulation and thins the uterine lining. That's why it's used in birth control.

At the same time, levonorgestrel is not entirely similar to progesterone. When you look at levonorgestrel and progesterone side by side, you can see that they are, in fact, different molecules.

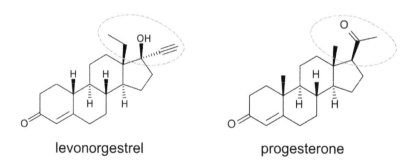

levonorgestrel   progesterone

image 2 - levonorgestrel is not progesterone

Different molecules have different effects in the body.

Progesterone, for example, improves brain health and cognition.

[7] As a progestin, levonorgestrel has been linked with depression and anxiety.[8]

Another example is hair. Progesterone is great for hair health, and promotes hair growth. Its counterpart levonorgestrel causes hair loss because it's similar to the male hormone testosterone.

Levonorgestrel is actually more similar to testosterone than it is to progesterone.

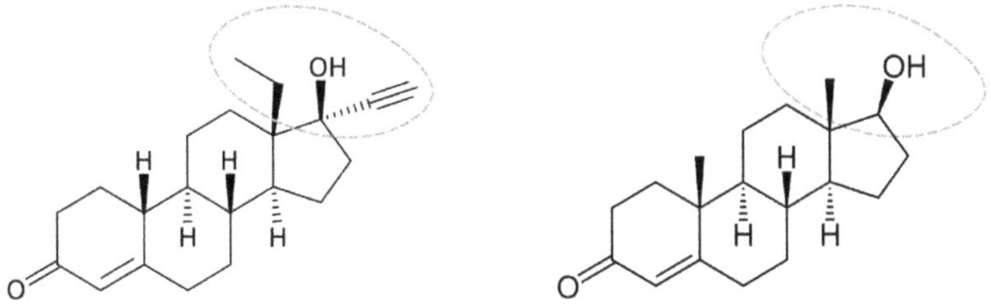

levonorgestrel   testosterone

image 3 - levonorgestrel is almost testosterone

---

progestin

Progestin is a general term for drugs that are similar to progesterone. Progestin drugs include levonorgestrel and drospirenone, which have some of the same effects as progesterone but also have many opposite effects. The terms progestin and progesterone cannot be used interchangeably.

Later in the chapter, we'll look at the many side effects of progestins. For now, let me say that their biggest side effect is that they rob you of your own beneficial progesterone. They do so by suppressing ovulation, which is, of course, their purpose, but unfortunately, without ovulation, you cannot make progesterone.

Special Topic: What's in a Word?

Some of my patients are reluctant to stop the pill, and I don't pressure them. I do, however, insist on one thing. I insist that we not use the word "period" when referring to their pill bleeds. Instead, we say "withdrawal-bleed" or "pill bleed."

The Pill Is Nothing Like Pregnancy

One of the arguments put forward in defense of hormonal birth control is that it's like pregnancy and that, therefore, any side effects are better than pregnancy—as if the pill or pregnancy were the only two options. Furthermore, the argument goes, the pill is "natural" because it mimics the continuously pregnant state of our ancestors.

That argument doesn't hold up.

For one thing, the pseudo-hormone drugs of hormonal birth control are *not* the hormones of pregnancy. Drugs such as ethinylestradiol, levonorgestrel, and drospirenone do not have the same effects as the pregnancy hormones hCG, estradiol, and progesterone.

And as for the continuously pregnant state of our ancestors, it's a little more complicated than that. Yes, your great-grandmother may have had relatively few periods compared to you. If she had many children, then she had only 40 periods in her life compared to your 400. Your hundreds of periods may put you at greater risk of fibroids and ovarian cysts, but then, *so does hormonal birth control*. And so does the modern onslaught of hormone-disrupting environmental toxins.

Any way you look at it, your health is going to be different from your great-grandmother's. And if 400 periods are the trade-off for living in the modern world, then I invite you to embrace your periods. The best part is, with the right support, you can be happy and healthy with all of them.

> ## Special Topic: Hormonal Birth Control Does Not Preserve Fertility
>
> Your doctor may have told you that hormonal birth control can preserve fertility and delay menopause. It's not true. Your doctor is referring to the outdated notion that ovaries run out of eggs—a myth we'll debunk in Chapter 10. Quite simply, the pill *cannot* delay menopause. If anything, it can bring menopause earlier.[9]

Is There Ever a Time to Take Hormonal Birth Control?

I would never say that no woman should ever take hormonal birth control.

My main goal is to speak the truth about what hormonal birth control is. Namely, that it shuts down hormones and functions as a type of synthetic hormone replacement.

Knowing this, there are two situations when you could consider taking hormonal birth control.

1. You understand the physiological reality of what the pill is. You are aware of your other options, but you still decide as a grown woman that hormonal birth control is the best method of contraception for you. Of course, that's fine. But in that case, you do not need this book. This is a book about periods and remember: pill bleeds are not periods.
2. You suffer debilitating symptoms from a serious condition such as endometriosis or adenomyosis. We'll look at natural treatments for those conditions in Chapter 9, and I hope they will work for you. If not, then you may need to resort to some type of hormonal birth control— preferably the Mirena® IUD discussed below.

Different Types of Hormonal Contraception

Combined Pill (Estrogen plus Progestin)

The classic pill is a combination of two synthetic hormones: ethinylestradiol plus a progestin such as levonorgestrel. All combined pills are the same stuff, but they're branded differently according to the amount and timing of estrogen, and the type of progestin. Drug companies give them cutesy girl brand names such as Brenda® and Yaz®, so they'll seem more benign and personable. (You might take Yaz® but are you as happy to take a drug called drospirenone?) The brand names are different in different countries.

Readers always ask me about the pill Zoely® and Qlaira® which use the natural estrogen estradiol instead of the usual synthetic ethinylestradiol. Yes, estradiol is better, and those pills do have slightly fewer side effects and risks compared to other pills, but they still shut down ovulation and hormones just like other types of hormonal birth control. And they still use a progestin rather than natural progesterone. I don't see them as a great improvement.

NuvaRing® (Estrogen plus Progestin)

NuvaRing® is similar to the combined pill in that it delivers both ethinylestradiol and a progestin called etonogestrel. Just like the pill and most methods of hormonal birth control, it works by suppressing ovulation.

When NuvaRing® was launched in 2001, it was touted as easier (because it's a monthly insert rather than a daily pill), and safer (because it's lower dose). The safety claim was extraordinary, given that a worrying blood clot risk had already emerged in the first clinical trials. The blood clot risk from NuvaRing® is higher than the pill because the ethinylestradiol goes directly into your blood without first passing through your liver. The high clot risk of NuvaRing® was concealed by the manufacturer during the FDA approval process, and that concealment has subsequently been the target of several lawsuits.

Contraceptive Patch (Estrogen plus Progestin)

The patches Xulane® and Evra® are also similar to the combined pill in that they deliver both ethinylestradiol and a progestin called norelgestromin. Just like the pill and most methods of hormonal birth control, they work by suppressing ovulation. Just like Nuvaring®, they carry a higher risk of blood clot compared to the pill.[10]

Mini-Pill or Progestin-Only Pill

The word "mini" means that the pill contains one drug (a progestin), not two (ethinylestradiol plus a progestin). Also, the dose of the progestin is lower than it is in a combination pill because the mini-pill does not work primarily by suppressing ovulation. Instead, the progestin-only pill works by thinning the uterine lining and impairing cervical fluid. It does also inadvertently suppress ovulation in the majority of cycles.[11]

The mini-pill still has many of the same side effects as the combined pill because progestins cause side effects. In fact, the first pill ever tested in 1956 was progestin-only.[12] It had so many side effects that estrogen was added to make the drug more tolerable.

Implants (Progestin-Only)

Arm implants, or rods, are another type of progestin-only birth control. They contain either the progestin levonorgestrel (Jadelle® or Norplant-2®) or etonogestrel (Nexplanon® or Implanon®). Like the mini-pill, implants work primarily by thinning the uterine lining and impairing cervical fluid, and like the mini-pill, they also inadvertently suppress ovulation in the majority of cycles. Implants can also cause weight gain and erratic bleeding.

Special Topic: What's with All the Crazy Bleeding on Implants and Injections?

Progestin-only methods of birth control are known to cause "irregular menstruation," which I would argue is a misnomer. Progestin bleeds are not real periods. Instead, they are anovulatory cycles or "breakthrough bleeds," which occur when the uterine lining has been exposed to estrogen, but not progesterone. Anovulatory cycles are also a feature of period problems such as PCOS, which we'll discuss in Chapters 4, 5, and 7.

The breakthrough bleeds that occur on progestin-only birth control are different from the pill bleeds of the combined pill, which are scheduled withdrawal bleeds from the synthetic estrogen and progestin.

Injection (Progestin-Only)

The injection Depo-Provera® delivers a high dose of the progestin medroxyprogesterone acetate, which completely suppresses both estrogen and progesterone. The profound hormone deficiency induced by Depo-Provera® can cause a number of troubling side effects, including seemingly unstoppable weight gain[13] and temporary bone loss.[14] It has also been associated with an increased breast cancer risk.[15]

Mirena® and Skyla® Intrauterine Devices (IUDs) (Progestin-Only)

Mirena® and Skyla® are intrauterine devices (IUDs) that release a small amount of the progestin levonorgestrel into the uterus. Like other progestin-only methods, they work primarily by thinning the uterine lining and impairing cervical fluid. Like other progestin-only methods, they also inadvertently suppress ovulation—but not as often. The hormonal IUD suppresses ovulation in 85 percent of cycles in the first year, but then only 15 percent of cycles after that.[16]

Because Mirena® does not completely suppress ovulation, I view it as the least harmful of all hormonal birth control. That said, it is still the progestin drug levonorgestrel. The hormonal IUD has been linked to depression[17] and may reduce your ability to cope with stress.[18]

On the plus side, Mirena® has the benefit of reducing flow by 90 percent and so can treat serious period problems such as flooding, adenomyosis, and endometriosis (Chapter 9).

There is also a non-hormonal type of IUD, which we'll look at in the next chapter.

Special Topic: Do You Need a Period?

Mirena® stops periods in some women, which of course raises the question: "Do you even need a period?"

No, you don't need a menstrual bleed per se, and you certainly don't need a pill bleed, which is not a period anyway. But you do need ovarian hormones, and a menstrual cycle is the only way to make them.

Mirena® is unique in that it suppresses a bleed but permits ovulation and hormones. So, if "menstrual suppression" is your goal, then Mirena® is your only reasonable option.

 With most hormonal birth control, you bleed but don't cycle. With a Mirena® IUD, you cycle but don't bleed.

Risks and Side Effects of Hormonal Birth Control

Cancer

Hormonal birth control slightly increases your risk of breast cancer. This is true of all modern methods including low-dose pills, implants, and the hormonal IUD.

Scientists had long known that the old high-dose estrogen pills increased the risk of breast cancer, but had hoped that the modern lower dose pills and progestin-only devices were safer. Unfortunately, a large 2017 study discovered that modern methods carry the same cancer risk as the old high-dose estrogen pills.[19]

On the plus side, the pill reduces your risk of colorectal, ovarian, and uterine (endometrial) cancers.

The protection from uterine cancer is important if you have PCOS and are therefore at greater risk of uterine cancer. Fortunately, there are other, better options for preventing uterine cancer. They include: 1) reversing your PCOS with natural treatment, and 2) taking natural progesterone to protect your uterine lining. See Chapter 7 for more information.

Blood Clots

All hormonal birth control carries a risk of blood clot, and that risk was known almost from the beginning. Barbara Seaman wrote about it in 1969 in her book *The Doctor's Case Against the Pill*.[20] Five decades later, not much has changed. Again and again, the blood clot risk is downplayed. Again and again, the solution has been to find a new and better pill.

We're told that each new generation of the pill is better and safer, but not unlike the "low-tar" advertising used by the cigarette industry, the terms "low-dose" and "new generation" are mostly just advertising.

"New generation" refers merely to the decade in which that

particular progestin was invented. And oddly, some modern progestins such as drospirenone have the highest risk of a fatal blood clot of any progestin so far.

The absolute risk of a blood clot from any hormonal contraceptive is small. Even NuvaRing®, which carries the highest risk, has an absolute risk of only 9.7 clot-events per 10,000 women per year[21] compared to 2.1 clot-events in non-users of hormonal birth control. The clot risk goes way up if you smoke, which you're not supposed to do if you take hormonal birth control.

Chances are, the pill will not give you cancer or a blood clot. However, it will give more likely you one or more of these "minor" side-effects: depression, loss of sex drive, hair loss, and weight gain.

So-called minor side effects are so common that they are the rule rather than the exception. The way they've been downplayed and ignored for the last three generations is perhaps the biggest tragedy of hormonal birth control.

Depression

Anyone who treats women knows that hormonal birth control affects mood. The fact that it remained "unproven" for fifty years is basically because no one was bothering to research it.

That all changed in October 2016 when the prestigious medical journal JAMA Psychiatry released a groundbreaking study called "Association of Hormonal Contraception With Depression."[22] In the study, researchers from the University of Copenhagen tracked one million women over thirteen years and found that girls and women who use hormonal birth control are significantly more likely to be diagnosed with depression. The risk was greatest for teens using progestin-only methods such as an implant or Mirena® IUD.

Researcher Professor Øjvind Lidegaard pointed out that his results may be an *underestimation* because he looked only at birth control users who went on to be diagnosed and take antidepressants. In reality, many women who experience mood changes on birth control simply stop taking it and don't say anything to their doctor.

"All women, doctors, and contraception advisers should realize we have this potential side effect in the use of hormonal contraceptives."[23]

Professor Øjvind Lidegaard

A follow-up study from the same group of researchers found that women taking hormonal birth control had triple the risk of suicide.[24]

How can birth control affect mood? One way is by making your nervous system more sensitive to stress.[25][26] Another is by changing the structure of your brain. In 2015, UCLA Neuroscientist Nicole Peterson found that women who take hormonal birth control have altered brains compared to women who cycle naturally. She says:

"The change in the lateral orbitofrontal cortex may be related to the emotional changes that some women experience when using birth control pills."[27]

Neuroscientist Nicole Peterson

Birth control could be causing or contributing to your depression. If this is the first time you've considered that possibility, then you're not alone. Professor Jayashri Kulkarni from Monash University in Melbourne, Australia put it this way:

"The onset of depression can happen within a day of taking (the pill) or within a year of taking it. Women often tend to blame themselves for feeling depressed and forget to consider the effect of the daily hormone they are taking."[28]

Professor Jayashri Kulkarni

That happened to my patient Lizzy.

Lizzy: Lifting the fog of depression

I met Lizzy when she was 21. By that point, she had been on antidepressants for five years, ever since she was 16. She'd tried coming off but felt terrible and had to go back on. Lizzy told me she had no real hope of ever getting off antidepressants, and that was not why she had come to me.

She'd come for help with chronic yeast infections. Hormones are often a contributing cause of yeast infections, so I asked about her periods. "They're fine," she told me. She did not mention the pill, and she hadn't listed it in the medication section of her intake form.

I had to ask outright. "Do you take hormonal birth control?"

"Oh, yes," she replied. "I started Yasmin for skin when I was fifteen."

Me: "Just before you developed depression?"

Lizzy: "Yes, I guess six months before."

I asked Lizzy if she had ever considered taking a break from the pill to see if it would improve her mood. It had never occurred to her and had never been suggested by her doctor. But she was happy to have a break and so stopped the next day. I also gave her a probiotic to help with the yeast infections.

I met with Lizzy again three months later, and two things had happened. First, her chronic yeast infections had gradually improved. But also, much to her surprise, her mood had dramatically improved after she stopped Yasmin.

"I felt different almost immediately," she told me. "Like a fog had lifted."

Lizzy still takes her antidepressant but is now hopeful that with the help of her doctor, she may eventually wean herself off it.

Loss of Libido or Sex Drive

Hormonal birth control can be bad for your sex life because it switches off the testosterone you need for libido. It can also cause vaginal dryness and put you at risk of a condition called vaginismus, which makes sex painful.

According to one survey, women who take hormonal birth control report less frequent sex, less frequent feelings of arousal, less pleasure, fewer orgasms, and less vaginal lubrication.[29] Unfortunately, it can take months, or even years, for libido to return to normal once the pill is stopped.[30]

I often ask patients about libido. Many of them say that yes, they did notice a decline on the pill, and an improvement when they stopped. Many women cannot say how their libido was before they started the pill because they were too young at the time.

Because really, who thinks to ask a teenage girl if she's suffered a drop in libido? Would she even know?

If you've had low libido ever since you started the pill at fifteen, then, of course, you'll think it's normal for you. Or worse, you'll think it's something that's wrong with you, rather than something that's wrong with the drug you've been taking.

You have the right to a libido, and that's true even if you are not planning to have sex anytime soon. Why? Because your libido is not just for sex. It's also an important part of your vitality and motivation for life.

You may have a high libido, or you may have a low libido, and that's fine. Everyone's libido is different. What matters is that your libido is the one that's normal for you and not the side effect of medication.

> ## Special Topic: Why Men Won't Take Hormonal Birth Control
>
> The technology exists for male hormonal birth control, but those drugs have not yet gone to market. Developers seem to think men would never agree to switch off their hormones and suffer the resulting depression and low libido. And, honestly, why should they? Why should women?

Hair Loss

Some progestins such as levonorgestrel cause hair loss because they have a *high androgen index*, which means they are testosterone-like.

The American Hair Loss Association (AHLA) warns about the risk of hair loss from hormonal birth control. In 2010, it stated:

> "It is imperative for all women especially for those who have a history of hair loss in their family to be made aware of the potentially devastating effects of birth control pills on normal hair growth."[31]

Have you been taking a testosterone type of birth control? Read the ingredients.

Progestins with a *high androgen index* include medroxyprogesterone acetate, levonorgestrel, norgestrel, and etonogestrel. They cause hair loss by shrinking (or miniaturizing) hair follicles, which is a slow process. You could be on the birth control for many months—or even years—before you start to notice hair loss. Progestins with a high androgen index can also cause acne.

Progestins with a *low androgen index* include drospirenone, norgestimate, and cyproterone. They do not cause hair loss when you take them, but they can cause hair loss when you stop them because they cause a rebound surge in androgens and androgen sensitivity.

Once your hair follicles have miniaturized on hormonal birth control, you will likely end up with the diagnosis of "androgenic" or "androgenetic" alopecia (female pattern hair loss), which is not easy to reverse. You'll find more information about androgenetic alopecia and how to treat it in the Treatment of Female Pattern Hair Loss section in Chapter 7.

 androgen

An androgen is a male hormone that promotes male characteristics.

 alopecia

Alopecia means hair loss.

Weight Gain

Hormonal birth control can cause weight gain because it interferes with a hormone called insulin. We'll learn more about insulin in Chapters 7 and 11. The pill also causes sugar cravings and prevents the muscle gain that you would expect to see with exercise.[32] Finally, the pill's synthetic estrogen causes fat to be deposited on the hips and upper thighs and can worsen cellulite.

But Wait, There's More

We've seen that hormonal birth control can cause depression, loss of sex drive, hair loss, and weight gain. That's just the tip of the iceberg.

Hormonal birth control can also cause high blood pressure, nutrient deficiency, and reduced thyroid function. Hormonal birth control alters both your intestinal and vaginal bacteria and that can lead to digestive problems, yeast infections, and abnormal PAP smears. Finally, studies have shown that hormonal birth control may prevent you from forming healthy bones.[33][34]

As if all those side effects were not enough, there are also the problems you may face when you stop hormonal birth control.

Coming Off the Pill

You will probably feel better when you stop hormonal birth control. Better mood, more energy, and regular cycles. That is the most common experience. You may, however, develop problems such as post-pill acne, PMS, or amenorrhea (lack of periods).

Post-Pill Acne

The steroid drugs in hormonal birth control work extremely well to clear acne. Both ethinylestradiol (synthetic estrogen) and the progestins drospirenone, norgestimate, and cyproterone strongly suppress sebum (skin oil). In fact, cyproterone suppresses sebum to "childhood levels,"[35] which is a bit unsettling when you think about it. Adults are supposed to have more sebum than children, so it's an abnormal situation.

In response to the drugs, your skin has to up-regulate sebum, and that upregulation will continue even once you stop the pill. The result can be more sebum than you ever had before.

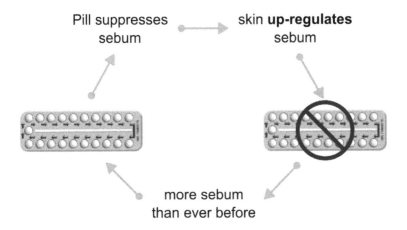

image 4 - pill addiction and withdrawal

At the same time, coming off the pill can trigger your ovaries to temporarily make more androgens as they kick back into action.

So, post-pill acne is the result of a double-whammy of rebound sebum as you withdraw from a sebum-suppressing drug, and rebound androgens as your ovaries become active again.

Fortunately, your ovaries should also start to make the hormones estrogen and progesterone, which are both *good for skin.*

Post-pill acne typically peaks after about six months—just when you might be ready to give up. After that, your skin should start to improve.

If you're prone to acne, or if you suffered acne the last time you tried to stop the pill, please start natural treatment at least one month *before* you stop the pill. That should reduce the severity of post-pill acne. See the Treatment of Acne and Anti-Androgen Treatment sections in Chapter 7.

Post-Pill PMS

If you're like many of my patients, you may encounter the new symptom of PMS when you stop the pill.

It's because you're having real cycles for the first time in what may have been years. Your pill "cycles" were associated with a fairly even dose of synthetic hormones, so you didn't feel much change day-to-day. Your real cycles, on the other hand, are associated with a natural up and down of hormones—and you have to adapt to that.

Which might lead you to ask: "If a real period can cause PMS, then why have a real period?" And my answer is: "For the hormones."

Your own hormones estradiol and progesterone are so beneficial that they're worth putting up with a little PMS. And fortunately, PMS need not impact your life too much, because it responds incredibly well to the treatments we'll discuss in Chapter 8.

Post-Pill Amenorrhea and PCOS

If you don't get your period after stopping the pill, the most important question to ask is: *what were your periods like before you took the pill?*

If your periods were irregular, then something was going on back then; coming off the pill has simply unmasked it. With the help of this book, you can now go back to the drawing board and figure out what that something is, and fix it.

If on the other hand, your periods were regular before the pill, then you now have a type of post-pill amenorrhea (post-pill syndrome) or post-pill PCOS, which we'll discuss in Chapter 7.

The Best Thing About Breaking Up with Hormonal Birth Control

Think of it this way: coming off the pill is the first test on your monthly report card—and that's a good thing. It's the first time your body has had a chance to show you what it can do. Getting a period right away—or not—gives you important clues about your health. With the help of this book, you should gain some ideas about what to do next.

In a way, this entire book is your guide to coming off birth control. I have also included a special section in Chapter 11, How to Come Off Hormonal Birth Control.

Going forward, you may need an alternative method of non-hormonal birth control. That's the topic of the next chapter.

Chapter 3

Better Birth Control. All the Options

THIS BOOK, as well as being a guide to healthy periods, is also a guide to enhanced fertility. The healthier your periods, the more fertile you will become. As soon as you start to get good marks on your monthly report card, you will have invited your body into full baby-making mode. If a baby is not what you're after right now, please read this chapter before you go any further.

If you feel daunted by the prospect of natural birth control, you are not alone. Natural methods are not as convenient as the pill. All of them require some compromise or effort by you and your partner. I wish I could offer a healthy, non-toxic, simple method of contraception that requires no compromise or effort, but I cannot. At this stage, that dream method of contraception simply does not exist. There is no herbal medicine, nutritional supplement, or natural hormone you can take to avoid pregnancy. Natural supplements can only make you *more* fertile—not less.

Hormonal methods of contraception damage your body because that is how they work. To avoid pregnancy, birth control has to fight against the very thing that your body is trying to do, which is to become pregnant. Put simply, when you're healthy, your body wants to be fertile. Therefore, there are really only two ways to avoid pregnancy: damage your body or outsmart your body.

You are a modern, smart woman. I assure you: you can outsmart your body. Avoiding pregnancy is not as mysterious or difficult as it has been made out to be.

You are fortunate to be a healthy, fertile, sexually active woman. And are fortunate to live in a time when contraception is legal and available to you. Hopefully, your partner is loving and liberated and willing to play his part in avoiding unwanted pregnancy. If so, then embrace your good fortune, and accept the task—as a couple—of avoiding an unwanted pregnancy.

In this chapter, I will outline three types of methods of contraception. Type 1 methods are the most natural but do require some responsibility by both partners. Type 2 methods are a little bit toxic, or potentially a little bit harmful, but are easier to use, and do not require any responsibility by your male partner. Type 3 methods are the types of hormonal birth control that I argued against in Chapter 2.

The advantages of Type 1 and Type 2 methods are that they do not suppress ovulation, so they permit you to make progesterone, which, as we'll see in the next chapter, is the hormone most important for period repair.

Disclaimer: This chapter is a brief survey of non-hormonal methods of contraception and not a complete how-to manual. Once you have chosen a method, please seek detailed instructions about its proper use. See the Resources section for more information and consider speaking to your healthcare professional.

Type 1 Contraceptive Methods

Type 1 contraceptive methods are non-hormonal, non-toxic, and carry no health risk. They do not suppress ovulation, and so permit you to make progesterone.

Fertility Awareness Method (FAM)

Here's something you might not have learned in sex education class. A man is fertile every day, but as a woman, you are fertile only six days per menstrual cycle.

To avoid pregnancy, you can determine *which* days you are fertile and then abstain from vaginal intercourse or use a barrier method. It's called *fertility awareness method* (FAM), and it can be surprisingly easy to do. Modern fertility awareness methods such as the *symptothermal method* are scientific because they use observations of up to three concrete signs of fertility: waking body temperature, cervical fluid, and cervix changes. They're different from the *rhythm method,* which is an old style of FAM that relies solely on dates on a calendar.

If your doctor scorns FAM, it's either because she thinks you're not smart enough to do it (you are!), or because she has confused the modern symptothermal method of FAM with the old rhythm method. Many doctors make that mistake. A recent Australian study found that the majority of family doctors "have significant knowledge deficits regarding physiological interpretation of fertility."[36] Help your doctor by directing her to the 2015 American College of Obstetricians and Gynecologists (ACOG) statement about FAM,[37] or consider finding a new doctor.

In short, your fertile days are the five days before ovulation (because that's how long sperm survive), and the one day after ovulation (because that's how long the egg survives). After ovulation, you have a short 24-hour window to ovulate once more, and maybe conceive twins. Your egg(s) survive for another 24 hours, and then you cannot ovulate again for the rest of that cycle. You should then enter the "safe" period for the rest of that cycle.

When used correctly, FAM can be as effective as the pill. One study of women trained in FAM found the method to have a perfect use failure rate of just 0.6 percent[38] which is pretty close to the 0.3 percent perfect use failure rate of the pill.

---

contraception failure rate

Contraception failure rate is the percentage of couples who experience an accidental pregnancy during one year of use. It is expressed as *perfect use* and *typical use*.

Perfect use means the failure rate for women who use the method perfectly. For most methods other than the IUD, perfect use is not as good as typical use, which allows for human error. For the pill, becoming pregnant after forgetting to take a pill would be a failure of typical use. For FAM, becoming pregnant after miscalculating your cycle and having unprotected sex on an "unsafe" day would be a failure of typical use. One study found that the typical use failure rate for the symptothermal method of FAM is 1.8 percent,[39] which is still better than typical use of the pill, which is 9 percent.[40]

So how does FAM work? First and foremost, you track your physical signs of ovulation—namely temperature.

Physical Signs of Ovulation

Temperature

Waking temperature, also called basal body temperature (BBT), is the cardinal sign for FAM. It's your under-the-tongue temperature first thing in the morning after you wake but before you get out of bed. You need a good quality thermometer (preferably a basal body temperature thermometer) that measures temperature to at least one decimal place (97.7°F).

How can temperature tell you about ovulation? It can detect progesterone, which, as you may recall, is the ovarian hormone you make *after* ovulation. Progesterone has many effects on your body, but it has the one very handy effect of raising your body temperature. For example, before ovulation, your waking temperature is between 97.0°F (36.1°C) and 97.7°F (36.5°C). After ovulation, progesterone increases your waking temperature by about 0.5°F (0.3°C), and maintains it at that higher level until your period. A few consecutive days of a small but significant increase in temperature is enough to know that you ovulated and cannot become pregnant for the rest of that cycle.

Your temperature goes up *after* ovulation, which makes it easy to identify your post-ovulation infertile or safe days. It's a bit harder to identify your *pre*-ovulation safe days, but it is possible. With the right training, you can predict your pre-ovulation safe days by interpreting your cervical fluid (see below). Alternatively, you can predict your safe days (both pre- and post-ovulation) with a computer algorithm from a medically certified device such as Daysy Fertility Monitor®.

With Daysy®, you do not need to be trained in FAM. Instead, you simply take your temperature, and the computer algorithm does the rest. It calculates your safe (infertile) and unsafe (fertile) days based on its database of five million cycles. It also learns the nuances of your own cycle the longer you use it. I like Daysy® because it undergoes independent quality testing every year and claims a failure rate of just 0.7 percent.[41] Daysy® doesn't use information about cervical fluid because it doesn't add to the effectiveness of their algorithm.

Of course, there are many other excellent FAM and period apps. Some, such as Kindara®, can assist you with your FAM calculations—but you still need to be trained in FAM. Others, such as Clue®, cannot be used to prevent pregnancy, but are still a great way to track your cycle.

I'm a big fan of period apps in general, but unless you're trained in FAM and taking your temperature and/or checking your cervical fluid, you cannot use a period app to prevent pregnancy.

To prevent pregnancy, you need training in FAM or the Daysy® device. You cannot rely on the "fertile window" of a standard period app.

Cervical fluid or fertile mucus

In the *symptothermal method* of FAM, you track your cervical fluid because it's the sign of ovulation that occurs *before* ovulation. Cervical fluid, also called cervical mucus or fertile mucus, is a unique type of vaginal discharge that looks and feels just like raw egg white. It is clear, stretchy, and slippery. You will see it on the toilet paper after you wipe or feel it at your vaginal opening.

You will usually see some form of fertile mucus during the days leading up to ovulation. The function of cervical fluid is to transport sperm rapidly through your uterus to your egg. If you are trying to prevent pregnancy, then fertile mucus is the red flag that you could be fertile.

Special Topic: Be Careful Interpreting Your Cervical Fluid

Cervical fluid is most obvious in the days before ovulation but you will see it any time you have high estrogen compared to progesterone. For example, you can see it early in your cycle if you have too much estrogen. You can even see it *after ovulation* if you do not make enough progesterone. You can, therefore, see fertile mucus more than once in your cycle. You cannot ovulate more than once.

Cervix position

The softness and position of your cervix are the final physical signs of ovulation. Remember, your cervix is the bottom part of your uterus, where the opening is, and where the menstrual blood comes out. Normally, your cervix is low (about one finger length inside your vagina) and has a surprisingly hard texture, like a smooth donut or the tip of your nose. In the days just before ovulation, your cervix will be higher and softer.

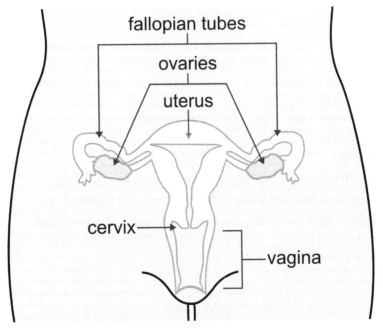

image 5 - female reproductive anatomy

Ovulation test strips

Another sign of ovulation is a surge in luteinizing hormone— known as a *LH surge or peak*— which you can detect with a urine test strip. Start testing by at least day 8 of your cycle, and when you see a positive LH test, it usually means you will ovulate within the next 36 to 40 hours.

---

luteinizing hormone (LH)

Luteinizing hormone is the pituitary hormone that signals your ovary to release an egg.

Measuring LH surge can be helpful when you're trying for pregnancy, but it is not usually used as part of FAM for several reasons. First, LH testing can miss up to 20 percent of LH peaks. [42] Also, by the time you detect an LH surge, it is too late to abstain from unprotected sex, because you will have already been fertile for several days. Finally, if you have PCOS, your LH readings may not correlate at all with ovulation. Instead, you may detect what appears to be an LH surge on almost every day of your cycle.

Other Signs of Ovulation

Other physical signs of ovulation include a mild twinging pain (*mittelschmerz*), light bleeding or spotting, abdominal bloating, fluid retention, and breast tenderness. You may or may not experience these signs, but you cannot rely on them for FAM.

Tracking Your Monthly Report Card

The best thing about FAM is that it gives you better clues about your period. For example, you can confirm that you ovulate, and *when* you ovulate. And once you ovulate, you can know exactly —almost to the day—when your period will come. That's true even if you have irregular cycles.

Knowing if and when you ovulate is essential for understanding your periods and your health.

If you do ovulate, then you already have a pretty good result on your period monthly report card. You also have a new kind of body awareness which is called *body literacy* (a lovely term coined by my colleague and reproductive health advocate Laura Wershler).

If you do *not* ovulate, then you are alerted to the fact that something is wrong. Not ovulating could mean that you are under stress or not eating enough. It could also mean that you have an underlying medical problem such as PCOS or thyroid disease, and that you need to see your doctor. Hopefully, your doctor is responsive to the information, and more helpful than the doctor of my patient Sylvia.

Sylvia: Why do you care if you ovulate or not?

Sylvia had been trying to use the FAM device Daysy®
but was not seeing any green or *safe days*. She knew that
meant she was not ovulating, so she showed her charts to her
family doctor. Unfortunately, he was not particularly
interested.

Doctor: "Do you want another baby?"

Sylvia: "No."

Doctor: "Then why do you care if you ovulate or not?"

Sylvia also had the problem of irregular cycles, but her doctor
had a simple solution for that. "You should be happy to have
fewer periods," he said. "If you're worried, you can take the
pill."

I ordered blood tests for Sylvia and discovered that she had
elevated male hormones and therefore qualified for the
diagnosis of PCOS. She had a small amount of the facial hair
typical of the condition, but her main symptoms were lack of
ovulation and irregular cycles.

"I'm glad I was tracking my cycle," she said. "Or I would
never have known."

Sylvia started natural treatment for PCOS, and after three
months she ovulated and finally saw some safe days on her
Daysy® FAM device.

Stories like Sylvia's are common, but fortunately, they're not the
rule. Most doctors will be more helpful when presented with the
right information and questions. Please see the How to Talk to
Your Doctor section in Chapter 11.

In summary, FAM is a great way to prevent pregnancy. I would
say it's the best. It's effective, and suitable for every age and
situation—even if you do not have regular cycles. The only
downside to FAM is that you'll have to abstain from vaginal

intercourse or use a barrier method on your fertile days. If that's not something you want to do, then please consider a copper IUD discussed below.

And just a reminder: With the exception of the Daysy Fertility Monitor®, all FAM methods require some training. Please read Toni Weschler's book *Taking Charge of Your Fertility*, or seek training from one of the several organizations and online trainers listed in the Resources section.

Male Condoms

Worldwide, male condoms are the most popular form of birth control, and it's easy to understand why. Condoms are simple, inexpensive, and don't present a health risk to either partner. You simply put a condom over your partner's penis before intercourse. It catches the ejaculated sperm and prevents it from entering your body.

Condoms are a barrier method. They are the best barrier method because 1) they reduce the risk of sexually transmitted infection, and 2) they can be used without toxic spermicide.

Special Topic: Avoid Condoms Packaged with Spermicide

Condoms packaged with spermicide offer no advantage over condoms packaged with normal lubricant. They are no more effective than normal condoms for preventing pregnancy or sexually transmitted disease. In fact, the spermicide could make you more susceptible to infections, especially bladder infections. If you suffer frequent bladder infections, read your condom package to see if spermicide is the problem.

Condoms need not mean a loss of pleasure. There are new, more comfortable brands of condoms such as the crowd-sourced (allegedly unbreakable) condom Hex™ and *myONE Perfect Fit*®, who provide 60 different sizes. Finding the right size condom is as important as finding the right size shoe!

The male condom has a *perfect use* failure rate of 2 percent and a *typical use* failure rate of about 18 percent.[43]

Female Condoms

The female condom is a latex tube or sheath with a flexible ring at each end. One ring is inserted into your vagina and lodged there during intercourse. The outer ring remains outside your vulva.

The main advantage of the female condom is that you are in control. You can insert it hours before sex, which means no distraction during foreplay. Because the outer ring of the female condom covers your entire vulva, it offers better protection against sexually transmitted disease than the male condom. The outer ring may also enhance your sexual pleasure by rubbing against your clitoris.

The female condom has a *perfect use* failure rate of 5 percent and a *typical use* failure rate of 28 percent.[44]

Diaphragm Without Spermicide

A diaphragm is a soft latex or silicone dome that seals against your vaginal wall and prevents sperm from entering your uterus. You can insert up to two hours before sex, but then you must leave it in for six hours after. Unlike the female condom, your partner will not feel a diaphragm.

The old latex style of diaphragm had to be fitted by a doctor. It also had to be used with a spermicide gel, which would put it into the Type 2 category of contraception that does some harm (discussed below).

The new silicone Caya® diaphragm is used with a non-toxic gel, and is one-size-fits-all so does not need to be fitted by your doctor. You can buy Caya® directly online or from your local family planning clinic or pharmacy.

A diaphragm has a *perfect use* failure rate of 6 percent and a *typical use* failure rate of 12 percent.[45] It does not protect against sexually transmitted disease.

Cervical Cap Without Spermicide

The cervical cap is similar to the diaphragm but smaller. It shaped like a little sailor's cap and fits around your cervix. You can leave a cervical cap in place for up to two days, and use it with a non-toxic gel.

The cervical cap Femcap® comes in three different sizes and is available in some countries without a prescription. In the U.S., it must be fitted and prescribed by a doctor.

Femcap® has a *typical use* failure rate of 8 percent.[46] It does not protect against sexually transmitted infections.

For links to Femcap® and the Caya® diaphragm, please see the Resources section.

Withdrawal or Pull-Out Method

In this method, your partner withdraws his penis and ejaculates outside of your vagina. Withdrawal has been popular for more than 2,500 years and is still widely used today. Withdrawal, also known as *coitus interruptus*, is controversial because it's considered less effective than other methods. The *typical use* failure rate is as high as 28 percent, but when used properly, withdrawal has a *perfect use* failure rate of just 4 percent, which is comparable to some of the barrier methods.

Success with withdrawal depends on the skill and commitment of your partner, so I do not recommend it for new, young, or inexperienced couples. It also offers no protection against sexually transmitted infection.

> **You cannot rely on withdrawal** if you have sex twice in a row. That's because sperm remains in the penis after ejaculation and can seep into your vagina during your second session. If you want to have sex a second time, then ask your partner to urinate to wash out the sperm and clean his penis, or use a barrier method.

Type 2 Contraceptive Methods

Type 2 contraceptive methods are less preferred methods because they carry some toxicity or health risk. However, they are better than Type 3 methods because they do not suppress ovulation. They permit you to make progesterone.

Type 2 methods are not ideal, but they are a still a reasonable choice.

Copper Intrauterine Device (IUD)

The IUD is a device made of plastic and copper. It looks a bit like an earring and is inserted into your uterus. Insertion is a simple procedure that happens in your doctor's office. It can be a little uncomfortable, but it's quick. It is not surgery and usually does not require sedation or general anesthesia.

One woman described IUD-insertion this way:[47]

> It's like a PAP smear test but a little weirder and more uncomfortable.

To remove the IUD, your doctor will find the removal string and pull it back out through your cervix. Removal is simple and something you can request from your doctor at any time. A patient once told me she'd like to try an IUD but didn't want to have to "convince her doctor to remove it" one day. Just to clarify: there should be no convincing involved. It's your body. If and when you want your IUD out, your doctor will take it out.

The best thing about the copper IUD is that it does not change your hormones. It does not prevent ovulation. Instead, the IUD prevents pregnancy in two ways:

- The copper ions impair sperm motility.
- The simple physical presence of something in the uterus changes the uterine lining so that a fertilized egg cannot implant and develop.

The copper IUD is highly effective, with a failure rate of 0.6 percent. And it's simple. Once inserted, it can stay in your uterus for ten years or more. When your doctor finally removes the IUD, you should regain full fertility within just one menstrual cycle.[48]

Special Topic: Dark Memories of the Dalkon Shield

Like many women, you may have a vague unease about the safety of a copper IUD. It's a dark memory from a terrible time more than 40 years ago. Back then, a poorly designed IUD called the Dalkon Shield caused 18 deaths and thousands of pelvic complications among its 2.8 million users. The problem was the multifilament string of that particular IUD, which grew bacteria. Modern IUDs have a different string and carry no significant risk of infection.[49]

Many women love the copper IUD, and it currently has the highest rate of user satisfaction of any method.[50] It's can also be used as emergency contraception if it is inserted within five days after unprotected intercourse.

Modern IUDs are potentially suitable for women of any age, including teenagers and women who have not yet had children. In 2014, the American Academy of Pediatrics stated that IUDs are a first-line contraceptive choice for teenagers, and overturned the previous opinion that IUDs should not be used until after childbirth.

There are, however, several downsides to the copper IUD.

Pain

You will probably experience some pain with insertion and for a few days after. You may also notice that your periods are more painful for the first twelve months after insertion. They should then return to normal.[51]

Heavy periods

A copper IUD will increase the volume of your menstrual flow by 20–50 percent. For example, if your flow is normally 50 mL per month, then it will increase to between 60 and 75 mL. It may then decrease again by the end of the first year.[52] Heavier periods can be managed by treatments discussed in the Heavy Periods section of Chapter 9.

Expulsion

An IUD can come out, and if you don't realize it's happened, then you could become pregnant. Signs of expulsion include pain, spotting, and the absence or lengthening of the string. The risk of expulsion is highest during the first three months after insertion.

New frameless IUDs such as GyneFix® and Ballerine® are easier to insert and has a lower risk of expulsion.[53]

Infection

If you have a pre-existing infection with gonorrhea or chlamydia, then you are at risk for pelvic inflammatory disease (PID) during the three weeks after IUD insertion.[54] Your doctor should screen for those common infections before inserting an IUD.

Bacterial vaginosis

The copper IUD disrupts the vaginal microbiome and doubles the risk of bacterial vaginosis (BV),[55] which causes vaginal discharge with a fishy odor.

Copper toxicity

Some women report anxiety after IUD insertion and attribute it to possible copper toxicity. Like so many aspects of women's health, there is very little research, but one study *did* find higher blood levels of copper in IUD users.[56] In theory, that elevated copper could affect mood and other aspects of health.

You are more likely to suffer symptoms from copper if you are deficient in zinc, so I recommend testing for zinc deficiency before inserting an IUD. And keep in mind that you also obtain quite a lot of copper from your diet, including dark chocolate, which contains about 1 mg per square.

 The pill can also cause copper excess because synthetic estrogen causes the body to retain copper.

Hormonal Intrauterine Device (Mirena® IUD)

Mirena® and Skyla® are hormonal IUDs that releases the progestin levonorgestrel into your uterus. As such, they could be included in the Type 3 hormonal contraception section, but I've included them here for comparison's sake.

With the hormonal IUD, levonorgestrel acts locally in your uterus to prevent pregnancy in three ways:

- It thickens cervical mucus.
- It inhibits sperm survival.
- It prevents the build-up of your uterine lining.

Mirena® users have a blood level of levonorgestrel which is about one-tenth that of pill users.

The hormonal IUD does not aim to suppress ovulation, which is why I view it as the least harmful of all the hormonal contraceptive methods. Unfortunately, as we saw in the last chapter, it does suppress ovulation at least some of the time.

You can leave Mirena® in place for five years until the progestin runs out. Then it must be replaced.

Mirena® will make your period very light—almost non-existent. That's why it's used to treat heavy periods.

Spermicide

Spermicide (or sperm-killer) prevents pregnancy by killing sperm.

Historically, people have tried many substances to kill sperm. The list includes crocodile dung, wool soaked in acacia, lemon juice, and—in the 1940s—Lysol (which caused burning and inflammation). None of those substances were terribly effective, and the modern spermicide nonoxynol-9 is not much better. When used alone as a foam or jelly, nonoxynol-9 has a failure rate of around 20 percent.[57] To improve its effectiveness, spermicide is typically used with a sponge or diaphragm. We discussed diaphragms in the Type 1 section above.

Nonoxynol-9 is a surfactant found in cleaning products. There's no question that it's toxic—that's its job! Regular exposure to nonoxynol-9 can cause itching, burning, and an increased frequency of vaginal infections and sexually transmitted disease.

Female Tubal Ligation

Tubal ligation or "having your tubes tied" is permanent blockage of your Fallopian tubes so that eggs can no longer pass into your uterus. Ligation requires keyhole surgery under general anesthetic. The surgeon cuts into your pelvic cavity and then severs, clamps, cauterizes, or removes your Fallopian tubes. The current recommendation is to remove the tubes entirely to reduce the long-term risk of ovarian cancer.[58]

There is also a non-surgical method of tubal ligation called Essure® which involves the insertion of fiber coils up through the uterus and into each tube. There are serious safety concerns about Essure, so I do not recommend it.

Tubal ligation is highly effective, long-term contraception. Ligation reversal can be attempted but is not usually successful, so the method is suitable only if you are 100 percent certain you do not want more children.

Tubal ligation carries the risks of surgery and general anesthetic. Officially, it does not interfere with ovulation or hormonal balance, but women with a history of tubal ligation are more likely to go on to suffer irregular and heavy periods.[59]

Vasectomy

Vasectomy is the male equivalent of tubal ligation. It involves the cutting, clipping, or cauterizing of the vas deferens tubes— tubes which carry sperm from the testicles to the penis. Unlike female tubal ligation, vasectomy is not surgery. It's done in a doctor's office with local anesthetic.

Vasectomy is highly effective, long-term contraception. Reversals can be attempted, and, according to the Mayo Clinic, are successful 40 to 90 percent of the time.

Up to 10 percent of men undergoing vasectomy can develop post-vasectomy pain syndrome.[60]

Vasalgel

A new method of reversible male contraception is under development by the non-governmental organization, the Parsemus Foundation. It is called Vasalgel and is a one-time injection of gel into the vas deferens. The gel blocks sperm in a way similar to vasectomy but can be flushed out with a second injection when a man wishes to restore his fertility.

Vasalgel is currently undergoing clinical trials and may soon be available.[61]

Type 3 Contraceptive Methods

Hormonal contraception includes all pills, implants, patches, injections, and vaginal rings. They use steroid drugs to suppress ovulation. As we saw in Chapter 1, ovulation is the key event in a healthy menstrual cycle. For that reason, drugs that suppress ovulation are all equally unsuitable for period health.

Chapter 4

➤──────────➤

WHAT SHOULD YOUR PERIOD BE LIKE?

M ENSTRUAL BLEEDS are nicknamed "periods" because they arrive *periodically* in a regular monthly pattern.

Why monthly? The timing of a healthy cycle is determined by three important events in your ovaries. First, your ovarian follicles enter a final race to ovulation. This stage—called your follicular phase—takes approximately two weeks, though it can be shorter or significantly longer. Then, you have ovulation, which takes about one day. Finally, you have your luteal phase, which takes pretty close to 14 days.

The timing of a healthy period is the sum of three main phases:

- the follicular phase, which can last anywhere from 7 to 21 days
- ovulation, which lasts one day
- the luteal phase, which lasts 10 to 16 days.

If you're an adult, it all adds up to a healthy menstrual cycle of anywhere between 21 and 35 days. Twenty-eight days is the average, but not the rule.

If you're a teenager, your cycle will be longer because you can have a follicular phase as long as 32 days. Your luteal phase is the same 10 to 16 days. It all adds up to a healthy menstrual cycle of anywhere between 21 and 45 days.

To determine the length of your menstrual cycle, start counting from your first day of heavy bleeding. Call this "day 1" and enter it as the first day of your period on your period app. The days of light spotting that come before your heavy day are not part of this cycle. They are the final days of your previous cycle.

 As an adult, it's normal to have a cycle of anywhere from 21 to 35 days.

Let's now look at your three phases in more detail.

Follicular Phase and Estrogen

A healthy period starts with healthy follicles. Your follicular phase begins when a few follicles (usually six to eight) enter the final days of their race to ovulation. It's important to understand that the total lifespan of each follicle is much longer than just the two or three weeks of your follicular phase. Your follicles actually started their race to ovulation months before.

 follicle

An ovarian follicle is a sac that contains one egg (oocyte). It is the part of your ovary that produces estrogen, progesterone, and testosterone.

It takes 100 days for your follicles to mature from their dormant state all the way to ovulation. If your follicles were unhealthy for any part of that maturation process, the result could be a period problem *months later*. When you see it this way, you can understand why period health is a long-term project. Your period problem now could be the result of something that was happening with your health months ago.

When your follicles enter the final stage of their development—your follicular phase—things really start to heat up. That's when the pituitary hormone FSH (follicle-stimulating hormone) pushes you closer to ovulation and stimulates your follicles to make estrogen.

FSH

FSH or follicle-stimulating hormone is a pituitary hormone that stimulates ovarian follicles to grow.

---

pituitary gland

The pituitary gland is a small endocrine gland attached to the base of the brain.

FSH is like the whip that snaps over your follicles. When you are young, you have a lower level of FSH, so your follicular phase will tend to be longer. When you are older (in your forties), you have more FSH, so your follicular phase will tend to be shorter.

Estradiol, Your Queen Estrogen

Your developing follicles release an important estrogen called *estradiol*. Estradiol is not your only estrogen. You also have estrone from fat tissue and a number of estrogen metabolites made by your gut bacteria. But estradiol is the estrogen made by your developing follicles, and it's your best estrogen.

Estradiol is your happy hormone or "yang hormone." It stimulates mood and libido because it boosts the neurotransmitters serotonin (which promotes feelings of well-being and happiness) and dopamine (which is associated with motivation and pleasure).

Estradiol has many other benefits for bones, muscles, brain, heart, sleep, skin, and metabolism. For example, estradiol enhances your sensitivity to insulin,[62] and so helps to prevent a pre-diabetic condition called *insulin resistance,* which we'll discuss in Chapter 6 and the insulin-resistant PCOS section in Chapter 7.

One of estradiol's main jobs is to stimulate your uterine lining to grow and thicken and prepare for a baby. It's quite simple: the more estradiol you have, the thicker your uterine lining, and the heavier your period will eventually be.

Estradiol also stimulates a unique type of vaginal discharge called *fertile mucus.*

Special Topic: Vaginal Discharge or Cervical Fluid

It's normal to see white stuff in your underwear. It's a combination of shed cells from your vaginal wall, healthy bacteria and—most importantly—fluid or mucus made by your cervix. In addition to its role in fertility, vaginal discharge keeps your vagina moist and healthy and free from infection.

Healthy vaginal discharge is white or light yellow and has a mild salty odor. If your vaginal discharge has a bad smell or causes discomfort or itching, you might have an infection and should see your doctor.

If your vaginal discharge is a copious slippery blob, it's something normal and healthy called *fertile mucus.*

Fertile Mucus

Cervical fluid or fertile mucus is the creamy and then wet and slippery kind of discharge you see when you have a lot of estrogen. At its peak, fertile mucus looks and feels like raw egg white and can occur in a fairly large quantity. You'll notice fertile mucus on your panties or toilet paper after you wipe, and it can be a bit disconcerting when you see it for the first time.

Fertile mucus is stimulated by estrogen, which is why it normally occurs when your estradiol is high just before ovulation. Its main purpose is to help sperm survive and get where they're going. Fertile mucus contains microscopic "sperm escalators" that hasten sperm into your uterus. If sperm had to swim unassisted, they would take hours to reach your waiting egg. Inside fertile mucus, sperm are propelled to your Fallopian tubes in just minutes. Progestin-only birth control methods such as the Mirena IUD work primarily by preventing the formation of fertile mucus.

As we discussed in the previous chapter, fertile mucus is an important part of the fertility awareness method of birth control (FAM), but please be careful. Fertile mucus *usually* occurs during the days before ovulation, but it can actually occur *anytime* that estrogen is high. For example, if your follicular phase is particularly long and drawn-out as might happen during stress, then your estrogen will rise and fall, and you could see several episodes of fertile mucus before you finally ovulate. You could also see fertile mucus without ever ovulating at all. See the Abnormal Timing of Fertile Mucus section in Chapter 5.

Ovulation

As your follicular race proceeds, eventually, one (or more rarely, two) of your follicles reach the finish line. Your winning, dominant follicle swells, and then—triggered by luteinizing hormone (LH)—finally ruptures to release its egg.

The release of the egg is ovulation. The final stages of swelling can take a few hours, but the event itself occurs over just a few minutes. As the egg ruptures out of your ovary, you may notice *mittelschmerz*, a twinge or mild pain on one or both sides of your lower pelvis.

Ovulation is an all-or-nothing event. You cannot *sort of* ovulate. You either ovulate, or you don't. Once you have ovulated, there is no going back. Your egg has been released, and it cannot be recalled. It's like the release of doves at your wedding. You are committed. After ovulation, you will either be pregnant *or* you will get your period approximately two weeks later. There's no third option. It's not possible to ovulate but then not be pregnant or get your period.

> (tip) **The average day** of ovulation is day 14, but don't worry if it doesn't happen then. If you have a longer cycle, then you have a later ovulation. To estimate when your next ovulation *might* occur, count back approximately two weeks from the first day of your next expected period.

After your egg is released, it's swept up into one of your Fallopian tubes, where it can be fertilized if sperm is present. The other follicles that lost the race to ovulation are reabsorbed by your ovary.

Ovulation is a momentous event, even if you're not trying for pregnancy. Why? Because ovulation is how you make progesterone.

Luteal Phase and the Rise of Progesterone

After ovulation, things start to get interesting. That's when your emptied follicle restructures itself into a progesterone-secreting gland called the *corpus luteum.*

> *corpus luteum*
>
> The corpus luteum is a temporary endocrine gland that forms from the emptied ovarian follicle after ovulation.

> *luteal phase*
>
> The luteal phase of a menstrual cycle is the 10 to 16 days between ovulation and the bleed, and is determined by the lifespan of the corpus luteum.

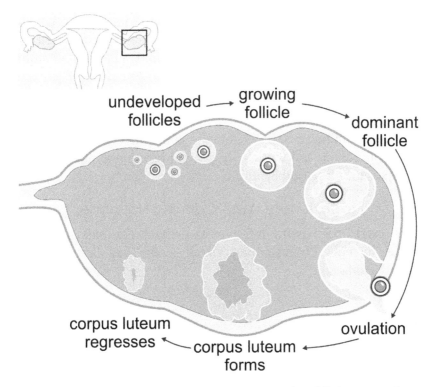

image 6 - the journey from follicle to corpus luteum

Your corpus luteum forms rapidly, and it's an amazing feat. The tissue grows from virtually nothing to a fully vascularized, 4-centimeter structure in less than one day. Researcher Dr Sarah Robertson at the University of Adelaide in Australia says this about the process:

> "There isn't anywhere else in the body where you have to develop a tissue from scratch in such a short period of time and get a blood supply in so fast."[63][64]

> *Dr Sarah Robertson*

Your corpus luteum is dynamic, vital tissue. And, remember, it is the final stage of your follicle's 100-day journey to ovulation. The health of your corpus luteum is affected by everything that affected your follicles during all of those 100 days.

For example, your corpus luteum can be affected by inflammation, thyroid disease, or a problem with insulin, which we will explore in the coming chapters. It can also be affected by a deficiency of nutrients such as magnesium, B vitamins, vitamin D, iodine, zinc, and selenium.

Your follicle requires good health and nutrition for a solid 100 days, and then, it must still have enough oomph and vitality to form a 4-centimeter corpus luteum gland in one day. It's an ovarian triathlon, and that's why general health and nutrition are so important for period health.

Progesterone, Your Calming Hormone

Your reward for passing the ovulation finish line and making a corpus luteum? Progesterone, which is the key hormone for period health.

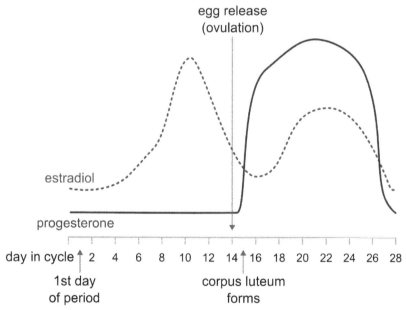

image 7 - menstrual cycle estrogen/progesterone levels

Progesterone is made by your corpus luteum, and it's a startlingly beneficial hormone. Progesterone's biggest job is to hold and nourish a pregnancy, which is how it got its name: progestation hormone, shortened to progesterone.

But progesterone does a lot more for you than just pregnancy.

Progesterone counterbalances estrogen. It is the yin to estrogen's yang. For example, progesterone thins your uterine lining, while estrogen thickens it. Progesterone prevents breast cancer,[65] while estrogen promotes it. Progesterone boosts thyroid hormone, while estrogen suppresses it. Progesterone's stimulating effect on thyroid[66] is how it raises your body temperature in your luteal phase.

> **By thinning your uterine lining,** progesterone can lighten your period.

Progesterone has many other benefits (I call them superpowers):

- reduces inflammation[67]
- builds muscles[68]
- promotes sleep[69][70]
- protects against heart disease[71]
- calms the nervous system and makes it easier to cope with stress[72]

Progesterone calms the nervous system because it converts to a *neurosteroid* called allopregnanolone (ALLO).

> 📖 *allopregnanolone (ALLO)*
>
> Allopregnanolone is a calming neurosteroid that acts like GABA in your brain.

> 📖 *gamma-Aminobutyric acid (GABA)*
>
> GABA is a neurotransmitter that promotes relaxation and enhances sleep.

One of the worst things about hormonal birth control is that it robs you of the calming, mood-enhancing effects of progesterone and allopregnanolone. Remember, the progestin drugs in hormonal birth control are progestins, *not* progesterone. Progestins do *not* convert to calming allopregnanolone, which could be why they cause anxiety and alter the shape of your brain.[73]

Progesterone has many other benefits, which we'll discuss throughout the book. *When it comes to healthy periods, it's mostly about progesterone.*

Anovulatory Cycles

Sometimes, none of your follicles reach the ovulation finish line. You do not ovulate, so you do not form a corpus luteum, and you do *not* make progesterone. But you can still bleed. Why? Because your follicles still make estrogen as they grew and tried to ovulate. And remember, estrogen stimulates fertile mucus and thickens your uterine lining. And, eventually, that uterine lining will have to shed.

Anovulatory cycles are not true menstrual cycles with all the steps of ovulation, corpus luteum, and a luteal phase. Instead, they're like one long continuous follicular phase interspersed with bleeding.

With an anovulatory cycle, you have *unopposed estrogen*, which means you have estrogen, but no progesterone.

Anovulatory cycles are common with PCOS (Chapter 7) and perimenopause (Chapter 10), but they can occur occasionally under normal conditions.[74]

Finally, anovulatory bleeds are the kind of bleed you get with the implant and injection methods of hormonal birth control because they suppress ovulation, but permit estrogen. They're different from pill bleeds which are drug withdrawal bleeds from synthetic estrogen and progestin.

Take the pill? Then you have no follicular phase, no ovulation, no corpus luteum, no luteal phase, and no progesterone.

Lifespan of Your Corpus Luteum

If you become pregnant, then your corpus luteum will survive three months until your placenta takes over the job of making progesterone. If you do not become pregnant, then your corpus luteum has the tiny lifespan of a butterfly. It will survive only ten to sixteen days, which is what defines your luteal phase. That is why (unless you are pregnant), your luteal phase can never be longer than sixteen days.

Your corpus luteum and progesterone are like beloved friends who come but rarely stay. You enjoy their company for a precious two weeks, and then they're gone again.

At the end of your luteal phase, your corpus luteum shrinks and your progesterone drops. That stimulates your uterus to contract and shed its lining.

The Grand Finale: Your Period

If you had a healthy corpus luteum and made enough progesterone, then your uterine lining should be in good shape. For example, it should be well-formed and not too thick or inflamed, and fairly easy to shed.

With enough progesterone, your period will arrive smoothly, with no premenstrual spotting or pain.

Here are some things to understand about the bleed itself.

Menstrual fluid is not all blood

Menstrual fluid contains some blood, but also cervical mucus, vaginal secretions, and bits of the uterine lining (endometrial tissue). Interestingly, two-thirds of your endometrial lining is not shed but is reabsorbed by your body.

Your menstrual fluid should be mostly liquid, with no large clots

As your uterine lining breaks away and sheds, your body releases natural anticoagulants to thin it and help it to flow more easily. If you flow heavily, then you may form a few clots because the anticoagulants do not have time to do their job. Menstrual clots are normal, but they should be few and fairly small: about the size of a dime (1.8 cm).

Your menstrual fluid can range in color from red to brown

Blood turns darker when it's exposed to air, so your period will be light to bright red when you're flowing quickly and darker when you're flowing slowly or just spotting. Your menstrual fluid can look almost brown when it has been on your sanitary pad for a while.

You should lose about 50 mL

You should lose a total of about 50 mL (or three tablespoons) of menstrual fluid over the days of your period. Less than 25 mL is scanty flow. More than 80 mL is heavy flow. Of course, unless you use a menstrual cup, you may never have measured the actual volume of your menstrual flow. You can estimate volume by counting the number of menstrual products. One soaked regular pad or tampon holds 5 mL, or about one teaspoon. A super tampon holds 10 mL. So, 50 mL equates to ten fully soaked regular tampons or five fully soaked super-tampons, spread over all the days of the period. If your menstrual product is not filled, simply adjust the count. For example, a half-filled regular tampon equates to about 2.5 mL.

In simple terms, you shouldn't need to change your pad or tampon more frequently than once every two hours during the day. Your flow should slow during sleep, so you shouldn't need to be up in the night changing a pad.

Your period should last anywhere between two to seven days

Most women flow for three to five days, including a day or two of light spotting as it finishes up.

Count the first day of your heavy flow as "day 1"

When tracking your period, it doesn't matter how many days of bleeding you have. "Day 1" is the first day of your heavy flow and the beginning of your follicular phase. That's when your FSH starts to rise again, and your next batch of ovarian follicles start their final race toward the ovulation finish line.

Counting "day 1" to "day 1," your period should come every 21 to 35 days

As we discussed at the beginning of this chapter, a healthy menstrual cycle consists of a follicular phase of anywhere from seven to 21 days, followed by a luteal phase of between ten and sixteen days. That adds up to a normal menstrual cycle of 21 to 35 days for adults and 21 to 45 days for teenagers.

Special Topic: Why Do We Have Periods?

Blood loss every month seems a waste of resources and nutrients; most other animals simply reabsorb their uterine lining if they don't conceive. Human periods are unique, and scientists think it's something to do with the vigorous and metabolically active nature of the human fetus. To host such a fetus, we need an exceptionally thick uterine lining compared to other animals. Our uterine lining is therefore too thick to be reabsorbed completely and must be shed.

Menstrual Products

You need some way to collect and dispose of your menstrual fluid.

Menstrual Pads

Disposable menstrual pads are the oldest technology. Modern versions are made from absorbent cotton and adhere to the inside of your underpants. Pads are more user-friendly than tampons or cups, and they're a good choice when you're young and have just started menstruating. Pads come in different sizes and absorbencies, from light pads for light-flow days to substantial pads for heavier flow. You can use a pad on its own, or together with a tampon to catch the overflow. To prevent bacterial growth, you should change your pad every four hours. Pads aren't suitable for swimming or some types of exercise.

Reusable menstrual pads are made of cloth so they can be washed and reused.

Tampons

Tampons are a bundle of absorbent material that you insert into your vagina. Many women find them more comfortable than pads, and they can be used during exercise or swimming. Tampons come in different sizes and absorbencies and are usually made of cotton alone, or cotton and rayon combined. Please choose 100 percent cotton tampons, because shreds of rayon can cause vaginal irritation. To prevent bacterial growth, you should change your tampon every two to six hours.

Special Topic: Toxic Shock Syndrome

Toxic shock syndrome (TSS) is a serious condition caused by a bacterial toxin. Some cases have been linked to high-absorbency tampons, particularly to a brand called Rely in the late 70s. Rely used the absorbent materials carboxymethylcellulose (CMC) and compressed beads of polyester, which unfortunately grew bacteria. Those products were eventually pulled from the market.

TSS is rare with modern tampons. It is estimated to affect three out of every 100,000 tampon users per year.

Menstrual Cup

A menstrual cup is a little cup you insert into your vagina. It's soft silicone or natural rubber so you can fold it before and during insertion. After insertion, it springs open to form a seal against your vaginal wall and collect your menstrual fluid. You can leave a cup in place for up to 12 hours. To remove it, simply pull the stem, pinch the base to release the seal, and then empty the cup into the toilet. Wash it with water and then reinsert.

A menstrual cup is reusable, so it saves you money and is better for the environment. It's also a good choice for heavy periods because it doesn't leak and it holds more than a tampon. The average menstrual cup holds about 30 mL, which is equal to about three super-tampons. Finally, it's healthier than tampon use, because it doesn't dry out the mucous membrane of your vagina.

Periods Over All Your Lifetime

Your period probably started when you were about 12 or 13. The average age is 13, but anywhere between 10 and 16 is normal. Your period may have been irregular or heavy for the first few years, but that was just your body finding its way. As we saw with Christine's story in Chapter 1, too many girls are put on the pill to "regulate their periods," when all they need is a little more time.

By the time you reach your reproductive years (age 20 to 45), your ovulation and menstruation should be fairly regular.

For about ten years before menopause, you will be in perimenopause, and your periods will start to change. They will become shorter or longer; heavier or lighter. You could make more estrogen than ever before and at the same time a lot less progesterone. It's a tricky time. Many of the strategies discussed throughout the book are helpful for perimenopause, but we'll also look at some specific strategies in Chapter 10.

Your periods will stop with menopause. The normal age for menopause is anywhere between 45 and 55. The average age is 50.

If menopause occurs earlier than age 40, it is *premature menopause*.

If menopause occurs due to surgical removal of your uterus and ovaries (total hysterectomy), it is called *surgical menopause*.

---

hysterectomy

Hysterectomy is the surgical removal of the uterus. Surgical removal of both the uterus and the cervix and possibly the ovaries is called *total hysterectomy*. Surgical removal of the uterus, but not the cervix or the ovaries, is called *partial hysterectomy*.

Removal of the uterus does not cause menopause. If you still have ovaries, then you still ovulate and make hormones. You may still benefit from many of the treatments in this book.

Period Tracking

You should now have a pretty good idea of what you can expect from your period. Your cycle should be 21 to 35 days with two to seven days bleeding. You should see fertile mucus and ovulate, and then progress to a moderate, painless bleed.

You now have some data for your period app or menstrual cycle diary:

Period tracking 101:

- first day of your heaviest day of bleeding ("day 1" of your cycle)
- number of days between "day 1" and your next "day 1" (length of your cycle)
- number of days of bleeding
- amount of blood (menstrual fluid) lost
- cervical fluid
- pain.

How is your monthly report card looking? If it's different from what I described in this chapter, then you need treatment. Please read on.

Chapter 5

What Can Go Wrong with Your Period? Looking for Clues

Now that you've had a good look at how your period *should* be, you can start to think about how it *really* is. Is it regular? Is it heavy? Is it painful? These are your clues. How can you interpret them?

Let's take a closer look at your monthly report card.

Do You Ovulate?

As you learn to interpret your period clues, please always come back to this one essential question: do you ovulate?

Knowing *if* and *when* you ovulate is the best way to understand your period. That will tell you if and when you make progesterone, which as we've seen, is an essential hormone for period health.

If you discover that you do *not* ovulate, then your next step is to figure out why not—and what you can do to fix that.

How do you know if you ovulate? As we saw in Chapter 3, signs of possible ovulation include fertile mucus, a positive urine ovulation stick, and a regular cycle. Evidence of definite ovulation includes a rise in waking temperature and an increase in progesterone as measured by a mid-luteal phase blood test to be discussed later in this chapter.

> *(tip)* **Your period app may indicate ovulation,** but it's only guessing. To truly *know* if and when you ovulate, you need to track your temperature as described in the Fertility Awareness Method section of Chapter 3.

A period is *not* a definite sign of ovulation because, as you may recall from the last chapter, it could have been an *anovulatory bleed*. An anovulatory cycle is like a continuous follicular phase followed by breakthrough bleeding.

You know you've had an anovulatory cycle if your temperature does *not* go up in the two weeks before your period. It's okay to have the occasional anovulatory cycle because they're actually pretty common even in healthy women.[75] An anovulatory cycle is only a problem if that's all you have—in other words, if you *never* ovulate.

Keeping the question of ovulation always in mind, let's now consider some common period problems.

No Periods or Irregular Periods

An absence of periods is called *amenorrhea*. More precisely, an absence of periods when you used to have them is called *secondary amenorrhea*, which is what we'll be discussing here. You could also have something called *primary amenorrhea*, which means you have never had a period. That is beyond the scope of this book. If you are aged 16 or older and have never had a period, then please see your doctor.

Pregnancy

First of all—and not to be overlooked—your lack of periods could simply mean pregnancy. It's an obvious possibility if you've had regular periods, and they then stop. It's a less obvious possibility (but still possible) if you have not had periods. For example, perhaps you have not had a period for many months after coming off the pill. You could still be pregnant. Maybe you did a pregnancy test a few months ago, and it was negative, and you have not had a period since. You could still be pregnant now.

How could it happen? Remember, first you ovulate, and *then* you bleed two weeks later. If you have not been ovulating, but then you *do* ovulate, you could become pregnant on that very first ovulation. In that case, you could be pregnant without ever seeing a period.

If you have irregular periods (and you want to avoid pregnancy), it is still possible to use the fertility awareness method with the right training; however, further precautions in the form of a barrier method may be necessary.

 No periods? Don't forget to rule out pregnancy, even if you frequently go for months without a period.

Another confusing thing is that light bleeding is a common symptom of early pregnancy. Take care that you do not mistake that for a strangely light period. If in doubt, do a pregnancy test.

Menopause Transition or Perimenopause

Your lack of periods could be the beginning of menopause.

The timing of menopause is for the most part genetically programmed. You cannot delay menopause with the pill or any natural treatment. If you want to know when your periods might stop, ask your mother, aunts, or older sisters when *their* periods stopped. You will likely be the same.

If you are younger than 40, then your lack of periods is probably not menopause. Only one in 100 women undergo premature menopause or primary ovarian insufficiency. Your doctor can easily rule out menopause with a blood test for follicle stimulating hormone (FSH). If your FSH is higher than 40 IU/L on two occasions a month apart, then you are beginning the menopause transition—see Chapter 10.

Stress or Illness

Emotional or physical stress, illness, trauma, or surgery are all common reasons to miss a period or two. It happens when your hypothalamus, which is the command center of your hormones, makes the executive decision to temporarily suppress reproduction and halt your period. It's a smart strategy because stress could mean you're in a dangerous situation such as illness or war, which would not be a good time to make a baby. You're probably not in a war, but your hypothalamus doesn't know that. When this kind of menstrual suppression becomes chronic, it is called *hypothalamic amenorrhea* (HA), which we'll cover in Chapter 7.

---

hypothalamus

The hypothalamus is the part of the brain just above the pituitary gland. It sends messages via the pituitary to all the other endocrine glands including ovaries, thyroid, and adrenal glands.

Undereating

Undereating is another kind of stress that can stop your periods and cause hypothalamic amenorrhea. Again, it's a smart decision by your hypothalamus—if you're not eating enough, then it could mean you're in a famine and would have a hard time making a baby. This is true even if you don't want a baby. From your body's perspective, having a healthy period is fundamentally about being healthy and nourished enough to reproduce.

Undereating can stop periods—even if you are a healthy body weight.

We used to think that amenorrhea occurred only below a certain body weight or body mass index (BMI). We now understand that the hypothalamus cares less about body weight and more about whether you're eating enough to keep up with your activity. This is called energy availability and is the ratio between energy intake, body mass, and energy expenditure or exercise.[76]

So, you can be normal weight or even slightly *over*weight and still lose your period due to undereating.

---

 body mass index (BMI)

Your BMI is your weight in kilograms divided by the square of your height in meters. A normal BMI is between 18.5 and 24.9.

Too few calories can trigger a starvation response in your hypothalamus that disrupts luteinizing hormone (LH) and shuts down ovulation. Too few carbohydrates (but enough calories) can do the same thing.[77] You can, therefore, lose your period to a low-carb diet. That's what happened to my patient Zarah.

Zarah: Have you lost your period to a low-carb diet?

Zarah came to me because she'd not had a period for four months. She was confused because her periods had always been as regular as clockwork.

Her doctor had run all the usual tests and found nothing abnormal.

"I don't understand it," said Zarah. "I eat super healthy. Actually, healthier than ever before."

The phrase "super healthy" caught my attention.

"How healthy?" I asked.

As it turned out, Zarah and her boyfriend Sam had been "eating clean" for the last ten months on the advice of Sam's personal trainer. They started each morning with a green smoothie and then limited their other two meals to meat and non-starchy vegetables. Sam was doing very well. He'd lost 10 centimeters around his waist and had never felt better.

Zarah had lost some weight too, but not too much. She assured me that she was getting enough to eat and I believed her. She ate plenty of high-calorie foods such as meat and avocado and eggs and butter. She just wasn't eating enough starchy foods.

"You need more carbs than your boyfriend," I said. "As a woman, you need a certain amount of carbohydrate to be able to ovulate and have a period."

I reassured Zarah that she did not need to eat "bad carbs," like sugar and flour, but she did need to eat rice or potatoes every day. Somewhat reluctantly, Zarah reintroduced starch, and three months later, she got her period.

Did you notice that Zarah's period didn't come back right away? It took three months because the ovarian follicle takes 100 days on its journey to ovulation.

Some women need quite a lot of carbohydrate to ovulate. Some need less. It all depends at what point the starvation response is triggered in your hypothalamus.

Medical Conditions

Lack of periods or irregular periods can be caused by medical conditions such as celiac disease (gluten sensitivity) or thyroid disease. We'll discuss thyroid disease in a few places in the book, including a special section in Chapter 11.

Final Diagnosis

After all the other things have been ruled out, your doctor will most likely give you the diagnosis of polycystic ovary syndrome (PCOS) or hypothalamic amenorrhea (HA).

Just a comment about diagnosing PCOS: the condition cannot be diagnosed or ruled out by pelvic ultrasound. In other words, you could have a normal ultrasound but still have the hormonal condition PCOS. Please see Chapter 7.

> *ultrasound*
>
> A pelvic ultrasound is an imaging study to view your ovaries and uterus. It uses sound waves (not radiation) and is safe, noninvasive, and painless.

Late Periods

Your period should come at least every 35 days. If it comes later, then you've had a long cycle. Long cycles are a type of irregular period. They can indicate either an anovulatory cycle or a very long follicular phase. They do not indicate a long luteal phase because that is not possible. Unless you're pregnant, your luteal phase can never be longer than sixteen days. You can have the combination of a long follicular phase and a short luteal phase. That's why it's so helpful to know if and when you ovulate.

A long follicular phase can occur at any age. If you're younger than 45, it can result from stress, illness, undereating, or PCOS. If you're over 45, your long follicular phase could also be due to thyroid disease or the final transition to menopause.

> *(tip)* **If you've always had cycles longer than 35 days,** you probably have PCOS. Many PCOS sufferers are not aware they have the condition.[78]

Early Periods

Your period should come no sooner than 21 days. If it does, then you've had a short cycle. Like long cycles, short cycles are a type of irregular period. They indicate either an anovulatory cycle, a short follicular phase, or a short luteal phase.

A short follicular phase is most common during perimenopause. It happens then because your pituitary starts making more FSH, which speeds up the race to ovulation. More FSH can also cause you to make more estrogen than you did when you were younger.

Early in perimenopause, you will probably have a short follicular phase. Later in perimenopause, you may swing to having a long follicular phase interspersed with a short follicular phase interspersed with anovulatory cycles.

What appears to be a short cycle could also be bleeding between periods, discussed later in this chapter.

Short Luteal Phase

As mentioned in Chapter 3, you can measure the length of your luteal phase by tracking the rise of your basal body temperature. When you see a rise in temperature for at least three consecutive days, then you ovulated *at the start of that rise*. With a healthy corpus luteum, you will then see between eleven and sixteen high-temperature days between ovulation and the first day of your period.

If you do not see a consistent rise in temperature, then you did not ovulate. If you go on to bleed, then you had an anovulatory cycle.

If you see a temperature rise, but it does not last at least ten days, then you had a short luteal phase.

A short luteal phase can be caused by many of the same things that cause lack of periods, stress being the most common. Stress-induced menstrual disturbance ranges from a short luteal phase as the mildest version to anovulatory cycles as the more severe, followed by amenorrhea as the most severe.[79]

A short luteal phase results in low progesterone.

Low Progesterone

There are two kinds of low progesterone.

- With an anovulatory cycle, you make no progesterone at all—at least for that cycle.
- With a short luteal phase, you make a less than optimal amount of progesterone.

How do you know if your progesterone is less than optimal? Symptoms of low progesterone include no luteal phase or a short luteal phase, fertile mucus during the premenstrual phase, PMS, premenstrual bleeding or spotting, and prolonged or heavy menstrual bleeding.

Testing for low progesterone

You can ask your doctor to measure progesterone with a blood test. The best day to test is in the *middle* of your luteal phase which is sometimes called a "day 21" progesterone test. Of course, your mid-luteal day may not be day 21. It depends on the length of your cycle. For example, if you have a 21-day cycle, then your mid-luteal day is approximately day 14. If you have a 35-day cycle, then your mid-luteal day is approximately day 28. By definition, your mid-luteal day is approximately seven days *after* ovulation and seven days *before* your next expected period.

 Your doctor may not know when to test progesterone.

If you test progesterone at the right time (after ovulation), then it should be at least 3 ng/mL (9.5 nmol/L).[80] If it's below that, then you either *did not ovulate*, or you tested at the wrong time. Avoid interpreting your progesterone result before your period comes. Wait for your period, and then ask: "Was the test done within the 14 days before my period?" If not, the test is meaningless.

A good progesterone reading is 10 ng/mL (30 nmol/L), and it can be much higher. In fact, the higher, the better. But don't worry too much if it's a bit on the low side. Progesterone fluctuates widely in bursts 90 minutes apart, so a low-normal reading may simply mean that your sample was taken at a low point between bursts.

 Take hormonal birth control? There's no point testing progesterone because you have none.

Charting your waking temperature is another, equally scientific way to measure your progesterone. If you see a consistent temperature rise and a luteal phase of at least eleven days, then you know you made enough progesterone.

Special Topic: Roadmap to Progesterone

You probably want more progesterone, and if so, you're not alone. Low progesterone is associated with PCOS, heavy periods, fibroids, acne, hair loss, premenstrual syndrome (PMS), and perimenopause.

This entire book is about boosting progesterone because this entire book is about ovulating. Healthy ovulation is *how* you have a regular cycle. It's also how you make progesterone.

Healthy ovarian follicles → healthy ovulation → healthy corpus luteum → more progesterone.

And remember, your ovarian follicles need to be healthy for *all* of their 100-day journey to ovulation. If they're unhealthy for even *part* of their journey, the result will be low progesterone months later.

Heavy Periods or Heavy Menstrual Bleeding

A heavy period is blood loss greater than 80 mL or lasting for more than seven days. That 80 mL equates to sixteen fully soaked regular tampons or eight fully soaked super-tampons, spread over all the days of your period.

Prolonged bleeding

If you flow for more than seven days, you have prolonged bleeding. It can be due to different things, including uterine polyps or fibroids, so please start with a visit to your doctor. The most common cause of prolonged bleeding is an anovulatory cycle, which typically occurs with PCOS (Chapter 7) or perimenopause (Chapter 10), but it can happen in other situations.

Menstrual clots

When menstrual flow is heavy, your body's natural anticoagulants don't have time to keep up with the flow, and so you will see menstrual clots. A few clots are fine, but if you regularly see clots larger than a quarter (2.4 cm), then check with your doctor.

What causes heavy menstrual bleeding?

Heavy menstrual bleeding and large menstrual clots can be caused by many things, including the copper IUD, perimenopause, anovulatory cycles, thyroid disease, coagulation disorders, endometriosis, and adenomyosis. We'll discuss those conditions in the later chapters.

(tip) **Periods suddenly much heavier or more painful?**
You could have the gynecological condition adenomyosis, which affects one in five women, and worsens with age. See the Adenomyosis section in Chapter 9.

---

adenomyosis

Adenomyosis is a gynecological condition in which uterine lining grows within the muscle of the uterine wall. It can cause pain and heavy periods.

The most common cause of heavy periods is a *hormonal imbalance,* which is a combination of 1) low progesterone (discussed earlier) and 2) estrogen excess.

Estrogen Excess

How do you know if you have estrogen excess? Symptoms include heavy periods, breast tenderness, PMS, and fibroids.

You can ask your doctor to measure estradiol with a blood test. I recommend you test in the middle of your luteal phase. That way, you can assess progesterone at the same time. At its highest point, estradiol should not exceed 270 pg/mL or 1000 pmol/L. If it does, then you have too much estrogen. As you interpret your result, understand that estradiol fluctuates greatly throughout your cycle, and even throughout the day. It's lowest on day 3 of your period. It's highest about four days before ovulation (day 10 in a standard cycle), and then again in the middle of your luteal phase (day 21 of a standard cycle).

Special Topic: Estrogen Dominance

Estrogen dominance means you have too much estrogen and not enough progesterone. Most commonly, estrogen dominance describes estrogen excess (as discussed in this section), but it can also refer to a situation of normal estrogen, but low progesterone.

I do not use the term estrogen dominance, because I prefer the more precise terms of *estrogen excess* and *low progesterone.* You can suffer both problems simultaneously.

The term "estrogen dominance" is popular online, but it may not be familiar to your doctor. For that reason, I recommend you don't use the term when speaking with your doctor (see the How to Talk to Your Doctor section in Chapter 11).

Estrogen excess is caused by a combination of 1) higher

production by your ovaries, and 2) impaired metabolism or detoxification. Higher production by your ovaries usually only occurs during perimenopause, which we'll discuss in Chapter 10. Impaired estrogen metabolism or detoxification can happen anytime.

Estrogen Metabolism

Estrogen metabolism is the healthy removal or detoxification of estrogen from your body. It's a two-step process.

First, your liver inactivates estrogen by attaching a little molecule or "handle," which is called *conjugation*. To do that effectively, your liver needs a good supply of nutrients such as folate, vitamin B6, vitamin B12, zinc, selenium, magnesium, and protein. Your liver also needs to be relatively free from the toxic effects of alcohol or endocrine disrupting chemicals. Even one drink per day can increase your blood level of estrogen.

Special Topic: Endocrine Disrupting Chemicals

Endocrine disrupting chemicals (EDCs), or endocrine disruptors, are the many different industrial chemicals that interfere with hormone action and metabolism. Common EDCs include pesticides, solvents, fire retardants, mercury, and plastic softeners such as bisphenol A (BPA). These chemicals can impair the healthy metabolism or detoxification of estrogen. They also alter hormone levels and interfere with hormone receptors.

EDCs have been linked with an increased risk of women's health conditions such as PCOS and endometriosis. See the Environmental Toxins section in Chapter 11.

The second step of estrogen metabolism or detoxification is the elimination of conjugated estrogen through your gut. It requires you to have healthy intestinal bacteria or a healthy gut *microbiome*.

> 📖 *microbiome*
> The genetic material of the microorganisms in a particular environment such as the body or part of the body.

When healthy bacteria are present in your gut, they assist with the safe removal of conjugated estrogens via your stool. When unhealthy bacteria are present, they impair estrogen metabolism by making an enzyme called *beta-glucuronidase*, which deconjugates and reactivates estrogen. The reactivated estrogen is then reabsorbed into your body by a process called *enterohepatic recirculation* or "gut-liver recirculation." The result can be estrogen excess.

To prevent estrogen excess, you want to maintain healthy gut bacteria. We'll look at ways to do that in Chapter 11.

Hypersensitivity to Estrogen

It is not just how much estrogen you have, but how *sensitive to it* you are. For example, you can be hypersensitive to estrogen when you have chronic inflammation or when you are deficient in the mineral iodine.[81] Replacing iodine can be a helpful treatment for estrogen excess symptoms such as heavy periods, breast pain, and more.

We'll look at the treatment of estrogen excess in Chapter 8 and heavy periods in Chapter 9.

Light Periods

A light or scanty period does not necessarily mean that something is wrong. You can lose as little as 25 mL of menstrual fluid, and that is still normal. That equates to five regular tampons, spread over all the days of your period.

If you see less than 25 mL of menstrual fluid, it raises the question: is it a true period or is it an anovulatory cycle? Remember, a true period is one that follows a follicular phase, ovulation, and luteal phase.

If you are confident that you *do* ovulate, then things are going pretty well with your periods, despite your scanty flow. You have enough estrogen, or you would not be able to reach ovulation. You just don't have as much estradiol as many women, and that can be the result of several factors. The most common reasons for lower than average estrogen include smoking, undereating, and high amounts of soy or other phytoestrogens in your diet. For more information about the estrogen-lowering effect of phytoestrogens, see the Soy section in Chapter 6 and Sam's patient story in Chapter 9.

 Remember that estrogen fluctuates. It's normal for estrogen to be *very low* on day 2 or 3 of your cycle.

If you find no evidence of ovulation or a luteal phase, then you are not ovulating, and that's the significant thing about your light period. The solution is not to boost estrogen but to restore regular ovulation. That may mean reducing stress or eating more or correcting a condition such as PCOS—for more on this subject, see Chapter 7.

Pain

Pain is an important clue on your period report card. It can mean a lot of different things—anything from benign run-of-the-mill period pain to more serious conditions such as infection and endometriosis. Let's have a look.

Period Pain

Normal period pain (*primary dysmenorrhea*) is a bit of cramping in your lower pelvis or back. It's also called menstrual cramps, and occurs just before your period or on the first day or two of your period. It can be relieved by ibuprofen, and should not interfere with your daily activities.

Normal period pain is caused by the release of prostaglandins in your uterus. Having more estrogen and less progesterone can cause a higher level of prostaglandins and more period pain.[82]

Normal period pain will usually improve as you get older. And normal period pain should disappear with the diet changes and supplements discussed in Chapter 9. Put it this way: if it doesn't disappear, then it's not normal period pain. I would consider it *severe* period pain.

---

dysmenorrhea

Dysmenorrhea is the medical term for painful menstruation.

---

prostaglandins

Prostaglandins are hormone-like compounds that have a variety of physiological effects, such as the constriction and dilation of blood vessels.

Severe period pain (*secondary dysmenorrhea*) is throbbing, burning, searing, or stabbing pain that lasts for many days and can even occur between periods. It's not relieved by ibuprofen, and can be so bad you vomit and need to miss school or work.

Severe period pain is caused by an underlying medical condition such as endometriosis or adenomyosis, which we'll discuss in Chapter 9. It can get worse as you get older.

Special Topic: A Missed Diagnosis

Endometriosis is a condition in which bits of tissue that are *similar to the endometrium* (uterine lining) grow in places other than inside your uterus. It is a very common condition and affects up to one in ten women. Unfortunately, endometriosis is not easy to diagnose. For example, endometriosis *cannot* be diagnosed by ultrasound. You could have a perfectly normal ultrasound and still have the disease. Also, some doctors miss the signs of endometriosis in young women and so fail to mention it as a possibility. That's why it typically takes up to ten years to diagnose.

Do not let that happen to you. Don't suffer a decade of crippling pain and be told that it's "just period pain," and there's nothing you can do.

Please read the Endometriosis section in Chapter 9, and then speak to your doctor. Tell her how many painkillers you take, and ask her outright if you should speak to a gynecologist about endometriosis.

Pain During Sex

A rubbing or friction pain during intercourse is common and probably means you do not have enough lubrication which can be the result of stress or not being adequately aroused. If you are approaching menopause, then vaginal dryness can be the result of declining estrogen.

Pain during intercourse can also be a sign of mild vaginal infection such as vaginosis or yeast infection (see below).

Deep, stabbing pain during sex is more serious and can be a sign of an ovarian cyst, endometriosis, adenomyosis, or an infection. Check with your doctor.

Pain from Infection (Pelvic Inflammatory Disease)

Pelvic infections are usually caused by sexually transmitted disease, but they can be caused by other types of infections. Some infections cause constant pain and fever, but some cause only occasional pain, or itchy, bad-smelling discharge. Some infections (such as chlamydia) cause *no* symptoms, which is why your doctor may want to screen you for chlamydia.

Do not ignore a possible pelvic infection—if left untreated, it can lead to complications and infertility. If you think you might have an infection, then see your doctor. You may require antibiotics.

Mid-Cycle Ovarian Pain

A little pain with ovulation is normal because your egg has to rupture out the side of your ovary, and that is a mildly violent event. Normal ovulation pain feels like a little twinge in your lower pelvis. It should be brief—no more than an hour or two—and it should not require a painkiller or interfere with your routine. Ovulation pain is called *mittelschmerz*, which is German for "middle pain."

You may experience stronger ovulation pain if it has been some time since you last ovulated, such as might occur if you've just come off the pill or are recovering from PCOS. In that case, you can expect your first ovulation or two to be painful, but then the pain should subside in subsequent cycles.

If you consistently experience severe pain with ovulation, please see your doctor. You could have an infection, ovarian cyst, adenomyosis, or endometriosis.

Ovarian Cysts

Your ovaries are filled with ovarian follicles, and follicles are essentially small, normal "cysts" (although they're not usually called that). Every month, those normal cysts grow, burst, and are reabsorbed. Occasionally, there is a glitch, and one of your follicles becomes abnormally large and fluid-filled, forming an abnormal ovarian cyst.

There are many different types of ovarian cysts. They may be symptomless, or they may cause pain. They may be hormonally neutral, or they may release estrogen and disrupt your menstrual cycle. Most of the time, ovarian cysts are benign and resolve on their own. Very occasionally, they require surgery.

The multiple small "cysts" of PCOS are not ovarian cysts in the true sense of the word. They are not abnormally large follicles.

Instead, they are abnormally *small* follicles that are in a state of partial development. The treatment of PCOS is different from the treatment of ovarian cysts.

For more information about the types of ovarian cysts and their treatment, please see Chapter 9.

Abnormal Vaginal Discharge or Cervical Fluid

As we saw in the previous chapter, it's normal to see white stuff in your underwear. Normal vaginal discharge is white or light yellow and has a mild salty odor. You will probably also see a few days of clear, slippery fertile mucus leading up to ovulation.

No Fertile Mucus

What if you do not see fertile mucus? Does that mean you did not ovulate? Not necessarily. You might be producing a small amount of fertile cervical fluid, but just not enough to notice unless you actively check for it. Or your fertile mucus might be masked by a yeast infection or bacterial vaginosis.

Yeast Infections or Bacterial Vaginosis

If you notice itchy or bad-smelling discharge, check with your doctor because you might have an infection and require antibiotics.

If your doctor says you have a yeast infection or bacterial vaginosis, then antibiotics is not necessarily the best treatment. Instead, it's time to think about your vaginal microbiome. Earlier in this chapter, we discussed the gut microbiome which is the community of bacteria living in your intestine. The vaginal microbiome is the community of bacteria living in your vagina.

One of the many benefits of the vaginal microbiome is to protect you from the overgrowth of unwanted yeast and bacteria. If your vaginal bacteria fail at their job, then yeast or certain strains of bacteria get the upper hand, and cause a yeast infection or bacterial vaginosis. Both conditions may be best described as an "ecological disorder of the vaginal microbiome."[83]

---

bacterial vaginosis

Vaginosis is an overgrowth of one or more species of normal vaginal bacteria.

To maintain a healthy vaginal microbiome, you want to avoid as much as possible those things that disrupt good bacteria, including antibiotics, hormonal birth control, and the use of a vaginal douche or wash.

For more information and treatment of yeast infections and bacterial vaginosis, please see the Yeast Infection and Bacterial Vaginosis section in Chapter 11.

Abnormal Timing of Fertile Mucus

What if you see fertile mucus more than once? You might think stop-and-start fertile mucus means you're ovulating several times —but that is not what is happening. You can ovulate only once, and you can detect that by your rise in basal body temperature. Stop-and-start fertile mucus means you're having a long, drawn-out follicular phase and a stuttering attempt to ovulate.

You can also see fertile mucus but then never actually ovulate. That is an anovulatory cycle.

Finally, you can see fertile mucus *after* ovulation. It doesn't mean you're going to ovulate again. It means you did not make enough progesterone to dry up the fertile mucus.

Bleeding Between Periods

Mid-Cycle Bleeding

Light spotting on the day of ovulation is common and normal. It's caused by a mini-estrogen withdrawal as your estrogen dips after its pre-ovulation surge. Ovulatory spotting is more likely if you have lower than average (but still normal) estrogen.

If you experience spotting at other times in the cycle, then ask yourself: *Is it mid-cycle spotting or is it a light anovulatory bleed?* Because what you experience as bleeding "between" periods may simply be the random breakthrough bleeding of an anovulatory cycle. That brings us back to the central question when it comes to period health: *Do you ovulate?* Knowing if and when you ovulate will help you to understand the pattern of your bleeding.

Mid-cycle bleeding can also be a sign of a more serious gynecological condition such as uterine fibroids, endometriosis, pelvic infection, or uterine polyps. If you are unsure as to the cause of your bleeding, check with your doctor.

---

uterine polyps

Uterine polyps or endometrial polyps are outgrowths from the uterine lining (endometrium). They are usually benign or non-cancerous.

Bleeding After Sex

There are several potential explanations for light bleeding or spotting directly after intercourse. It could simply be from inadequate lubrication, but it could also be the result of underlying infection or inflammation. It's best to see your doctor.

Premenstrual Bleeding

It's common to see a bit of spotting or light bleeding in the day or two before your period starts. Two days of premenstrual bleeding is normal. If you spot for more than two days, then your progesterone may be dropping away too soon, or you have something else going on. For example, premenstrual spotting can be a symptom of thyroid disease, fibroids, endometriosis, or uterine polyps.

> **Remember that "day 1" of your cycle** is the first day of your heavy bleed. The days of premenstrual spotting are the final days of your previous cycle.

Theresa: Two kinds of spotting

Theresa noticed a lot of spotting when she first came off the pill. She would bleed for a few days, which she thought was her period. Then, just ten days later she would spot again for a week. And then have another period. This went on for six months until she saw her doctor, who ordered blood tests and a pelvic ultrasound and said that everything was normal.

I asked Theresa to track her temperatures, and we discovered that she did *not* have a luteal phase temperature rise which meant she was not ovulating. Instead, she was having anovulatory cycles or breakthrough bleeding.

With further testing, we were able to detect that Theresa had high androgens or male hormones, which meant she had PCOS, a common cause of anovulatory cycles.

I asked Theresa to reduce sugar in her diet and take the herbal medicine peony and licorice combination, which we'll discuss in Chapter 7. Over the next seven months, she started to ovulate and see a nice temperature rise in her luteal phase.

The spotting, however, did not improve, which surprised me. Theresa was now ovulating and making progesterone which should have improved the spotting. What was going on?

I asked her to have another pelvic ultrasound.

"But I had an ultrasound over a year ago," she said. "And it was normal. I don't see the point of testing again because nothing has really changed."

But something *had* changed. "You weren't ovulating before," I said. "And now you are. So, there must be something new that's masking your improvement."

Theresa had a second ultrasound which this time showed the presence of a uterine polyp. Her gynecologist removed the polyp, and finally, the spotting stopped.

Premenstrual Symptoms

You may experience a wide variety of symptoms during the week or two before your period. Common symptoms include irritability, headaches, acne, breast tenderness, fluid retention, food cravings, and acne. Premenstrual symptoms are clues from your luteal phase, and, as we'll see in Chapter 8, they stem from a combination of high estrogen, low progesterone, and inflammation.

 Acne can flare during PMS, but it often stems from an underlying cause such as PCOS or coming off the pill. Refer to Treatment of Acne in Chapter 7.

Postmenstrual symptoms

If you notice "postmenstrual" symptoms, it may indicate that you've had an anovulatory cycle such as occurs with PCOS.

 Mood symptoms that occur on hormonal birth control are side effects. They are not premenstrual symptoms.

Advanced Period Tracking

Now that we've had a good look at what can go wrong with your period, you have more data for your period app. You're ready for advanced period tracking which can include any or all of the following.

Advanced period tracking:

- "day 1" of your cycle
- length of your cycle
- number of days of bleeding
- quantity of menstrual fluid
- bleeding between periods (spotting)
- cervical fluid
- result of an LH test stick
- waking temperatures
- duration of luteal phase
- pain and number of painkillers
- premenstrual symptoms such as irritability, headaches, acne, or breast tenderness
- unusual stress or illness.

You don't have to track every sign and symptom on an ongoing basis. You can, if you enjoy it, but you can also just track the basics like "day 1." And then track other data if and when you notice that something is wrong, and you want to gather data to communicate to your doctor.

When should you see your doctor?

- If you have no periods at all, or if your cycle is shorter than 21 days or longer than 35 days. (Please read Chapter 7 before talking to your doctor about irregular periods.)
- If you suspect you do not ovulate.
- If you bleed for more than seven days or lose more than 80 mL of menstrual fluid.
- If you experience pain between periods or pain so severe you cannot carry out your normal activities.
- If you notice bad-smelling vaginal discharge.
- If you observe bleeding after sex or bleeding between periods that is not ovulation spotting.

I hope this chapter has given you the beginning of an idea of what might be wrong with your period. We'll dive deeper into assessment and diagnosis in the second half of the book and we'll also look at all the many options for treatment.

Your Period Report Card

A summary of your clues.

No periods at all

Possible significance: pregnancy, menopause, stress, illness, thyroid disease, celiac disease, coming off hormonal birth control, PCOS, HA, high prolactin.

Late periods

Possible significance: anovulatory cycle, long follicular phase, stress, illness, thyroid disease, PCOS, HA, high prolactin.

Early periods

Possible significance: anovulatory cycle, short follicular phase, short luteal phase, low progesterone, PCOS, perimenopause, stress, mid-cycle bleeding.

Heavy periods

Possible significance: perimenopause, adolescence, anovulatory cycle, estrogen excess, low progesterone, PCOS, copper IUD, thyroid disease, fibroids, endometriosis, adenomyosis, coagulation disorders.

Prolonged bleeding

Possible significance: anovulatory cycle, perimenopause, uterine polyps, PCOS.

Menstrual clots

Possible significance: heavy menstrual bleeding, low progesterone, perimenopause, thyroid disease, endometriosis, adenomyosis, fibroids.

Light periods

Possible significance: anovulatory cycle, PCOS, excess phytoestrogens, mid-cycle bleeding mistaken for a period.

Severe period pain

Possible significance: copper IUD, endometriosis, adenomyosis, infection.

Pain before periods

Possible significance: normal period pain, endometriosis, adenomyosis, ovarian cysts, infection.

Pain during sex

Possible significance: insufficient arousal causing lack of lubrication, low estrogen, infection, fibroids, endometriosis, adenomyosis.

Mid-cycle ovarian pain

Possible significance: normal ovulation pain (mittelschmerz), temporarily worsened ovulation pain (during first few cycles off the pill), infection, endometriosis, ovarian cysts.

No fertile mucus

Possible significance: anovulatory cycle, low estrogen, yeast infection, bacterial vaginosis.

Abnormal timing of fertile mucus

Possible significance: anovulatory cycle, long follicular phase, low progesterone.

Yeast infections or bacterial vaginosis

Possible significance: hormonal birth control, problem with the vaginal microbiome, antibiotics.

Mid-cycle bleeding

Possible significance: normal ovulation spotting, anovulatory cycle, endometriosis, adenomyosis, uterine polyp, ovarian cysts, infection.

Premenstrual bleeding

Possible significance: anovulatory cycle, low progesterone, endometriosis, thyroid disease, uterine polyps.

Bleeding after sex

Possible significance: inflammation of cervix, cancer of cervix, infection, cervical or uterine polyp, endometriosis.

Premenstrual symptoms (PMS)

Possible significance: estrogen excess, low progesterone, inflammation, histamine intolerance, stress.

Postmenstrual symptoms

Possible significance: anovulatory cycle, PCOS.

Acne

Possible significance: PMS, PCOS, hormonal birth control, coming off hormonal birth control.

PART TWO

➤————→

Treatment

Healing is a matter of time, but it is
sometimes also a matter of opportunity.

~ Hippocrates ~

Chapter 6

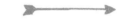

General Maintenance for Periods

WELCOME TO the treatment section of the book. In the coming chapters, I will provide you with targeted treatment strategies for your specific period problem. To get the maximum benefit from those treatments, you must first have some general maintenance.

I know you want to read ahead to the nitty-gritty of your particular period problem, but please don't skip this chapter. *It is the most important chapter in the book.* General maintenance lays the groundwork for all the treatments that come later. If you do not first implement these basic principles, you will not reap the benefits from those targeted treatments.

What is "general maintenance" for periods? It's all the different things that you can do to soothe, cool, and nourish your body.

Soothe Your Hormonal System

Stress

Stress has a huge impact on period health. For one thing, it directly affects your hypothalamus, which is your brain's hormone command center. Under stress, your hypothalamus reduces its signals to your pituitary, which, in turn, reduces production of FSH and LH—the two hormones that promote ovulation. In simplest terms: stress leads to reduced pituitary signaling, which leads to fewer ovulatory cycles. We'll discuss this more in the Hypothalamic Amenorrhea section in the next chapter.

Cortisol

The problem of stress doesn't stop there. Stress also increases *cortisol*, which is the stress hormone made by your adrenal glands. Cortisol is a life-saving, fight-or-flight hormone that gets you through acute challenges such as infection or danger. It changes your physiology in ways that improve short-term survival such as increasing heart rate and raising blood pressure. Cortisol makes you more alert and increases your blood sugar to provide your muscles with energy. Short-term activation of cortisol is beneficial.

Long-term, chronic activation of cortisol is *not* beneficial. When your cortisol stays high day after day, it steals protein from your muscles and reduces your sensitivity to insulin. It also weakens your immune system and impedes ovulation and ovarian steroid production.[84] And finally, it damages the hippocampus which is the part of the brain that calms the hypothalamic-pituitary-adrenal (HPA) axis. Chronic stress, therefore, can lead to dysregulation or dysfunction of your HPA axis.

HPA Axis Dysfunction

HPA axis dysfunction or dysregulation is impaired

communication between your hypothalamus, pituitary, and adrenal glands. It causes symptoms such as fatigue, anxiety, insomnia, low libido, low blood pressure, salt cravings, poor immunity, brain fog, PMS, and irregular periods.

 HPA axis dysfunction

HPA axis dysfunction is a pattern of chronic stress and abnormal regulation of cortisol. It's the correct medical term for what some clinicians used to call "adrenal fatigue" or "adrenal exhaustion."

HPA axis dysfunction is caused by stress and other factors such as sleep deprivation, circadian disruption (jet lag or staying up late), undereating, nutrient deficiency, and illness.

Female hormones *improve* HPA axis function because both estrogen and progesterone stabilize the HPA axis.

So, if you have a problem with ovulation, then it can become a vicious cycle: HPA axis dysfunction causes period problems, which further increase HPA axis dysfunction. The way to improve things is to treat HPA axis dysfunction with the strategies discussed here. You may then require additional strategies when your hormones and HPA axis start to change dramatically in your forties, as we'll discuss in Chapter 10.

---

tip **The synthetic progestins** in hormonal birth control may worsen HPA axis dysfunction.[85]

How to test for HPA axis dysfunction

At this stage, there is no reliable way to assess HPA axis dysfunction. A recent study surveyed all possible methods including salivary cortisol tests and concluded that none are accurate predictors of fatigue or symptoms.[86] Better testing methods may become available in the future,[87][88] but in the meantime, I assess HPA axis dysfunction based on symptoms and sometimes a blood test for the adrenal hormone *DHEAS*, which can become deficient during chronic stress.

DHEAS

DHEAS (dehydroepiandrosterone sulfate) is a steroid hormone made by the adrenal glands. It's often high with PCOS and low with HPA axis dysfunction. DHEAS naturally declines with age.

(tip) **Your doctor may not be familiar** with the terms "adrenal fatigue" and HPA axis dysfunction. If you mention "adrenals" to your doctor, she may test for Addison's disease, which is a rare autoimmune disease of the adrenal glands.

Diet and Lifestyle to Regulate Your HPA Axis

Rest and joy are the best treatments for your HPA axis. In the pursuit of period health, you now have permission to take time away from your work and other duties, and instead, spend time doing the things you love. Maybe you like sports, athletics, swimming, or dancing. Make time to do that. Or maybe your thing is to head to the art gallery or go walking with friends. Make time to do that. Or maybe you love yoga or reading novels, or cooking. Whatever it is that you love to do, commit at least two hours per week to that activity. Put it on your calendar like you would a meeting or an appointment. It's an appointment with yourself! Within two months, you will see the results on your monthly report card.

Meditation, massage, and yoga are all helpful relaxation techniques. Please choose the style that appeals to you.

Finally, **maintaining stable blood sugar** is a simple way to improve the function of your HPA axis. The best way to do that is to eat a small portion of protein with every meal, especially breakfast.

Supplements and Herbal Medicines to Regulate Your HPA Axis

Magnesium is the key nutrient for calming your nervous system and regulating your HPA Axis. We'll look at magnesium later in this chapter as The Miracle Mineral for Periods.

Zinc improves the health of the hippocampus,[89] which is the part of the brain that calms the HPA axis. Please see the Zinc section later in this chapter.

B vitamins can help reduce perceived stress and improve anxiety.[90]

> **How it works:** B vitamins boost levels of the calming neurotransmitters GABA and serotonin.

> **What else you need to know:** For stress and HPA axis dysfunction, choose a B-complex that contains choline and vitamin B5, the "anti-stress factor."[91] For PMS and perimenopause, you may require additional vitamin B6.

Rhodiola rosea is a herbal medicine that was traditionally used as an energy and fertility tonic in Iceland, Norway, Sweden, and Russia.

> **How it works:** It calms your HPA axis by sheltering your brain from cortisol and excitatory neurotransmitters.[92] In one Swedish placebo-controlled study,[93] participants given Rhodiola had measurably lower cortisol levels and scored better on scales of burn-out and cognitive function. Rhodiola can also relieve symptoms of depression.[94]

> **What else you need to know:** The exact quantity of the herb depends on the concentration of the formula, so please take as directed on the bottle. You can take Rhodiola on its own or combined with other *adaptogen* herbs such as Siberian ginseng and ashwagandha; for best results, take an adaptogen formula twice daily for at least three months. Be aware that Rhodiola is endangered in some parts of the world, so try to

choose a product that's been sustainably sourced.

 adaptogen

In herbal medicine, an adaptogen is a plant extract which helps the body adapt to stress. The term is not recognized by the scientific community.

Sleep

Sleep is another priority strategy for period health. Getting seven or eight hours of quality sleep each night will do more for you than almost any supplement or herb we discuss in this book.

Why is sleep so important for hormones? For one thing, it stabilizes your HPA axis and cortisol. It also improves insulin sensitivity and regulates the release of luteinizing hormone (LH), estrogen, and progesterone.

(*tip*) **Sleep is more important** than exercise. Hopefully, you have time in your day for both. If you have to choose between sleep and exercise, choose sleep!

Aim for at least seven hours each and every night. If you have trouble sleeping, then please take a minute to consider the underlying reason. Here are the possible causes of insomnia:

- chronic stress
- HPA axis dysfunction and elevated cortisol
- low blood sugar
- lack of evening wind-down time
- too much caffeine
- magnesium deficiency
- thyroid disease
- perimenopause
- grief

- anxiety
- depression
- evening exposure to blue light.

> (tip) **Blue light is the glare** from your TV or phone, and it's bad for sleep because it interferes with the sleep hormone melatonin. A simple solution is to dim your phone and use one of the tools to reduce blue such as the computer plugin *f.lux* or the phone apps Twilight or Night Shift.

Supplements and Herbal Medicines to Aid Sleep

Magnesium is the best supplement for promoting healthy sleep. Please see the Magnesium section later in this chapter.

Melatonin promotes sleep and works particularly well when insomnia is due to aging, depression, or jet lag. I recommend 0.5 to 3 mg at bedtime. It is non-addictive, so safe for long-term use.

Ziziphus spinosa is a herbal medicine from traditional Chinese medicine. It is a non-addictive sedative[95] which is typically combined with magnolia (*Magnolia officinalis*) for a stronger effect.[96] *Ziziphus* is particularly helpful for perimenopause because it can relieve palpitations and night sweats. The exact quantity of the herb depends on the concentration of the formula, so please take as directed on the bottle.

Other effective herbal medicines for sleep include kava, valerian, magnolia, passionflower, and hops.

Exercise

Regular exercise is highly beneficial for period health. Here are just some of the ways in which exercise improves period health:

- modulates your stress response and reduces cortisol
- improves your sensitivity to insulin so can prevent or

treat period problems like PCOS

- improves circulation to your pelvic organs, strengthens your pelvic floor muscles, and aligns your uterus inside your pelvis.
- reduces chronic inflammation.[97]

What type of exercise should you do? Bottom line: choose the type you enjoy. That will make it much easier to commit to exercise on an ongoing basis. For example, you may enjoy team sports. Or you may prefer swimming, dancing, walking, or yoga. Any and all of those activities are beneficial for period health.

Special Topic: Is Too Much Exercise Bad for Periods?

There's an old idea that too much exercise can stop periods. It's because some athletes develop what used to be called "female athlete triad," which is amenorrhea in combination with an eating disorder and decreased bone mineral density. The updated term is *relative energy deficiency in sport* (RED-S) which is defined as "energy deficiency relative to the balance between dietary energy intake and energy expenditure required for health and activities of daily living, growth and sporting activities."[98]

In other words, the problem is not exercise per se, but rather not consuming enough energy (food) to sustain that level of activity. As we'll see in Chapter 7, the solution is to *eat more*.

Cool Inflammation

Chronic Inflammation

Now we come to an important topic in period health, as chronic inflammation is a major factor in *all* types of period problems. Does that surprise you? When you think of inflammation, you probably think of the pain and redness that occur in parts of the body like joints or skin. It might also make sense that inflammation causes certain types of period problems, such as period pain.

But chronic inflammation is about more than just pain and redness. Much, much more. Chronic inflammation is about *whole-body communication.*

The different parts of your body need to talk to one another. They need to communicate, and your hormones are a big part of that communication. For example, your pituitary gland talks to your ovaries with your hormone FSH. In turn, your ovaries talk to the rest of your body with your hormones estradiol and progesterone. For example, there are estradiol and progesterone receptors in *all* your body's tissues including breasts, uterus, brain—but also bones, muscles, liver, and intestine. Even your gut bacteria respond to hormones.

Your hormones are important messengers for your period health, but they are not the only messengers. You have other chemical messengers made by your immune system. They have names like *TNF-alpha, IL-6,* and *IL-8.* You don't need to learn all the names of your immune system's chemical messengers—we'll leave that to the biochemists. From now on, we will simply refer to them as *inflammatory cytokines.*

---

cytokines

Inflammatory cytokines are chemical messengers that your body uses to fight infection. They are part of your body's inflammatory response.

The primary job of inflammatory cytokines is to protect you against infections and cancer. That's a good thing.

Unfortunately, inflammatory cytokines also insert themselves into the conversation between your hormones and your hormone-sensitive tissues—and their contribution to the conversation is mostly obstructive. For example, inflammatory cytokines slow the response of your ovarian follicles to FSH. They impede ovulation and impair progesterone production. Inflammatory cytokines also block the receptors for your beneficial hormones, progesterone and thyroid hormone, and can hyperstimulate your receptors for estrogen and testosterone.

All things considered, inflammatory cytokines are a profound hindrance to period health.

How do you reduce inflammatory cytokines? You avoid as much as possible anything that over-activates your immune system. You avoid sources of inflammation, such as:

- smoking
- stress
- lack of exercise
- lack of sleep
- unhealthy gut microbiome
- environmental toxins
- inflammatory foods.

Smoking is the most inflammatory thing you can do because cigarette smoke contains cadmium and pesticides and other hormone-damaging, immune-activating toxins. If you are a smoker, your first step is to quit.

Another source of inflammation is environmental toxins such as plastics, pesticides, and mercury. Toxins can be tough to avoid entirely, so don't worry too much. I have provided some tips in the Environmental Toxins section in Chapter 11.

Finally, your diet can be a source of inflammation because certain foods stimulate your immune system to make inflammatory cytokines. That means your diet can be inflammatory.

Your diet can be *anti*-inflammatory, which is exciting. Change your diet, and you can dramatically reduce inflammation.

How do you get started? Which foods are inflammatory? Based on my reading of the research, and my experience with patients, I have identified the five foods which are most likely to cause inflammation. They include:

- metabolic disruptors: sugar and alcohol
- digestive and immune disruptors: wheat and dairy

products
- processed vegetable oils.

Sugar, alcohol, wheat, dairy and vegetable oil—these are the top five potentially inflammatory foods. Let's now look at each food in detail, and let's be sensible about it.

The following recommendations are guidelines, not hard and fast rules. Depending on your individual situation, you may need to focus on just one or two of the foods. For example, if you have PCOS, then you probably need to focus on avoiding sugar (described below). If you have a gluten sensitivity like Meagan in Chapter 1, then you need to focus on avoiding gluten. Please read through the following discussion of inflammatory foods to discover which aspect of the anti-inflammatory diet is most important for you.

Also, remember that these are only five foods. That leaves you with a lot of other delicious foods to enjoy. I provide some menu suggestions at the end of the chapter.

Sugar and alcohol generate *metabolic inflammation*, which is the activation of inflammatory cytokines in metabolic tissue such as body fat and the liver.

Inflammatory food #1: Sugar

Sugar causes inflammation in a couple of different ways. First, it causes tissue damage. Sugar gloms onto your cells like little bits of chewing gum, and your immune system does not like that. It perceives this kind of "sugar-damage" as an attack and makes inflammatory cytokines to defend against it.

The second way that sugar causes inflammation is that it causes *insulin resistance*.

---

insulin

Insulin is a hormone made by your pancreas. It stimulates your liver and muscles to take up sugar from your blood and convert it to energy.

What is insulin resistance? Under normal conditions, your hormone insulin rises briefly after eating. It stimulates your liver and muscle cells to take up food energy from your blood and convert it to energy. That causes your blood sugar to fall, and then your insulin to fall. When you are *insulin sensitive*, both your sugar and insulin are low on a fasting blood test.

When you are *insulin resistant*, your blood sugar may be normal, but your insulin is high. Why? Because your pancreas has to make more and more insulin to try to get its message through. Too much insulin generates inflammation and causes weight gain. It can also lead to diabetes and heart disease. Finally, too much insulin can impair ovulation and stimulate your ovaries to make testosterone, which is why insulin resistance is a major driver of PCOS, as we'll see in Chapter 7.

---

insulin resistance

Insulin resistance is a condition of high insulin, in which the cells of the liver and muscles fail to respond properly to insulin. It is the precursor to Type 2 diabetes. And if you have Type 2 diabetes, you still have insulin resistance.

You can easily diagnose insulin resistance with a blood test. Please refer to Chapter 7 for testing and treatment.

How does sugar cause insulin resistance?

Sugar, or more specifically, *fructose* causes insulin resistance by generating inflammation in the liver that impairs insulin sensitivity.[99] High-dose fructose in the form of sweet drinks has been found to cause insulin resistance in as little as eight weeks. [100] Fructose is also a potent appetite-enhancer,[101] which is why sugar makes you feel hungry and overeat.

But wait. Isn't fructose in fruit? How could fruit be unhealthy? Yes, there's fructose in fruit, but it's a small amount. A small amount of fructose does *not* cause inflammation or insulin resistance but instead *improves* insulin sensitivity and health. A small amount of fructose is less than 25 grams per day, which is about what you'd get from three servings of whole fruit.

In contrast, a large amount of fructose is what you get from the Standard American Diet, also called the Western pattern diet, or "normal" diet. If you eat this so-called "normal" diet, you're eating at least 100 grams of *added* fructose per day, and probably more. You're getting it from all the sweet things like soft drinks, candy, chocolate bars, desserts, sweetened yogurts, and breakfast cereals. That's true whether they're sweetened with high fructose corn syrup (55 percent fructose), table sugar (50 percent fructose), or honey (40 percent fructose).

Did you see honey on that list? "Natural sugars" such as honey, agave syrup, date balls, and fruit juice are a big source of fructose. They're a big source of sugar because *natural sugars are still sugar*. Dates, for example, are among the most sugary foods you can eat, and a single 8-ounce glass of orange juice contains 18 grams of fructose.

> (tip) **The impact of fructose** on your health depends on the amount you consume. The small amount in whole fresh fruit is fine. The large amount in fruit juice and dried fruit can cause or worsen insulin resistance.

Need a quick way to know if a food item has too much sugar? Ask yourself: does it taste really sweet? If it does—if it is essentially *dessert*—then it has too much sugar.

So how much sugar should you eat? Put it this way: *not* the 100 grams of added sugar of the Western pattern diet. Instead, you can most certainly have the 25 grams that occur naturally in a whole food diet. That's true regardless of your health. Beyond that, it depends.

If you have normal insulin sensitivity, you might be able to get away with the 25 grams of *added* sugar recommended by the World Health Organization.

If you have insulin resistance or insulin-resistant PCOS, you'd do better to avoid all added sugar.

I understand that quitting sugar is not easy, especially if you're addicted. For a full discussion and treatment ideas, please see the Quit Sugar section in Chapter 7.

Aren't rice and potatoes just as bad as sugar?

Sugar is a carb, so what about other carbs such as rice and potatoes? Aren't they just as bad? In a word: no. Starchy foods contain mostly glucose and very little fructose. Glucose does not impair insulin sensitivity as profoundly as does fructose.

Glucose and starch do *increase* insulin, so they could cause or worsen insulin resistance if you were to eat lots and lots of starch and nothing else. Hopefully, that's not what you're doing. Hopefully, you're eating a moderate amount of starch together with other foods such as meat and vegetables (protein, fat, and fiber) which slow the absorption of glucose into your body and thereby help to keep insulin low.

 Adding vinegar to a meal is an easy way to slow the absorption of glucose.[102]

Suffice to say: sugar is inflammatory and can cause insulin resistance. In moderation, starch does not. According to researcher Richard Johnson from the University of Florida:

> "Starch-based foods don't cause weight gain like sugar-based foods and don't cause the metabolic syndrome like sugar-based foods. Potatoes, pasta, and rice may be relatively safe compared to table sugar. A fructose index may be a better way to assess the risk of carbohydrates related to obesity."[103]

Professor Richard Johnson

Inflammatory food #2: Alcohol

For a long time, we thought a small amount of alcohol might be good for health. That wishful thinking seems to have come to an end as we discover that even a few drinks per week can have long-term negative effects on health.[104]

Why is alcohol inflammatory?

For one thing, it's often mixed with sugary beverages such as pop, tonic water, or fruit juice. If that's what you're doing, then you're getting a double whammy of inflammatory food #1 (sugar) *plus* inflammatory food #2 (alcohol).

 If you want to enjoy the occasional alcoholic beverage, then at least choose a non-sugary kind such as dry wine or beer.

Secondly, long-term consumption of alcohol shrinks the brain including the hippocampus, which is the part of the brain that regulates the HPA axis or stress response system. The result can be a dysregulation of your stress response or HPA axis.[105]

There's more. Alcohol impairs the healthy clearance of estrogen, which could be why even moderate drinkers have a greater risk of breast cancer compared to non-drinkers.[106] Also, alcohol causes insulin resistance,[107] damages gut bacteria,[108] prevents nutrient absorption, impairs detoxification, and depletes an important anti-inflammatory molecule called glutathione.

Glutathione is a powerful antioxidant and immune-regulator. Every cell in your body makes glutathione, and every cell needs it. Its primary job is to quench free radicals and eliminate toxins, but it also reduces inflammatory cytokines. One of the best ways to support glutathione is to cut back on alcohol or avoid it altogether. We'll consider other ways to support glutathione in Chapter 11.

What's the verdict on alcohol? You can enjoy the occasional wine or beer, but, as a woman, do not exceed five standard drinks per week and two standard drinks per sitting.

> ### standard drink
>
> In the US, a standard drink contains 0.6 ounces (18 mL) of alcohol which equates to a 12 ounce (350 mL) glass of beer or a 5 ounce (150 mL) glass of wine.

Sugar and alcohol generate metabolic inflammation because of their effects on insulin and glutathione. Food sensitivities such as wheat and dairy are different. They're inflammatory because of their effects on digestion and the immune system.

To understand this kind of inflammation, you must first understand that your immune system and digestion are *not separate things*. They are, in a sense, one continuous entity. Eighty percent of your immune system is clustered around your digestion, where it's in constant communication with your gut and gut bacteria. A "food sensitivity" or a "food intolerance" occurs when a food upsets your gut bacteria or inflames your gut lining—thereby causing your immune system to make inflammatory cytokines.

A food sensitivity is any adverse reaction to a food. It is a broader and more complex reaction than a food allergy.

> ### food sensitivity
>
> Food sensitivity is a broad category of adverse reactions to food. It is often a delayed reaction that involves inflammatory cytokines. Food sensitivity is different from a true food allergy.

> ### food allergy
>
> Food allergy is an immediate reaction to food. It is mediated by a part of the immune system called IgE antibodies and causes symptoms such as hives or swollen airways.

Common symptoms of food sensitivity include headaches, joint pain, digestive bloating, and food cravings. Of course, many of those symptoms can be attributed to other causes which is why "food sensitivity" is a controversial topic.

Did you notice that food cravings are a symptom of food sensitivity? Very often, the craving is for the food that causes the sensitivity (wheat or dairy), but it can also express itself as a craving for sugar (inflammatory food #1).

Intestinal permeability

You are more at risk for food sensitivity if you have a digestive condition called *intestinal permeability,* which means your intestinal wall is "leaky" and permits food proteins to enter your body. The result of that "leakiness" is chronic inflammation.[109] For more information, please see the Intestinal Permeability section in Chapter 11.

Which foods cause food sensitivity?

Any food can potentially trigger a food sensitivity reaction, but the most common reactive foods are wheat and dairy products. Based on clinical signs (which I'll explain below), wheat and dairy are the inflammatory foods that I most commonly ask my patients to avoid. Much of the time that gets a result within three months. If not, then I consider other common food sensitivities such as eggs, soy, and high histamine foods (see below).

 Removing an inflammatory food from your diet can do far more for you than any supplement.

Inflammatory food #3: Wheat

You've probably heard conflicting opinions about wheat and gluten, with some people claiming that gluten is the root of all evil, and others saying it's just fine. There's a reason for the controversy: wheat affects some people more than others. It all depends on your genetic susceptibility, and also on the state of your gut microbiome and whether you have intestinal permeability.

For a lucky few of you, wheat is not inflammatory and not a problem for period health. For many of you, however, wheat *is* a problem. Consider Meagan from Chapter 1, who had irregular periods because of wheat. Wheat is also a contributing cause for premenstrual migraines (Chapter 8) and endometriosis (Chapter 9).

Based on my experience with thousands of patients, I can say this: when wheat is a problem, it is a big problem. I predict that wheat is a major issue for at least one in ten of you. That's why I've listed it as the third most inflammatory food. Wheat is a minor issue for about six in ten of you. For the rest of you, wheat is probably not an issue.

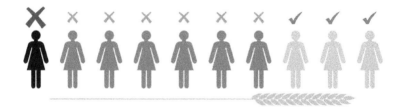

image 8 - wheat sensitivity

What is the problem with wheat?

First, you could have a true IgE-mediated allergy to one of several wheat proteins. A wheat allergy can be picked up by a standard allergy "scratch test." Symptoms of wheat allergy come on quickly— within minutes or hours—and can progress to anaphylaxis.

Alternatively, you could be reacting to gluten, which is an inflammatory protein in wheat and other gluten grains. If your reaction to gluten is severe enough, you will test positive for celiac disease on a blood test. For the test to be accurate, you have to consume gluten for a few weeks. That's why it's important to rule out celiac disease *before* you eliminate gluten.

There is gluten in wheat, spelt, rye, barley, and possibly oats. There is *no* gluten in rice, corn, millet, quinoa, or potatoes.

Celiac disease is becoming more common but it still only affects about one in 100 people. Unfortunately, many of you who test negative for celiac disease may still have a significant problem with gluten. You may have something called *non-celiac gluten sensitivity,* or NCGS.

For a long time, doctors and researchers did not acknowledge the existence of NCGS, but that's all changed. Most experts now recognize that it exists and that it's an inflammatory condition which can manifest with digestive and, more commonly, *non-*digestive symptoms.[110][111][112] In other words, you can have a serious problem with gluten but have *no* digestive symptoms.

Non-digestive symptoms of NCGS include: [113]

- depression[114]
- mouth ulcers
- migraines
- brain fog
- joint and muscle pain
- leg or arm numbness
- eczema
- psoriasis
- autoimmune disease.

 Symptoms of non-celiac gluten sensitivity (NCGS) can occur days or even *weeks* after gluten exposure.

Researchers are scrambling to understand gluten sensitivity and to come up with a way to diagnose it. In the meantime, the best way to assess yourself is to try avoiding wheat for *at least* eight weeks and see how you feel. It's eight weeks because that's how long it takes for the inflammatory reaction to subside

For some of you, the problem may not be gluten at all, but rather another component of wheat called *fructan* or *fructooligosaccharide*. Fructooligosaccharide is one of the several carbohydrates that together are called *FODMAPs*.

 FODMAPs

FODMAPs (Fermentable, Oligo-, Di-, Mono-saccharides, And Polyols) are short-chain carbohydrates that are poorly absorbed in the small intestine. The term FODMAP is an acronym invented by researchers at Monash University in Australia.

FODMAPs occur in wheat, legumes, fruit, and some vegetables. If you cannot absorb them properly, they ferment in your small intestine and cause inflammation. The main symptom of a FODMAP problem is digestive bloating and symptoms of irritable bowel syndrome (IBS). That is more likely to happen if you have a digestive problem called small intestinal bacterial overgrowth (SIBO). For more information about SIBO and FODMAPs, refer to the Digestive Health section in Chapter 11.

small intestinal bacterial overgrowth (SIBO)

Small intestinal bacterial overgrowth (SIBO) is the overgrowth of normal gut bacteria in your small intestine.

tip **Spelt is a cousin of wheat** and a popular wheat substitute. Spelt does contain gluten but it does not contain FODMAPs, so it is easier to digest than wheat.

Inflammatory food #4: Dairy products

Second only to wheat, dairy is the next most common food

sensitivity.

The problem with dairy is not the fat or the lactose—although some people do have difficulty digesting lactose. The problem with dairy is a protein called A1 casein (also called casomorphin or BCM7). For some of you, A1 casein is inflammatory because —like gluten—it stimulates your immune system to generate inflammatory cytokines.[115][116] A1 casein can also reduce your production of the natural anti-inflammatory molecule glutathione.[117]

Fortunately, A1 casein does not generate inflammation in everyone. If you have no signs of casein sensitivity, then you probably do not have the enzyme that converts A1 casein into its inflammatory metabolite (BCM-7). You can, therefore, consume normal cow's dairy.

How do you know if you have casein sensitivity? The first clue is: did you suffer recurrent tonsillitis or ear infections when you were a kid? To me, that is a clear sign that casein may have been disrupting your immune function back then. You probably outgrew those childhood symptoms, but you did not outgrow the immune disruption. Instead, that same immune disruption might manifest now in adult symptoms such as hay fever, sinus infections, chest infections, eczema, and asthma. And that same immune disruption might manifest now in period symptoms such as acne, period pain, PMS, and heavy periods.

One of the ways that casein drives period problems is by contributing to something called *histamine intolerance*.

---

histamine intolerance

Histamine intolerance is the temporary state of having too much histamine, which is the part of the immune system that causes allergies and swelling. In addition to its role in immune function, histamine also regulates stomach acid, stimulates the brain, boosts libido, and plays a key role in ovulation and female reproduction.

Histamine is not bad. It's an important part of physiology, but too much histamine can cause a variety of unwanted symptoms including period symptoms.

Too much histamine can be the result of several different inputs. For example, your body *makes* histamine; food sensitivities like dairy *stimulate* histamine; and many foods like fermented foods *contain* histamine. That's a lot of histamine coming in, but if you're healthy, your body should be able to clear it all with an enzyme called diamine oxidase (DAO). If that enzyme is not functioning well or if there's just too much histamine coming in, you will develop symptoms of too much histamine or histamine intolerance.

There are times in your cycle when you are more vulnerable to histamine intolerance. For example, you may experience it at ovulation and just before your period. Why? Because that's when estrogen is high compared to progesterone, and *estrogen increases histamine*. It does so by stimulating your immune system to make more histamine[118] and by downregulating the DAO enzyme that's supposed to break it down.[119] At the same time that estrogen stimulates histamine, too much histamine stimulates your ovaries to make more estrogen![120] The result can be a vicious cycle of *estrogen → histamine → estrogen → histamine*.

Taking steps to lower histamine can dramatically improve PMS, period pain, and heavy periods. Such steps include avoiding cow's dairy (histamine-stimulating food), avoiding fermented foods (histamine-containing food), and taking vitamin B6 which clears histamine by upregulating the DAO enzyme.[121] We'll revisit the topic of histamine intolerance when we talk about PMS in Chapter 8.

And just a warning: histamine intolerance is not yet a recognized medical diagnosis, so your doctor may not be responsive when you ask about it.

For an example of just how dramatically dairy can affect periods, consider my patient Nina.

Nina: Dramatic improvement by avoiding dairy

Nina was not well. She came to me for bad premenstrual anxiety, but there were lots of other things going on. For example, she had hay fever, itchy ears, and recurrent headaches. She suffered constipation, fluid retention, and bad sugar cravings. She also found it hard to lose weight.

All of her blood tests were normal.

Me: "Did you suffer recurring tonsillitis or ear infections when you were a kid?"

Nina: "Yes, I had tubes in my ears." She meant the small tubes that are inserted in kids' ears to prevent the accumulation of fluid in the middle ear.

Me: "I need you to stop having all normal dairy products for a few months. That includes cheese, yogurt, milk, and ice cream. You can have butter and goat cheese".

Nina: "But I love those foods!"

Me: "Yes, I know." (It's common to crave a food sensitivity, especially dairy.) "But you are going to be amazed at how different you feel. Please try it."

I also prescribed magnesium and vitamin B6 for her PMS, and I then did not hear from Nina for four months.

When she came back, she was ecstatic.

"Almost from the first day I stopped having dairy, I felt better," she said. "The fluid retention went away and I literally *deflated*."

She went on to tell me that her digestion had improved immensely and she no longer needed her hay fever medication. She had no headaches, and she had lost 10 kilograms.

"How about the premenstrual irritability?" I asked.

"Non-existent."

Nina did not require any more appointments with me.

Nina had a fairly severe dairy sensitivity, which I estimate to affect about one in twenty patients. Her kind of dairy sensitivity is different from a true milk allergy, and there's no way to test for it.

Even if you don't have a severe sensitivity like Nina's, you could have a milder version of a sensitivity to A1 casein or cow's dairy —and that could be affecting your periods. Temporarily stopping normal cow's dairy is a simple thing to try and there is a very real possibility that it will improve your PMS, acne, endometriosis, or heavy periods.

If you discover you do have a problem with cow's dairy, you can change to non-dairy alternatives such as rice milk, coconut milk, and almond milk. You could even occasionally have a small amount of soy milk as long as you don't have a thyroid problem —see the Soy section below. Or you can change to Jersey, goat, or sheep dairy. Jersey, goat, and sheep dairy does not contain the inflammatory A1 casein that you get from normal Holstein Friesian cows. The other dairy foods that contain little to no A1 casein include cream, ricotta, and butter.

> (tip) **Whey is the other protein** in dairy products, and there is no evidence that it is inflammatory. Unless you have a whey allergy (which is rare), you can safely consume whey protein.

You don't need to worry about calcium because you can obtain all the calcium you need from Jersey, goat, or sheep dairy products. You can also obtain calcium from other foods such as almonds, leafy greens, and canned salmon with bones. The importance of dairy in our diet has been vastly overstated and a recent Harvard study concluded that humans have *no nutritional requirement for animal milk.*[122]

Finally, we come to processed vegetable oils.

Inflammatory food #5: Vegetable oil

Vegetable oil includes soy, corn, canola, and cottonseed oil. Those oils are inflammatory if they are processed or *hydrogenated* and therefore contain a toxic metabolite called trans fat. Trans fat is most likely to occur in deep-fried food. Fortunately, food regulators have moved to ban trans fat, but there's another problem with vegetable oil: omega-6 polyunsaturated fatty acids. Omega-6 oil is healthy and essential in the small amount you obtain from nuts, seeds, and brown rice. It is not healthy in the large amount you obtain from cooking with vegetable oil. At that dose, omega-6 promotes inflammatory prostaglandins. It's in direct opposition to another type of fatty acid called omega-3, which promotes *anti-inflammatory* prostaglandins.

To keep inflammation low, you want *less* omega-6 and *more* omega-3. And the best way to do that is to decrease omega-6 by avoiding vegetable oil. Instead, choose olive oil, butter, coconut oil, or avocado oil. At the same time, increase omega-3 by eating seafood, organic eggs, and grass-fed meat. You can also supplement 2000 mg of fish oil.

> **Olive oil is healthy.** Although technically a vegetable oil, olive oil is not a source of omega-6 fatty acids. Instead, it provides beneficial monounsaturated fatty acids. Take care to choose a quality brand as some olive oils are blended with other vegetable oils.

Special Topic: What About Coffee?

The milk and sugar in coffee can be inflammatory, but coffee itself—black, organic coffee—is not inflammatory. In fact, the polyphenols in coffee may *reduce* inflammation,[123] which can be good for periods. Other benefits of coffee are that it improves insulin sensitivity[124]and can promote healthy estrogen metabolism or detoxification in some women.[125] Moderate coffee consumption may even reduce the risk of breast cancer.[126]

On the other hand, high caffeine intake has been linked to heavy periods,[127] and caffeine is a stimulating drug. Too much coffee can cause anxiety and insomnia and worsen HPA axis dysfunction. Your response to caffeine depends on your genetic ability to metabolize caffeine and also whether you take the pill, which impairs caffeine metabolism.[128]

Anti-Inflammatory Vegetables

Vegetables reduce inflammation, and they do so in several different ways. First, they provide important nutrients such as vitamin C, folate, and magnesium. Vegetables also feed your gut bacteria and deliver a wonderful cocktail of anti-inflammatory phytonutrients.

Phytonutrients are naturally occurring plant chemicals. They have names such as polyphenols, flavonoids, lutein, and resveratrol. There are thousands of phytonutrients, and we are just beginning to understand all the ways they benefit health and prevent disease. For example, we used to think that phytonutrients were just antioxidants. We now understand that they talk directly to our cells and DNA. Phytonutrients modify hormonal metabolism and function. They switch *off* pro-inflammatory genes and switch *on* anti-inflammatory, anti-aging genes.

Phytonutrients are wonderful medicine. To harness their power, eat as many vegetables and fresh fruits as you can. Fill your fridge every week, and then your job is to eat it all.

Three ways to fill your fridge with vegetables:

1. Schedule a weekly trip to your local veggie market.

2. Sign up for a weekly delivery of a produce box.

3. Grow your own vegetables and herbs.

Some phytonutrients are available as supplements. Two examples discussed in this book are resveratrol and diindolylmethane (DIM).

Phytoestrogens (plant estrogens)

Phytoestrogens are a special group of phytonutrients. They're called phytoestrogens because they exert a weak estrogen-like effect—but they're not estrogen. Phytoestrogens bind so weakly to estrogen receptors that they act more as *anti*-estrogens, which can be beneficial for symptoms of estrogen excess such as heavy periods.

Phytoestrogens occur in plant foods such as nuts, seeds, whole grains, and legumes. In a moderate amount, they are healthy.[129] In a large amount, they can make periods lighter and sometimes even suppress ovulation. Please see A short light cycle: Sam's patient story in Chapter 9.

The best-known phytoestrogens are lignans from flaxseeds and isoflavones from soy.

Soy

Soy isoflavones are a strong phytoestrogen or *anti*-estrogen.

In a large amount, isoflavones can lighten or stop periods, but in a *small amount* (such as from edamame beans or tofu), the anti-estrogen effect of soy is *beneficial*. For example, it can prevent PMS, lighten periods, and has been associated with a reduced risk of breast cancer.[130]

Before menopause, phytoestrogens are *anti*-estrogenic because they block estradiol. After menopause, they're slightly *pro-*

estrogenic because there's less estradiol to block. That's why isoflavones and other phytoestrogens can relieve menopausal symptoms such as hot flashes.

Too much soy can inhibit an enzyme called thyroid peroxidase and affect thyroid function.[131] That's less likely to happen if you consume sufficient iodine.

Nourish Yourself

Good periods require good nutrition. In this section, we're going to look at all the macronutrients and micronutrients your body needs for a healthy menstrual cycle. Macronutrients are substances that you require in relatively large amounts and must be obtained from food (unlike micronutrients which you require only in small amounts).

Macronutrients for Period Health

The main macronutrients are protein, starch, and fat. You need an adequate supply of all three macronutrients each and every day.

Protein

Protein is essential for healthy periods because it provides amino acids to repair and maintain your hormones, muscles, organs, nervous system, and immune system. You need at least one gram of protein for every kilogram of ideal body weight. For example, if you are 65 kilograms (140 pounds), then you need at least 65 grams of protein per day. That equates to at least three servings of an animal protein (meat, fish, eggs, dairy) or six servings of a plant protein (lentils, nuts, tofu).

 Protein for breakfast is an easy way to improve insulin sensitivity, stabilize blood sugar, and calm your stress response or HPA axis.

There are a couple of things to consider if you're relying solely on plant protein. First, you'll need to combine grains plus beans to obtain the complete array of essential amino acids. Next, you should consider the phytoestrogen content of plant proteins and how too many phytoestrogens can have an *anti*-estrogen effect.

Special Topic: Are You Vegan or Vegetarian?

It's easier to be healthy if you eat animal products such as meat, eggs, fish, and goat cheese. That's because animal foods are the best source of protein, zinc, iron, choline, iodine, taurine, omega-3 fatty acids, preformed vitamin A, and vitamin K2. They're the *only* source of vitamin B12. Animal foods are also highly satiating, which prevents over-eating and keeps your insulin low.

If you feel better on a vegan diet, then ask yourself whether it might actually be because you're avoiding dairy. As we saw earlier in this chapter, A1 milk can cause inflammation and histamine intolerance—both of which are a big problem for periods. I've spoken to more than one former vegan who came to realize that the problem was not meat, but dairy products.

If you prefer to be vegetarian, then please eat eggs and non-inflammatory dairy products such as goat and sheep dairy.

If you prefer to be vegan, then I recommend supplementing with vitamin B12 and all or some of the following: zinc, iron, iodine, choline, taurine, vitamin D, preformed vitamin A, vitamin K2, omega-3 fatty acids, and protein. When choosing a vegan protein supplement, consider its phytoestrogen content and watch that it does not shut down your ovulation.

Starch

Complex carbohydrate or starch has many potential benefits for periods.

On the plus side, starch is a good source of energy and supports immune function. Starch also aids with the activation of thyroid hormone and calms your nervous system, which prevents excess cortisol. Finally, starchy foods are a source of fiber and resistant starch to feed your gut bacteria and promote the healthy metabolism of estrogen.

On the negative side, some starch is wheat, which is an inflammatory food for some of you. Also, *too much* starch may cause or worsen insulin resistance, as discussed earlier.

How much starch is too much starch? If you eat the Western pattern diet, you're likely eating cereal for breakfast, bread for lunch, and pasta for dinner. Adding in fruit juice and desserts, this can add up to more than 400 grams of carbohydrate per day, which is too much.

Instead, aim for at least 150 grams of carbohydrate which, for example, equates to a serving of porridge, two potatoes, a small serving of rice, and three pieces of fruit. Choose what I call "gentle carbs," which are *non-inflammatory* carbohydrate foods such as rice, oats, potato, sweet potato, gluten-free pasta, and whole fruit. If you can tolerate gluten, then you can also enjoy some good quality bread.

Yes, rice is a gentle carb. Many of my patients fear and avoid rice because it's a "carb," yet still consume breakfast cereal, muffins, and cookies. Rice is a better choice than any of those foods.

Should you follow a low-carb diet?

You almost certainly want to avoid sugar, the worst carb. Beyond that, you may also want to reduce your intake of starch, especially if you already have insulin resistance or diabetes.[132]

 One simple way to reduce carbohydrate is to have a low-carb breakfast of eggs or meat plus vegetables.

Please think carefully before restricting carbohydrate to less than

100 grams per day. Yes, it might make you feel quite well in the short term. But that could be because you stopped eating wheat —not because you stopped eating all carbs. Or it could be because you stopped eating difficult-to-digest types of carbohydrate called FODMAPs, which we discussed earlier. If your problem is FODMAPs, then a better plan is to fix your digestion so you can eat FODMAPs again. We'll discuss how to do that in the Digestive Health in Chapter 11.

If you follow a low-carb diet in the long term, you might run into problems. A low-carb diet can increase cortisol, slow down thyroid,[133] and cause insomnia, constipation, and hair loss. A low-carb diet can also cause you to eventually lose your period because women need carbohydrate to ovulate.[134] Some women need quite a lot of carbohydrate to ovulate, and some need less. If you are in menopause, then you don't need to ovulate, so you might fare reasonably well on a longer term low-carb diet.

To summarize, potential adverse effects of a low-carb diet include:

- anxiety
- insomnia
- underactive thyroid
- hair loss
- constipation
- amenorrhea (lack of periods).

In general, men do better on a low-carb diet. Remember Zarah from Chapter 5? Her boyfriend Sam thrived on a low-carb diet, but she lost her period.

You don't have to eat a lot of carbohydrate. About 150 grams is usually enough, and the best time to eat it is with dinner so it will stabilize your blood sugar overnight and help you sleep.

Fat

Fat and cholesterol are important for your period because they are the building blocks for your steroid hormones estrogen and progesterone. Certain types of fat, such as medium-chain and omega-3 fatty acids found in coconut oil and fish, have the additional benefit of being anti-inflammatory.

Satiety

You need all three macronutrients—protein, starch, and fat—for satiety. In other words, you need all three to feel full and satisfied and happy in your body. Please don't underestimate the importance of this. We'll look more closely at satiety later in the chapter.

You also need all three macronutrients to convince your hypothalamus that you have enough nutrition to ovulate and have a period.

Micronutrients for Period Health

Micronutrients are vitamins and trace minerals that are essential to period health. There are dozens of micronutrients. You need them all, but fortunately, you do not need to *supplement* them all. You only need to supplement those that are difficult to obtain from diet.

Let's start with the one I recommend most often: magnesium.

Magnesium: The Miracle Mineral for Periods

I prescribe magnesium for almost every patient, and for almost every period problem. As you'll discover in the coming chapters, magnesium is my front-line treatment for PCOS (Chapter 7), PMS (Chapter 8), and period pain (Chapter 9). I love magnesium because it gives fast results. My patients typically feel better almost immediately when they supplement magnesium.

Food sources of magnesium include nuts, seeds, and leafy green vegetables. For most of you, that food supply is not enough. Why? Because you live in the modern world, and the modern world is stressful. Stress causes your body to dump magnesium, which is unfortunate because it's during stress that you most need such a wonderful, calming mineral. It seems illogical, but your body has a plan. By actively excreting magnesium, your body revs up your nervous system, and that helps you to deal with whatever stressful situation you are experiencing. In a traditional, less stressful lifestyle, this magnesium-dump would not have been a problem. You would experience one acute stress but then have days to recoup your magnesium from leafy green vegetables.

In the modern world, you shift from one stressful situation to the next. Your body dumps magnesium again and again, and your leafy green intake can never keep up. On top of that, you are faced with environmental toxins that deplete you of magnesium.

How it works: Magnesium soothes and calms your nervous system and aids with sleep. It regulates your HPA axis and improves the function of both insulin and thyroid hormone. Finally, magnesium is anti-inflammatory and promotes the healthy metabolism of estrogen.[135] For all those reasons, magnesium is my #1 supplement for periods.

What else you need to know: You might be wondering if you can test magnesium to confirm that you are deficient. The answer is no. Most of your magnesium is *inside* your cells, so cannot be detected by a serum, urine, or hair test. A test for red cell magnesium is a bit better, but truly, there is no reason to test magnesium. If you live in the modern world, you need magnesium. It's that simple, and it's easiest to just try some and see how you feel.

Unless you have kidney disease, magnesium is safe for long-term use. Some forms of magnesium (such as magnesium chloride) cause diarrhea, but gentler forms such as magnesium chelate (magnesium glycinate) are usually fine. I recommend 300 mg directly after food.

Amy: Magnesium to the rescue

Amy was suffering bad PMS.

"I'm snappy for the ten days before my period," she told me. "And I need chocolate just to get through the afternoon." Otherwise, her health was pretty good, which surprised me considering how busy she was. She worked ten-hour days for a busy law firm and got home late most nights—just in time to eat, sleep, and do it all over again.

"I might need the herbal medicine Vitex," Amy said. "I've heard it's good PMS."

"I think you need something stronger," I replied. "Your body is under a lot of pressure from your long work hours."

I prescribed a tablet that contains 150 mg of magnesium glycinate and 35 mg of vitamin B6 and suggested she take two per day. I also recommended a 15-minute meditation audio to do at lunchtime.

"Let's give that one cycle," I suggested. "And then we'll talk about Vitex."

I met with Amy after her next period, and she estimated her premenstrual irritability was already 60 percent better. She had also noticed that her sugar cravings improved within just a few days of starting the magnesium.

We continued to work on a few things. For example, Amy removed sugar and dairy from her diet. Instead of milk chocolate, she changed to dark chocolate (85 percent cocoa). She also did take Vitex for a few months which improved her PMS even more. Of everything Amy tried, the magnesium plus vitamin B6 had the most dramatic impact on her PMS.

Amy's story shows the power of magnesium to stabilize the HPA axis. Magnesium is particularly helpful for PMS, as we'll see in Chapter 8.

The other micronutrients I prescribe most often are zinc, vitamin D, and iodine. Let's have a look.

Zinc

Zinc is a *huge* player in period health. For example, zinc deficiency has been demonstrated to play a role in irregular periods, facial hair, PMS, and period pain. Second only to magnesium, zinc is the supplement I prescribe most often for period problems.

How it works: Zinc is anti-inflammatory[136] and regulates your HPA axis or stress response.[137] It also nourishes ovarian follicles to promote healthy ovulation and progesterone. Finally, it's essential for the synthesis, transport, and action of *all* hormones including thyroid hormone, and it's a natural androgen blocker.
[138]

What else you need to know: Animal products, particularly red meat, are the best source of zinc. If you're vegetarian, you're likely to be deficient. Also, your body can't store zinc, so you need a small amount every day. Your doctor can test zinc with a blood test. If you're deficient, consider taking 30 mg of zinc citrate or zinc picolinate directly after food. Do not take zinc on an empty stomach or it may cause nausea.

Vitamin D

Vitamin D is not like other vitamins. It's actually a steroid hormone that regulates more than 200 different genes in your body. It's essential for both healthy insulin sensitivity and ovulation, so you can see why correcting a vitamin D deficiency might be pretty important for periods.

How it works: Vitamin D helps you to absorb calcium and deposit it in your bones, but that's just the tip of the iceberg. It's also a powerful regulator of both immune and hormone function.

What else you need to know: You normally synthesize vitamin D from a cholesterol precursor when your skin is exposed to UV light (sunshine). Several things can interfere with vitamin D synthesis, including obesity, chronic inflammation, and magnesium deficiency. Your doctor can test 25-hydroxy vitamin D, and your blood level should be between 30 and 50 ng/mL (75 and 125 nmol/L). If you're deficient, consider taking 2000 IU after food. Food sources of vitamin D include egg yolks and mackerel, but it's hard to get enough from food.

Iodine

Iodine is one of the most important treatments for estrogen excess symptoms such as breast pain, ovulation pain, ovarian cysts, and PMS. You might be thinking that iodine's benefits are indirect benefits from its role in thyroid hormone, but that's not the case. Iodine is essential for thyroid, yes, but iodine also has direct effects on both ovulation and estrogen.

How it works: Iodine promotes the healthy metabolism or detoxification of estrogen and also makes cells *less sensitive* to estrogen.[139] The ovaries need a lot of iodine[140] to stabilize estrogen receptors and promote a smooth and healthy progression to ovulation.

What else you need to know: There is no topic in natural medicine more controversial than the dosing of iodine. On the one hand, conventional medicine is conservative. The RDA for iodine is 150 mcg (0.15 mg) with a tolerable upper intake of 1,100 mcg (1.1 mg). Thyroid experts warn that doses greater than 500 mcg (0.5 mg) can trigger autoimmune thyroid disease and that doses greater than 225 mcg (0.25 mg) are not safe for pregnant women.[141]

On the other hand, some natural practitioners recommend mega-doses of up to 50,000 mcg (50 mg) which is 100 times (10,000 percent) greater than what your doctor considers safe.

I agree that the RDA of 150 mcg is too low. It's enough to prevent goiter (enlarged thyroid), but it's not sufficient for the health of your ovaries and breasts. At the same time, I do *not* think that mega-dosing is safe. Too much iodine can worsen acne, and it can also suppress thyroid function and trigger autoimmune thyroid disease.[142] Even the Japanese, who are the world's highest iodine consumers, do not consume more than 5280 mcg (5.2 mg) per day.

Testing for iodine

The most important test to have before taking iodine is a test for thyroid autoimmunity or "thyroid antibodies," a subject we'll revisit in Chapter 11. If you have autoimmune thyroid disease, then you need to stay low with the dose or avoid iodine altogether. There's a urine test for iodine, but it is not reliable. If your doctor does order the urine test, you can improve its accuracy by testing in the morning and by avoiding iodine-containing supplements, foods, or thyroid medication for 24 hours before the test. There is also something called an *iodine challenge test,* but I do not recommend this because it involves taking a single large dose of 50,000 mcg (50 mg) of iodine.

 Breast tenderness can be a sign of iodine deficiency. I personally find it more useful than any lab test.

When I prescribe iodine, I usually give a minimum of 250 mcg (0.25 mg) in the form of either potassium iodide (KI) or molecular iodine (I2). Compared to KI, I2 is absorbed more slowly into the thyroid and more quickly into breast tissue.[143] That makes it safer for thyroid and better for breast pain. Popular products such as Lugol's solution (which I do *not* recommend) provide a combination of high-dose I2 and potassium iodide.

I always give iodine together with selenium which protects the thyroid. You can also obtain iodine from food:

- iodized salt (400 mcg per teaspoon)
- seafood (10 – 190 mcg per 100 grams)
- butter from grass-fed cows
- plant foods such as mushrooms and leafy greens, but only if they're grown in iodine-rich soil

Seaweed also contains iodine, but I do not recommend it as a source of iodine because it contains bromine, which prevents the uptake of iodine.

The Best Diet

Patients and readers always ask me: What is the best diet? What exactly should I eat?

The bottom line is: the best diet is one that provides an adequate supply of macro- and micronutrients, and one that is not inflammatory for you. As long as you do those two things, you will find that you have a surprising amount of wiggle room regarding exactly what you eat.

Be satisfied

I encourage you to eat full, hearty meals—and to feel good doing it. It is only by eating full meals that you will experience satiety. My advice is that dinner is the most important time to eat a full meal, because that's when you tend to be the most hungry.

Avoid snacking

Satiety makes you feel good, and it prevents snacking. In general, snacking is something you want to minimize. Every time you eat, you go through a little pro and con trade-off.

Pro: food gives you the macro- and micronutrients you need. Food (especially starch) also calms your nervous system and regulates cortisol, so you feel less stressed.

Con: Food increases insulin and creates inflammation. Some foods are more inflammatory than others, but all food is a *little bit* inflammatory. For this reason, I recommend that you eat substantial amounts, but *less* frequently.

In general, I recommend three solid meals per day and no snacks. It's not a hard and fast rule. If you're stressed or have not slept well, and need to snack, then please do so. As your health improves, you should find it easier and easier not to snack.

Eight-hour eating window

One way to reduce snacking is to restrict eating to an eight or ten-hour eating window.

The way it works is that you eat a normal dinner by 6 or 7 p.m. Be sure to eat all three macronutrients (protein, starch, and fat) with that meal or you will be too hungry to fast overnight. After dinner, you can have unsweetened drinks—but no food—until about 9 a.m. the next morning.

An eating window is a gentle type of *intermittent fasting*, which has been shown to reduce inflammation[144] and reverse insulin resistance.[145] Research has also indicated that intermittent fasting may also help to prevent the recurrence of breast cancer. [146]

You will, of course, be hungry during your eating window, so please eat what you need in the form of full, satisfying meals. An eating window is *not* a calorie-restricted diet.

Don't be afraid of hunger, don't be afraid of food

I'm disturbed by the way our popular culture portrays dieting and low appetite to be a desirable trait in women. For example, when a man has a hearty appetite, it's a sign of virility and strength. When a woman has a hearty appetite, it's a character flaw. We hear things like: "She eats like a bird," and that is supposed to be a good thing. I reject that. Hunger is normal, natural, and healthy. Hunger is how your body gets the nutrition it needs to have healthy periods. Don't fight your hunger. Instead, *honor* it by giving your body substantial, satisfying meals.

Special Topic: Do You Have an Eating Disorder?

Eating disorders such as anorexia, bulimia, and binge eating have a profound effect on period health. An eating disorder is defined as having extreme emotions, attitudes, and behavior toward body weight and food.

Eating disorders are complex conditions with a diverse set of causes including physical, emotional, and social factors. Diagnosis and treatment are beyond the scope of this book. If you think you might have an eating disorder, then know you're not alone. Be gentle with yourself and reach out for professional help. See the Eating Disorders section in the Resources.

I want to say a word here about a possible pitfall inherent in diet modification for health. As soon as you remove inflammatory foods from your diet, you will come to realize how much better you feel. That's great, and you should rejoice in your results. But you do not need to view those foods as *dangerous*. Please do not fall into the trap of becoming too rigid or fearful of food. That can lead you into a downward spiral of undereating or being afraid to eat out or visit friends.

 If you start to feel anxious or lose your periods, ask yourself: "Am I getting enough to eat?" For further discussion of undereating, see the Hypothalamic Amenorrhea section in the next chapter.

I encourage you to be flexible and joyful in your eating. Your body is more resilient than you think. As long as you choose real, unprocessed foods, then you can be fairly flexible. You need not fear the occasional snack or meal that doesn't conform to a particular diet. And you need not beat yourself up if you stray to unhealthy foods every once in a while. As you regain your health, and particularly after you quit sugar, you should find that your cravings decrease and it becomes easier and easier to choose—to *prefer*—healthy, anti-inflammatory foods.

 If you have a serious problem with gluten then, of course, please do strictly avoid it. Fortunately, more and more restaurants offer gluten-free options.

Your diet doesn't have to have a name

Mediterranean diet, whole foods diet, Paleo diet. What do they have in common? They're all diets with fewer inflammatory foods than the typical Western pattern diet. In that way, they're all good places to start. They can guide you to your own best diet but you don't have to adhere rigidly to any one of them.

As you plan your menu, start by reducing the foods that are inflammatory for you. Then look to foods that provide the necessary macronutrients, and that are pleasurable and satiating.

Menu Ideas

What about specific foods? What exactly should your menu look like?

It entirely depends on what appeals to you. I invite you to honor your appetite. For example, you may enjoy a large cooked breakfast. Or perhaps you prefer something simple like sardines on toast. Your appetite will change according to your levels of activity, sleep, and stress. It's natural to want different foods at different times.

To inspire you, here are menu ideas that I eat myself and recommend to patients.

Breakfast:

- Eggs with mushrooms fried in butter, served with avocado and tomato. Unsweetened black coffee, or coffee with coconut milk or full-fat Jersey milk.
- Gluten-free bread with sardines or soft goat cheese. Fresh fruit. Tea.
- Fresh fruit with unsweetened granola and sheep yogurt.

 You need *protein* for breakfast. It can be meat, eggs, fish, cheese, nuts, or unsweetened yogurt.

Lunch:

- A large green salad with grated beet, goat cheese, and smoked salmon. Olive oil dressing. Gluten-free bread on the side. Sparkling water. Two squares of dark chocolate.
- Rice with a can of salmon and steamed broccoli and olive oil.
- Leftover dinner.

Dinner:

- Bolognese meat sauce with gluten-free pasta. Green beans with butter. A mandarin.
- Lamb chops with boiled potatoes and a green salad. Sparkling water. Two squares of dark chocolate. Two plums.
- Lentils and brown rice with broccoli and sheep yogurt. Frozen berries and coconut cream for dessert.

These are only ideas. I'm sure you can come up with many more.

My ideas are wheat-free and dairy-free options for those of you who need to avoid those inflammatory foods. If you are lucky enough to not be sensitive to wheat or dairy, then you can expand your menu to include cheese, bread, and pasta.

We'll explore diet changes for specific period problems throughout the book.

Chapter 7

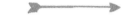

RESTORING REGULAR PERIODS

A RE YOU MISSING PERIODS? Maybe you haven't had one since you stopped the birth control pill. You have arrived at the treatment section for this problem.

Why Does It Matter?

No periods? Your doctor may have advised you just to take the pill and not worry until you're ready for a baby. That will give you fake drug-induced bleeds for now, and you can always take a fertility drug later.

You know that's not good enough. You want a real period, and you want a regular period. According to the American College of Gynecologists,[147] a regular period is a *vital sign* of health; according to me, it's a key indicator of your monthly report card.

A regular period is also a good sign that you ovulate. If you take it one step further and track your temperatures to *confirm* that you ovulate, then you know that all is well with your underlying health and metabolism.

And remember, you *want* to ovulate. It's how you make the wonderful hormones estradiol and progesterone and receive their many benefits for mood, metabolism, hair, and bone health.

> "Ovulatory cycles are both an indicator and a creator of good health."[148]
>
> *Dr Jerilynn Prior*

Let's take a closer look.

Healthy Mood

Together, estrogen and progesterone are the perfect yin and yang for mood. Estradiol lifts you up by boosting serotonin, oxytocin, and dopamine. Progesterone calms you down by acting like GABA in your brain.

Healthy Metabolism and Body Weight

Together, estrogen and progesterone support a healthy metabolism and body weight. Estradiol improves insulin sensitivity and so helps to prevent insulin resistance.[149] Progesterone enhances the production of thyroid hormone, and so increases your metabolic rate.

Healthy Hair

Together, estrogen and progesterone are very, very good for hair.

If you have irregular periods, you won't make enough of either hormone, and that can lead to hair loss—especially if you also have the excess testosterone of PCOS, discussed later in the chapter.

The pill's synthetic hormones are not a solution for hair loss, and, as we saw in Chapter 2, can actually *cause* hair loss.

Healthy Bones

Finally, estrogen and progesterone are essential for bone health. If you've had no periods for more than three months, then you are slowly increasing your lifetime risk of osteoporosis. You may have heard that the pill offers "bone protection." Unfortunately, the evidence is not clear that the pill does anything to help your bones.[150] The best solution for your bones is to re-establish regular ovulation make estradiol and progesterone.

How Regular Do Your Cycles Need to Be?

You do not have to have a perfect 28-day cycle. Different women have different bodies and different cycles, and that's okay. Count your cycle from your first day of heavy bleeding (day 1). It should range anywhere from 21 to 35 days. That is normal, and a good sign that you ovulate—which is what matters. As discussed in the physical signs of ovulation section in Chapter 3, you can confirm ovulation by tracking your body temperatures or with a blood test for progesterone.

If your cycles are longer or shorter than 21 to 35 days, then you may not be ovulating every cycle or *any* cycle.

Anovulatory cycles

If your cycles are within 21 to 35 days, then you probably are ovulating, but you still might not be. Remember, you can bleed without ever having ovulated, and that's called an anovulatory cycle. It's normal to have the occasional anovulatory cycle,[151] but if you have them regularly, then it could be a sign that you are under stress or undereating or have the hormonal condition PCOS.

From a hormonal perspective, anovulatory cycles are almost as big a problem as no cycles at all. This is the treatment chapter for irregular cycles, anovulatory cycles, and no cycles.

Working Toward a Diagnosis

The occasional irregular cycle is probably nothing to worry about. Temporary "menstrual disturbance" is common following illness, stress, or dieting, especially if you are still in your early twenties and have not yet established regular ovulation. Your periods should regulate again as soon as your life gets back to normal.

If you are consistently missing periods (or if you have never seen a period), then your starting place is your doctor's office.

To assist you with the diagnostic process, I have provided a list of questions in the How to Talk to Your Doctor section in Chapter 11. Your doctor will probably order blood tests to work through the following possibilities.

Are you pregnant?

As we saw in the Irregular Periods section of Chapter 5, your first step is to rule out pregnancy. This possibility would be obvious if you had regular periods and now they've stopped. But you might not think about pregnancy if you have not had a period in a long time or if you are used to them being irregular. Remember: ovulation comes first, and then your period. If you become pregnant the first time you ovulate, then you will not see a period. If in doubt, do a pregnancy test or visit your doctor.

Are you a teenager?

If you have just started your periods, it is normal to have 45-day cycles. They should reduce to the normal 21 to 35 days after a few years. If they don't, you may have PCOS, discussed later in the chapter.

Are you in perimenopause?

It's normal for your cycles to first shorten and then become less regular in your forties. It happens because you have more estrogen and more of the hormone FSH. The result is that you either ovulate earlier in your cycle, or you don't ovulate at all. If you don't ovulate, you cannot make progesterone and that can cause the perimenopausal symptoms anxiety, insomnia, and heavy periods. For more information and treatment ideas, see Chapter 10.

Are you breastfeeding?

Let's take a quick look at breastfeeding. Breastfeeding suppresses periods because it stimulates your pituitary gland to make a hormone called prolactin, which prevents ovulation. Your prolactin should drop within three months after you stop breastfeeding, but it can sometimes stay high. Prolactin can also be mildly elevated from thyroid disease and stress. We will explore different reasons for elevated prolactin at the end of this chapter.

---

prolactin

Prolactin is a pituitary hormone that stimulates breast development and breast milk. It suppresses normal cycling and ovulation.

Do you have a medical condition?

After ruling out pregnancy, menopause, and breastfeeding, your doctor should screen for some of the many underlying medical conditions that cause irregular or absent periods. One of the most common period-disrupting conditions is thyroid disease.

If your doctor has not yet screened for thyroid disease, ask her to do so, and do not accept the vague statement that it's "normal." Instead, look at your result and compare it to what I describe as normal in the Thyroid Disease section of Chapter 11.

If thyroid disease or another medical condition is the cause of your irregular or absent periods, then you need treatment for that particular condition. The treatments covered in this chapter will not help you.

Is it your medication?

Next, ask your doctor if your prescription medication could be causing your irregular periods. Common period-disruptors include stronger psychiatric medications such as antipsychotics, as well as anticonvulsants, and some blood pressure medications. If your medication is the cause of your irregular or absent periods, talk to your doctor about an alternative.

Do you eat enough?

Undereating is a common reason for lack of periods. And undereating means too little food in general or too few carbohydrates in particular. See the Eat More section later in this chapter.

Are you vegetarian?

You can be vegetarian and have healthy periods. But if you don't have periods and you don't know why, then please at least consider whether your vegetarian diet could be a factor.

There are two ways a vegetarian diet can cause amenorrhea or irregular periods. The first is that it can cause zinc deficiency, which is easy to test and correct. The second is that it can contain too many phytoestrogens such as soy and legumes, which can suppress ovulation. The solution is to switch to *non-*phytoestrogen vegetarian proteins such as goat cheese and eggs.

Phytoestrogens can also cause light periods, which is not a bad thing. We'll look at A short light cycle: Sam's story of light periods in Chapter 9.

Do you have a hormone imbalance?

Once all those possibilities have been ruled out, your doctor will check for an imbalance in your female hormones. She will order blood tests and possibly a pelvic ultrasound, and from those investigations, she should be able to offer you a diagnosis. Most likely, it will be either PCOS or hypothalamic amenorrhea (HA).

Great, you're thinking, you've finally got a diagnosis. Unfortunately, your problems are not over. What is your treatment? Your doctor will likely recommend the pill for either condition, which is the same treatment she would have offered before your diagnosis. If you're lucky, she may offer you the diabetes drug metformin for PCOS. That's a bit better, but is still not a complete solution.

If you look for natural treatments, you may be overwhelmed.

There are hundreds of proposed natural treatments for PCOS and irregular periods. How on earth do you select the one that's right for you?

It's time to go deeper. Look beyond the label of PCOS or HA. What is driving your PCOS? Why do you not ovulate?

It's called *deep diagnosis,* and this chapter is your guide.

Polycystic Ovary Syndrome (PCOS)

PCOS is a common diagnosis that affects up to 10 percent of women. It's best defined as *a group of symptoms* related to anovulation (lack of ovulation) and a high level of androgens or male hormones. The main symptom of PCOS is irregular periods, specifically late periods or too many days of bleeding. Irregular periods are typical of anovulatory cycles.

Other symptoms of PCOS include excessive facial and body hair (hirsutism), acne, hair loss, weight gain, and infertility.

---

hirsutism

Hirsutism is the excessive growth of hair on your face and body. A little hair on your upper lip is normal and is not hirsutism. True hirsutism is when you have excess hair on your chin, cheeks, belly, and around your nipples.

PCOS is essentially a problem with ovulation, which results in an overproduction of androgens (male hormones) such as testosterone.

Special Topic: Androgens

Androgens are male hormones such as testosterone, androstenedione, and DHEAS. It's normal to have *some* androgens. You need them for mood, libido, and bone health. Too many androgens cause acne, hair loss, and hirsutism.

In addition to the troubling symptoms of irregular periods, weight gain, and facial hair, PCOS is associated with a long-term risk of diabetes and heart disease. In that sense, PCOS is much more than just a period problem. It is a whole-body hormonal condition that can last a lifetime.

Diagnosis of PCOS

If you've been given the diagnosis of PCOS, your first question should be: "How was it diagnosed?"

PCOS cannot be diagnosed by ultrasound.

Does that surprise you? Polycystic ovary syndrome got its name from the way the ovaries look on ultrasound. Of course, you might therefore think that the polycystic appearance is an important feature of the condition. You'd be wrong.

In part, the confusion comes from the word "cyst." As we saw in Chapter 5, normal ovaries are filled with ovarian follicles, and those follicles are essentially small, normal "cysts." Every month, those normal cysts grow, burst, and are reabsorbed.

If you progress normally to ovulation, then your ovaries will have up to twelve developing follicles if you're an adult, and up to 25 follicles if you're a teenager. Then one of those follicles will become dominant and larger than the others, and will suppress the others for the rest of that cycle.

If you do not progress to ovulation (as occurs with PCOS), then you will not form a dominant follicle and suppress the other follicles. Instead, the other follicles will keep growing just a little bit, and you will end up with many small undeveloped follicles —now officially called "cysts." That's the finding on ultrasound. *Polycystic* comes from *poly* (meaning multiple) and *cystic* (meaning follicles). It means *multiple follicles*.

The problem was that you did not ovulate, and that led to a higher than normal number of follicles—at least for that month. There's no reason to think your ovaries will always look that way. Ovaries are dynamic, and they *change*. Every month, your ovaries make new follicles, and then every month, your ovaries reabsorb them again. That's why every month, your ovaries will look different on ultrasound. The appearance of polycystic ovaries simply means you did not ovulate *that month*. It does not explain *why* you did not ovulate, nor does it predict whether you will ovulate in the future.

Polycystic ovaries can occur with PCOS, but they're not *specific* to PCOS. Polycystic ovaries occur in other situations such as being on the pill, or even in normal, healthy women. For example, one study found that healthy women have polycystic ovaries about *25 percent of the time*.[152]

And this is important: polycystic ovaries *do not cause pain* like other types of large ovarian cysts (see Chapter 9). If pain is your main symptom, then there is something else going on.

Special Topic: Polycystic Ovaries Are Normal for Teenagers

As a teenager, you have more ovarian follicles than older women. In fact, you can have as many as 25 follicles on each ovary and still be "normal."[153]

Likewise, as a teenager, you have longer cycles than older women. Your cycles can be as long as 45 days for a couple of years before they shorten to the normal 21 to 35 days.

Polycystic ovaries, irregular cycles, and even mild insulin resistance (discussed later in the chapter) are all *normal* and healthy during puberty. Those symptoms are considered abnormal only if they continue for more than the first few years of cycling.

So, if PCOS cannot be diagnosed by ultrasound, how can it be diagnosed? Very subjectively.

There is no definitive test for PCOS because it's not a well-defined disease, but rather a group of symptoms. Those symptoms have been defined according to a couple of sets of diagnostic criteria.

Androgen Excess and PCOS Society Criteria

The Androgen Excess and PCOS Society (AE-PCOS) says a woman qualifies for a PCOS diagnosis when she meets *all three* of the following criteria:[154]

- ovarian dysfunction and/or polycystic ovaries
- clinical and/or biochemical hyperandrogenism
- exclusion of other conditions that would cause hyperandrogenism.

Put into simpler words, you must have all three of the following to be diagnosed with PCOS:

- irregular periods *or* polycystic ovaries on ultrasound
- high androgens on a blood test *or* symptoms of high androgens such as hirsutism
- other reasons for high androgens have been ruled out.

I like the AE-PCOS criteria because it emphasizes the two main aspects of the condition: failure to ovulate regularly and androgen excess.

Rotterdam Criteria

The Rotterdam Criteria is a broader and looser set of criteria that says a woman qualifies for a PCOS diagnosis when she meets *only two* of the following three criteria:

- oligo-ovulation or anovulation
- clinical and/or biochemical hyperandrogenism
- polycystic ovaries on ultrasound.

Plus the exclusion of other conditions that would cause excess androgen activity.

Put into simpler words, you could be diagnosed with PCOS if you have irregular periods and androgen excess, which makes sense). Or if you have androgen excess and polycystic ovaries, which is also okay. *Or,* you could be diagnosed with PCOS if you have only irregular periods and polycystic ovaries—but *not* androgen excess. Which makes no sense because, as we've seen, your irregular periods could be due to a lot of different reasons and the ultrasound finding of polycystic ovaries does not mean anything.

Under the Rotterdam Criteria, you could be given the diagnosis of PCOS when you do not have high androgens and so *do not have the condition.* Being told you have PCOS when you don't could subject you to a lot of unnecessary treatment and worry as described in a recent study called "Are expanding disease definitions unnecessarily labelling women with polycystic ovarian syndrome."[155]

I vastly prefer the AE-PCOS criteria to the Rotterdam criteria because it says that PCOS is, by definition, a condition of excess androgens. And as to the ultrasound finding, the AE-PCOS has this to say:

"The finding of polycystic ovarian morphology in ovulatory women not showing clinical or biochemical androgen excess may be inconsequential."[156]

Inconsequential means unimportant or insignificant, so this is saying that the presence of polycystic ovaries may not mean anything. As a sole finding, it cannot be used to diagnose PCOS.

At the same time, the absence of polycystic ovaries cannot be used to rule out PCOS. You can have a normal ultrasound and still have PCOS.

In conclusion, if you were diagnosed based solely on ultrasound, there's a real possibility you do not actually have the androgen excess condition currently known as PCOS. If you need help speaking to your doctor about this, please refer to the How to Talk to Your Doctor section in Chapter 11.

 PCOS may soon get a new name. A couple have been put forward including Metabolic Reproductive Syndrome (MRS) and Anovulatory Androgen Excess (AAE). I prefer the latter.

Defining androgen excess

Both the Rotterdam and AE-PCOS criteria agree on one thing: androgen excess can be defined as either 1) high androgens on a blood test or 2) physical signs of androgen excess.

Blood tests for androgen excess

The best blood test for androgen excess is *free testosterone*, but other tests include total testosterone, androstenedione, and DHEAS. If your doctor measures *total testosterone*, she should also measure SHBG (sex hormone binding globulin) which is a blood protein that binds to testosterone and estrogen. SHBG is typically low with PCOS.

Saliva testing cannot be used to diagnose PCOS because it's not accurate.[157]

Physical signs of androgen excess

- Facial or body hair (hirsutism) that is long and dark and occurs on your chin, cheeks, belly, and around your nipples is the most reliable sign of androgen excess. "Peach fuzz" on your cheeks or a bit of hair on your upper lip are not reliable signs of androgen excess.
- Acne, especially hormonal acne on your chin, can be a sign of androgen excess if you are an adult. Acne is not a reliable sign of androgen excess if you are a teenager.[158]
- Hair loss and hair thinning with miniaturized hair follicles is the third sign of androgen excess. This particular kind of hair loss is called *androgenetic alopecia*. There are other types of hair loss, which we'll discuss in the Hair Loss section in Chapter 11.

---

androgenetic alopecia

Androgenetic alopecia is also called androgenic alopecia or female pattern hair loss. It's caused by androgen excess or androgen sensitivity.

Rule out other reasons for androgen excess

PCOS is the most common diagnosis of androgen excess, but it's not the *only* diagnosis. Other diagnoses include:

- hormonal birth control with a "high androgen index"
- some types of psychiatric medications
- high prolactin
- hypothyroidism
- rare pituitary or adrenal diseases
- congenital adrenal hyperplasia.

---

congenital adrenal hyperplasia

Congenital adrenal hyperplasia is a genetic disorder that causes the adrenal glands to make too many androgens.

Nonclassic congenital adrenal hyperplasia (NCAH) accounts for up to 9 percent of cases of androgen excess[159] and is often misdiagnosed as PCOS. It can be diagnosed with the blood test 17-OH progesterone.

Conventional Treatment of PCOS

Hormonal birth control

The conventional approach to PCOS is to suppress ovulation with the pill, which seems odd when you consider that the central issue of PCOS is a failure to ovulate. The pill can also suppress androgens, which is more helpful, but unfortunately, it works for only as long as you take it. As soon as you stop, you'll have more androgens than ever before.

The biggest downside of the pill is that it can *worsen* insulin resistance, which is one of the primary drivers of PCOS, as we'll see later in the chapter.

Spironolactone

Spironolactone (Aldactone®) is almost the same drug as the progestin drospirenone used in the birth control pill Yasmin®.

Spironolactone suppresses androgens which can improve the symptoms of hirsutism and acne. Unfortunately, spironolactone can also prevent healthy ovulation and alter the activity of the HPA axis. And my observation is that stopping the drug can result in even worse acne.

Cyproterone acetate

Cyproterone acetate is another anti-androgen drug. It's given on its own as Androcur® or as one ingredient in the contraceptive pills Brenda-35® or Diane®. Cyproterone carries a higher risk of blood clot than other progestins and has never been approved for use as a contraceptive in the US.

Metformin

Your doctor may have offered you a diabetes drug called metformin, which is a reasonable treatment. It's a better approach than the pill because at least it works to correct insulin resistance, which is one of the primary drivers of PCOS.

If you want to take metformin, you can combine it with the natural treatments in this chapter.

Metformin can cause digestive problems and deplete your body of vitamin B12 so please speak to your doctor about testing your levels. You may need a B12 injection.

The Natural Approach to PCOS

I would love to now give you a simple list of what works for PCOS, but it's more complicated than that. To get results from natural medicine, you must first go deeper and understand the different possible drivers of PCOS.

PCOS is not one disease. Instead, it's a group of symptoms related to androgen excess. That's why it's described as a *heterogeneous endocrine disorder.*

A heterogeneous disorder is a group of symptoms that can result from several *distinctly different* underlying drivers.

In the case of PCOS, those drivers are insulin, inflammation, adrenal androgens, and a post-pill surge in androgens. We'll consider each driver in turn, but first, let's look at the underlying *susceptibility* to PCOS that can come from both genetics and exposure to environmental toxins.

Genetic susceptibility to PCOS

Are you born with PCOS? Well, yes and no.

You can certainly be born with genes that put you at risk of PCOS. For example, you can be born with genes that alter how your hypothalamus communicates with your ovaries, or genes that influence how likely you are to develop insulin resistance. You can also be born with genes that make your ovaries more likely to overproduce androgens under certain conditions.

Ultimately, your genes determine how *easily* you can ovulate and how likely you are to overproduce androgens. But the expression of those genes depends on your current environment.

For example, those genes put you at a disadvantage in your current environment of the Western pattern diet and environmental toxins, but those same genes may have given your ancestors an advantage during challenging times of stress or famine. As genes, they're not inherently bad. They're just not well adapted to our modern world.

 The good thing about PCOS genes: as a woman with PCOS, you may become more fertile as you get older.[160]

Exposure to endocrine disrupting chemicals

Another factor that can put you at risk of PCOS is early exposure to endocrine disrupting chemicals such as pesticides, phthalates, and bisphenol A (BPA).[161] By early exposure, I mean exposure when you were a child or even before you were born. Such exposure can alter how your hypothalamus communicates with your ovaries, or how sensitive you are to insulin, leading to a lifelong susceptibility to PCOS.

Modifying risk and reversing PCOS

Yes, both genes and toxins put you at risk of PCOS, but being at risk does not mean you will always have PCOS. You can modify your genetic expression and ovarian function with diet, lifestyle, and other natural treatments—and that will improve your symptoms.

> (tip) **Know when to let go** of your PCOS diagnosis. You qualify for a PCOS diagnosis based on your current symptoms. If you can reach the point of no symptoms, then you will no longer have PCOS. You may, however, always have a susceptibility.

Now, let's get to the nitty-gritty of natural treatment for PCOS. And let's break it down by which type of PCOS you have.

Types of PCOS (Drivers of Androgen Excess)

What do I mean by "type of PCOS?" I mean that if you have a susceptibility to androgen excess, then you can be pushed into full-blown PCOS by exposure to various *drivers*.

Based on my work with patients, I have identified those drivers to be: insulin-resistant PCOS, post-pill PCOS, inflammatory PCOS, and adrenal PCOS.

Identifying your driver or "type" of PCOS can be incredibly helpful for finding your best treatment. We'll now look at each driver in turn in the following sections, but, please first look at the questions in the following flow-chart. They are the questions I ask my patients to determine their type of PCOS.

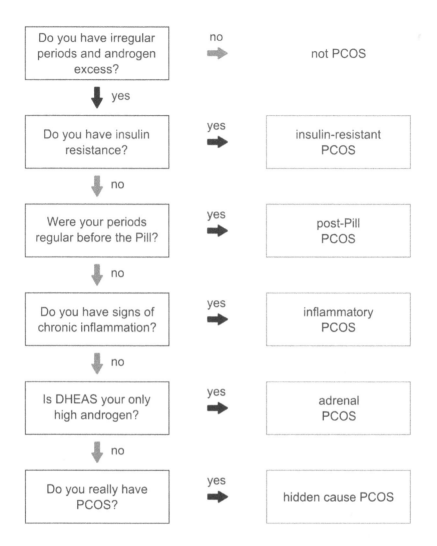

image 9 - flow chart for PCOS type

Insulin-Resistant PCOS

The most important question is "do you have insulin resistance?" because insulin resistance is by far the most common driver of PCOS.

You may recall that insulin resistance is the hormonal condition described in the Sugar section in Chapter 6. When you have insulin resistance, you may have normal blood sugar, but too much insulin. Too much insulin is not good for you. It can lead to weight gain, heart disease, osteoporosis, and eventually diabetes. It can also lead to high androgens if you have the genetic susceptibility to PCOS.

How does insulin resistance lead to PCOS? Too much insulin can impair ovulation and cause your ovaries to make testosterone instead of estrogen. Too much insulin also stimulates your pituitary to make more luteinizing hormone (LH), which stimulates even more androgens. Finally, too much insulin lowers the androgen-binding protein SHBG, which results in even more free testosterone or unbound testosterone.

 The insulin resistance of PCOS continues past menopause. If you don't treat insulin resistance, you will have it your entire life.

What causes insulin resistance? As we saw in the previous chapter, sugar is the biggest culprit. A small amount of fructose is healthy, but a large amount induces insulin resistance.[162]

Other potential causes of insulin resistance include smoking, stress, hormonal birth control, sleep deprivation, alcohol, trans fat, unhealthy gut bacteria, magnesium deficiency, and environmental toxins.

You have insulin-resistant PCOS if you meet all the criteria for PCOS (irregular periods and elevated androgens) *plus* you have insulin resistance.

How do you know if you have insulin resistance? First, look for the physical sign of apple-shaped obesity, which is weight gain around your waist.

> (tip) **Get out the tape measure.** To assess for apple-shaped obesity, take a measure at the level of your belly button. You're aiming for a waist measurement of about 35 inches (89 cm) or less. A more precise measure is to calculate your waist to height ratio—your waist should be less than half your height.

Apple-shaped obesity is a common symptom of insulin resistance, so if you are overweight, then your PCOS is likely the insulin resistant type.

At the same time, you could be *normal weight* and still have insulin resistance and the insulin-resistant type of PCOS.[163] In that case, the only way to know if you have insulin resistance is to do a blood test. A test for blood sugar or blood glucose is *not* a test for insulin resistance. Instead, you need one of the following:

- fasting insulin
- HOMA-IR index (insulin resistance index)
- insulin glucose challenge test (also called insulin assay with oral glucose tolerance test or glucose tolerance test with insulin)

Fasting insulin is a blood test for the hormone insulin. Your result should be less than 8 mIU/L (55 pmol/L). Fasting insulin can pick up severe insulin resistance. To detect milder insulin resistance, you'll need the more sensitive insulin glucose challenge test.

HOMA-IR index is a mathematical calculation using the ratio of glucose to insulin. For healthy insulin sensitivity, your HOMA-IR index should be less than 1.5.

Insulin glucose challenge test is a blood test that is similar to the two-hour oral glucose tolerance test, in which several blood samples are taken during the two hours following a sweet drink. The difference with this test is that insulin is tested in addition to glucose.

As previously mentioned, insulin resistance is the most common driver of PCOS. If you have PCOS, there's a 70 percent chance it's the insulin-resistant type. So please read this treatment section.

Diet and Lifestyle for Insulin Resistance

Quit sugar

The first thing to do is to stop having desserts and sweet drinks. I am sorry to be the bearer of bad news, but I mean stop completely. I don't mean drop back to a small amount of natural dessert.

If you have insulin resistance, then you are not hormonally equipped to handle any amount of dessert. Every time you eat something sweet, you're pushed deeper and deeper into insulin resistance —and deeper and deeper into the weight gain, acne, and hirsutism of PCOS.

 You can have whole fruit as long as you stay below the 25 grams of fructose discussed in Chapter 6.

You won't always have insulin resistance. Once your insulin is normal, you'll be able to go back to enjoying the occasional dessert. By occasional, I mean about once per month.

I understand it's not easy to quit sugar because sugar is in almost everything you're used to eating including cereal, yogurt, muffins, fruit juice, smoothies, and date balls. You may need to do some serious reorganizing of your pantry and shopping list.

You may also be faced with the problem of sugar cravings and sugar addiction.

Special Topic: Are You Addicted to Sugar?

Sugar addiction is real and common. Signs include:

- You crave sugar even when you are not hungry.
- You crave sugar in response to negative emotions.
- You hide your sugar eating from your loved ones.
- You feel angry or upset at the thought of giving it up.

If you are addicted to sugar, please do not feel guilty or ashamed. Like any addiction, sugar addiction can be overcome with the right support. Reach out for professional help.

Patients tell me that quitting sugar is as hard as quitting cigarettes. You need a plan. Here are some tips to make it easier:

- Get enough sleep, because sleep reduces sugar cravings.
- Eat full, satisfying meals that include all three macronutrients: protein, starch, and fat.
- Do not restrict calories.
- Pick a start date during a low-stress time of your life.
- Go cold turkey for four weeks.
- Know that intense cravings subside after twenty minutes.
- Know that all cravings should subside after seven days.
- Supplement magnesium, because it reduces sugar cravings.
- Know that you're okay. You're not a bad person just because you crave sugar.

 If you need a sweetener while you adapt to a low-sugar diet, try the natural sweeteners stevia or xylitol.

Quitting sugar is different from *going low-carb*. In fact, you'll find it easier to quit sugar if you allow yourself to eat potatoes and rice. Why? Because starch is highly satiating and reduces cravings.

That said, you could find it *harder* to quit sugar if you eat inflammatory foods such as wheat and dairy. Why? Because those inflammatory foods can cause food cravings.

Rose: Can I really eat potatoes?

Rose knew she had insulin-resistant PCOS, so she was doing her best to cut carbs. It wasn't working well. She hadn't lost any weight, and her PCOS symptoms were as bad as ever.

"I have an omelet every morning," she said. "And then salad plus meat for both lunch and dinner."

"That sounds good," I replied. "But was that enough food for lunch and dinner? Did you eat anything else yesterday?"

Rose then told me that she had a skim latte with sugar in the morning and five or six date balls in the afternoon.

"Anything else?"

Rose was hungry after dinner, so she ate two bowls of Paleo ice cream made with coconut milk and agave syrup.

"I know I have bad willpower," she said guiltily. "I have to try harder."

"No, you don't have a problem with willpower," I said. "You were just hungry."

I asked Rose to eat three full meals per day. "Please keep going with your low-carb breakfast and lunch, but I want you to have meat and potatoes for dinner," I said. "Plus some vegetables, of course, and butter or olive oil. And please eat as much as you need to feel full. But then don't eat again until morning."

Rose (incredulous): "Can I really eat potatoes? That can't be right. They're bad carbs."

"Sugar is the bad carb," I said. "I need you to stop having sugar in your coffee and also stop having the date balls and any kind of dessert."

I also prescribed a powder with 300 mg magnesium to relieve Rose's sugar cravings.

Rose was worried she would feel tired without the date balls to get her through the afternoon. But much to her surprise, she started to feel better, and her energy improved.

When she stopped having sugar, she stopped craving sugar.

Reduce other carbs

Once you've successfully quit sugar, you can think about reducing other carbs such as bread and potatoes and rice.

A simple strategy is to have a *low-carb breakfast*. That means eggs or meat plus non-starchy vegetables. By avoiding starch and sugar with breakfast, you will keep your insulin low and extend the benefits of your overnight fast.

If that feels good, you could also think about having a low-carb lunch.

At some point, however, you'll need *some* starch. Why? Because starch is satisfying and calms your nervous system so you can sleep. Starch also tops up your liver's glycogen stores to keep your blood sugar stable through the night.

For all those reasons, I recommend you eat at least a small portion of rice or potato with dinner.

> (tip) **Don't make the mistake** of reducing starch but continuing to eat sugar. In other words, there's no point forgoing potatoes with dinner only to binge later on a Paleo dessert.

Adhere to an eight-hour eating window

As described in Chapter 6, you can also restrict your eating to an eight- or ten-hour eating window. You will, of course, be hungry during your eating window, so eat what you need in the form of full, satisfying meals. An eating window is a gentle type of intermittent fasting which has been found to improve insulin resistance.[164]

Exercise

Exercise sensitizes your muscle to insulin. For example, just twelve weeks of strength training can improve insulin sensitivity by 24 percent.[165]

Sign up for some strength training or Pilates classes. Or start even smaller than that with a simple walk around the block. Climb stairs. Do some pushups.

For best results, choose the exercise you enjoy.

Avoid hormonal birth control

The birth control pill can cause or worsen insulin resistance,[166] in part because it prevents the muscle gain you would normally achieve with exercise.[167] One study found that just three months on hormonal birth control was enough to worsen insulin resistance in women with PCOS.[168]

Special Topic: How to Reduce the Risk of Uterine Cancer Without Birth Control

One of the reasons your doctor may want you to take hormonal birth control is to reduce the long-term risk of uterine cancer that comes with PCOS. Her reasoning is that the progestin will prevent the build-up of your uterine lining —which is true. Fortunately, there are other, *better* ways to prevent the build-up of your uterine lining, as follows:

- Reverse insulin resistance to prevent insulin's stimulating effect on your uterine lining. Reversing insulin resistance can also help you to ovulate.

- Find a way to ovulate so you can make progesterone, which will naturally protect your uterine lining—that's one of its main jobs. (All of the natural treatments discussed in this chapter will help you to ovulate.)

- Take micronized or natural progesterone, which can work as well as a synthetic progestin to thin the uterine lining.

Supplements and Herbal Medicines for Insulin Resistance and Insulin-Resistant PCOS

Before we get into the supplements, please know that *diet is more important than any supplement*. That is true for almost every condition in this book, but it's particularly true for insulin-resistant PCOS. You must quit sugar. You can then choose one or two of the following supplements. You don't need them all.

Magnesium is the wonderful Miracle Mineral for Periods we met in the previous chapter, and it's my front-line treatment for insulin resistant PCOS. Studies have shown that a high-magnesium diet is correlated with a lower risk of insulin resistance,[169] while a low-magnesium diet is correlated with a higher risk of insulin resistance. Some researchers have gone so far as to propose magnesium deficiency as one of the *causes* of insulin resistance.[170]

I prescribe magnesium to every PCOS patient. I call it "natural metformin."

How it works: It improves insulin sensitivity.[171]

What else you need to know: I recommend 300 mg magnesium per day taken directly after food. I prefer magnesium bisglycinate (magnesium joined to the amino acid glycine) because glycine has its own insulin-sensitising properties.[172] And I usually give it in combination with another amino acid taurine, which also improves insulin sensitivity. See Chapter 10 for more information about taurine.

Alpha-lipoic acid is a naturally occurring molecule involved in energy production. It's made by the body and can also be obtained from foods such as liver, spinach, and broccoli. As a supplement, alpha-lipoic acid is beneficial for PCOS.[173][174]

How it works: It improves insulin sensitivity and promotes the healthy development of the ovarian follicle. It also boosts glutathione.

What else you need to know: Alpha-lipoic acid is safe, but more than 1000 mg per day may decrease thyroid hormone. I recommend 300 to 600 mg per day with food. It combines well with the next supplement, myo-inositol.[175]

Myo-inositol is an intracellular messenger for insulin. Taking it as a supplement can improve PCOS.[176]

How it works: It improves insulin sensitivity, reduces androgens, and supports regular ovulation.[177]

What else you need to know: There are two types of supplementary inositol, which have different effects. D-chiro-inositol improves insulin sensitivity throughout the body. Myo-inositol improves insulin and FSH signaling *inside* the ovary, thereby improving ovarian function and promoting healthy ovulation. The inositol formula used in the clinical trials is a combined supplement of myo-inositol and d-chiro-inositol in a 40:1 ratio, which corresponds to the body's normal ratio. The standard dose is 2000 to 4000 mg and is generally safe for long-term use.

Vitamin D is the sunshine vitamin we met in Chapter 6.

How it works: It improves insulin sensitivity and promotes the healthy maturation of ovarian follicles.[178]

What else you need to know: Ask your doctor to test your vitamin D. If you're deficient, take 2000 IU with food.

Berberine has done well in PCOS clinical trials, outperforming metformin in two large studies.[179][180] It's a good treatment for PCOS generally and a great treatment for acne as we'll discuss later in the chapter. Berberine has the nice side benefit of reducing anxiety.[181]

How it works: It improves insulin sensitivity, possibly by its beneficial effect on gut bacteria.[182][183] Berberine also promotes ovulation[184] and prevents the ovaries from making too much testosterone.[185]

What else you need to know: Berberine is not a single herb. Instead, it's a *phytonutrient,* or active constituent, of a number of different herbs including goldenseal (*Hydrastis canadensis*), barberry (*Berberis vulgaris*), and the Chinese herb *Phellodendron amurense.* You can take a concentrated berberine extract or a preparation of a whole herb such as Phellodendron. Berberine-containing herbs taste bitter so are best taken as a tablet or capsule. The exact quantity depends on the concentration in the formula. The standard dose for a berberine extract is 350 to 500 mg twice daily.

There are a few precautions. Do not take berberine if you are pregnant or breastfeeding. And consult your doctor when combining it with prescription medication such as antidepressants, beta-blockers, antibiotics, or immunosuppressants because it can alter the levels of those medications.

Do not take berberine for more than eight weeks in a row, because its antimicrobial effects could alter the composition of your gut bacteria. In the short term, berberine's antimicrobial effects are probably beneficial. For example, berberine can improve digestive health and repair intestinal permeability.[186] In the long term, it could deplete gut bacteria. I'm cautious with berberine and usually recommend taking it only five days per week, with a two-day break. Then, after eight weeks, I recommend stopping the medicine for at least one month. If in doubt, seek professional advice.

The next two supplements are zinc and peony and licorice combination. They're special because, in addition to their many other benefits, they also have direct *anti-androgen* effects. That makes them a good addition to your other core PCOS treatments such as quitting sugar and taking magnesium. I'll refer again to zinc and peony and licorice combination later in the Anti-Androgen Treatments section.

Every natural treatment discussed in the PCOS chapter works indirectly or directly to reduce androgens.

Zinc is one of the key nutrients for period health we met in Chapter 6. As you may recall, it has many benefits including reducing inflammation and regulating the stress response. It's also involved in ovarian function. Zinc deficiency has been correlated with a higher risk of PCOS.[187]

> **How it works:** Zinc nourishes ovarian follicles to promote healthy ovulation and progesterone. It also has direct anti-androgen effects. In a recent clinical trial, zinc was demonstrated to improve hirsutism.[188]

> **What else you need to know:** I recommend 30 mg per day taken directly after a large meal. Do not take zinc on an empty stomach, or it may cause nausea.

Peony and licorice combination is a herbal medicine I frequently prescribe for my PCOS patients. It has undergone a couple of clinical trials, in which it was found to reduce testosterone and improve cycle regularity.[189][190]

> **How it works:** Peony (*Paeonia lactiflora*) inhibits the production of testosterone and promotes the activity of the enzyme aromatase, which converts testosterone to estrogen.[191] Licorice (*Glycyrrhiza glabra*) lowers testosterone in women[192] and blocks androgen receptors.[193] Together, the two herbs also have a synergistic normalizing effect on pituitary hormones.[194]

> **What else you need to know:** The exact quantity of the herb depends on the concentration in the formula, so please use as directed on the bottle.

Peony and licorice combination is a powerful medicine, so you need to be careful about how you take it. For example, do not take it in combination with fertility drugs. Do not take it if you are younger than 18, because your pituitary-ovarian communication is still developing. And do not take it for more than six months continuously except under professional guidance. If you are taking peony and licorice to regulate your periods, you should not need it for longer than six months because it should have worked within that time. You should then be able to stop it and your periods remain regular. If you're taking it to improve androgen symptoms such as hirsutism, take it for six months, then take a break for a month, then resume. *Watch your blood pressure!* Licorice raises blood pressure, so do not take it if you already have high blood pressure. If in doubt, please seek professional advice.

Special Topic: Natural progesterone for PCOS

Canadian endocrinologist Dr Jerilynn Prior recommends *cyclic progesterone therapy* for PCOS. It involves giving natural or micronized progesterone in a pattern that mimics the luteal phase. It works for PCOS because it suppresses luteinizing hormone (LH) and can thereby help to normalize communication between the hypothalamus, pituitary, and ovaries. For more information about cyclic progesterone therapy, visit the website for The Centre for Menstrual Cycle and Ovulation Research.[195]

Micronized progesterone also helps protect against uterine cancer and has a nice anti-androgen effect, which we'll discuss later in the chapter.

---

micronized progesterone

Micronized progesterone is a form of replacement hormone. It is natural or bioidentical progesterone rather than a synthetic progestin. It can be taken as a topical cream or a capsule such as the brand Prometrium®.

bioidentical hormone

A bioidentical or "body identical" hormone is a hormone that is structurally identical to your own human hormone.

That covers treatment for insulin-resistant PCOS— and remember, that's the type that applies to most of you. If you're *certain* you do not have insulin resistance, then please read on to the other types of PCOS.

(tip) **Remember, a test** for blood glucose is *not* a test for insulin resistance.

Checklist for insulin-resistant PCOS

- Quit sugar.
- Take magnesium.
- Consider an additional PCOS supplement listed above, such as myo-inositol, zinc, or peony and licorice combination.
- Consider an additional anti-androgen supplement, as discussed later in the chapter.

Post-Pill PCOS

Coming off the pill can cause symptoms that qualify you for a PCOS diagnosis. It happens for several reasons:

- Hormonal birth control can cause or worsen insulin resistance,[196][197] and is a major contributor to insulin-resistant PCOS.
- Hormonal birth control suppresses ovulation, which of course, it's meant to do. For most women, ovulation will resume once birth control is stopped. For some of you, ovulation will not return for months or even years. During that time, you may qualify for a PCOS diagnosis.

- Coming off a "low androgen index" pill such as Yasmin®
can cause a temporary surge in androgens. While your
androgens are high, you may qualify for a PCOS
diagnosis, but your androgens should come down again
after a year or two. We'll look more closely at the issue of
post-pill androgens in the How to Come Off Hormonal
Birth Control section in Chapter 11.

Post-pill PCOS is the second most common type of PCOS I see
with my patients. It's different from other types of PCOS in that
it is usually temporary. In other words, it's a situation of what Dr
Jerilynn Prior calls *adaptive anovulatory androgen excess*. It
doesn't necessarily stem from the underlying genetic tendency of
the ovary to overproduce androgens that characterizes other
types of PCOS.

Diagnosis of Post-Pill PCOS

Your PCOS is post-pill PCOS if you meet all the criteria for
PCOS (irregular periods and elevated androgens), *plus* you do
not have insulin resistance, *plus* you were fine before you started
the pill.

If you were *not* fine before you started the pill, you possibly had
PCOS back then, so you may not have post-pill PCOS.

Look at your LH to FSH ratio

With post-pill PCOS, you'll probably have high LH compared to
FSH. That's a common finding with *all* types of PCOS, but with
post-pill PCOS it's one of the *only* findings. LH prevents your
ovarian follicles from developing properly and stimulates them
to make androgens.

> (tip) **PCOS is not the only kind** of post-pill problem.
> Remember Christine from Chapter 1, who had post-
> pill amenorrhea (post-pill syndrome) but did not have
> high LH or androgens, and so did not qualify for a PCOS
> diagnosis.

If you find your PCOS is of the post-pill variety, the first thing to note is that there is no conventional treatment for post-pill PCOS. The standard advice is to go back on the pill. Therefore, we'll move on to natural treatments.

Diet and Lifestyle for Post-Pill PCOS

Post-pill PCOS is often temporary so your first step is to stay calm and give it time. And to know that it's not a problem with you, but rather with the ovulation-suppressing drug you were given.

Your next step is to eat well and eat *enough*. If you do not have insulin resistance, then you do not need to strictly avoid sugar (but you shouldn't have too much either). Follow the dietary guidelines discussed in Chapter 6 and please don't undereat.

If you restrict your food thinking it will help your PCOS, you may end up with another condition called hypothalamic amenorrhea (HA), which we'll discuss later. In fact, having PCOS puts you at greater risk of HA.[198] Be sure to eat enough food and enough carbohydrate—because your body needs starch to ovulate.[199]

 If you're avoiding carbs because you had polycystic ovaries on an ultrasound, you could be on the completely wrong track.

Supplements and Herbal Medicines for Post-Pill PCOS

Zinc suppresses androgen and supports ovarian function. As discussed above, it's good for any type of PCOS, but it's my first choice for post-pill PCOS because zinc deficiency is common after the pill.

Peony and licorice combination is a good way to break out of the "stalled hormones" that can occur post-pill. It helps to normalize pituitary hormones[200] and so can promote healthy ovulation. See the previous section for further information.

> (tip) **Vitex** is another popular herb for restoring periods, but it can raise LH and therefore worsen PCOS. *Vitex* is a better choice for prolactin-induced hirsutism and HA discussed later.

You can expect fairly rapid and permanent improvement of post-pill PCOS. The trick is to give your body the time it needs to recover from the pill. That's what happened with my patient Karla.

Karla: Post-pill PCOS

Karla was 33 when she stopped Yasmin® to try for pregnancy. She'd been on it for the previous seven years for birth control. Before taking the pill, her periods were regular with a 30-day cycle.

Karla got her period straight away, which was great, but her cycles were about 50 days long, and her skin broke out. Her fertility specialist thought she was having anovulatory cycles (not ovulating), and I agreed. He diagnosed her with PCOS based on the irregular cycles, the new symptom of acne, and high testosterone.

Karla was only ten months off the pill, but already looking at the ovulation-stimulating drug clomiphene.

"Whoa," I said. "You haven't been ovulating, but that doesn't mean you *can't* ovulate. You were fine before the pill. All this could improve on its own with just a bit more time."

I asked her about fertile mucus, and she thought she'd seen some just the week before.

"Sounds like you might have ovulated before you even came to see me," I said. "So, you'll probably get a period next week. In the meantime, I think we should wait on any herbal ovulation-promoting treatment. Instead, I suggest zinc, which will nourish your ovaries and skin."

I asked Karla to take 30 mg of zinc after dinner, and to temporarily remove both sugar and cow's dairy from her diet to help with her post-pill acne.

Karla got her period a week later, which meant she had probably ovulated when she saw the mucus. She had four more cycles and then became pregnant.

I do not expect Karla to have any PCOS symptoms after her baby. Her irregular periods, acne, and even elevated testosterone were all *temporary* as her body adjusted to coming off Yasmin®.

Checklist for post-pill PCOS

- Stay calm and give it time.
- Eat enough.
- Consider zinc or peony and licorice combination.
- Consider an additional anti-androgen supplement, as discussed later in the chapter.

Inflammatory PCOS

What if you don't fit into either of the previous types of PCOS? You could be quite frustrated by now. Your PCOS isn't driven by insulin resistance or coming off the pill. By what, then, is it driven?

Inflammatory PCOS is driven by inflammation and environmental toxins. Inflammation also plays a role in the previous types of PCOS—and indeed, in any period problem—but it is the *primary* driver of inflammatory PCOS.[201]

How does inflammation drive PCOS? As we saw in Chapter 6, inflammation disrupts hormone receptors and suppresses ovulation. It also stimulates both your adrenal glands and ovaries to make more androgens.[202]

Inflammation can come from insulin resistance, in which case, please see the insulin-resistant PCOS section. Inflammation can also come from smoking, inflammatory foods, environmental toxins, and digestive problems. In which case, this is the section for you.

Diagnosis of Inflammatory PCOS

Your PCOS is inflammatory PCOS if you meet all the criteria for PCOS (irregular periods and elevated androgens), *plus* you do not have insulin resistance, *plus* your periods were not affected by the pill, *plus* you have signs and symptoms of inflammation, as follows:

- digestive problems such as irritable bowel syndrome (IBS)
- unexplained fatigue
- headaches
- joint pain
- skin conditions such as eczema and psoriasis.

As for post-pill PCOS, there is no conventional treatment for inflammatory PCOS, so we'll turn to natural methods of treatment.

Diet and Lifestyle for Inflammatory PCOS

First and foremost, please follow the ***anti-inflammatory diet*** as outlined in Chapter 6. That means avoiding wheat and dairy, and possibly avoiding other common food sensitivities such as eggs.

 Avoiding inflammatory foods is more effective for inflammatory PCOS than any supplement.

Be sure to identify and treat any underlying digestive problem, and reduce your exposure to environmental toxins such as pesticides, plastics, and mercury. Refer to the Inflammation section in Chapter 11.

Supplements for Inflammatory PCOS

Both zinc and magnesium are once again my favorite prescriptions. In addition to their many other benefits, zinc and magnesium have been demonstrated to reduce the inflammation that drives PCOS.

Probiotic supplements are another treatment idea for inflammatory PCOS.

> **How they work:** Probiotics improve gut health and reduce inflammation. They also aid in the detoxification of mercury.[203]

> **What else you need to know:** if you have an underlying problem with IBS, consider the probiotic strain *Lactobacillus plantarum 299v*. For more advice about probiotics, refer to the Digestive Health section in Chapter 11.

N-acetyl cysteine (NAC) is a version of the amino acid cysteine. It's been trialed with PCOS patients and found to be successful at restoring regular ovulation.[204]

> **How it works:** It reduces inflammation and promotes the detoxification of environmental toxins. NAC also improves insulin sensitivity.

> **What else you need to know:** NAC has the nice side benefit of reducing anxiety. Too much can thin your stomach lining so do not take it if you have gastritis or stomach ulcers. I recommend 500 to 2000 mg per day.

Melatonin is the sleep hormone we met in the last chapter. It's made by the pineal gland in your brain, but it's also made by your ovaries. Melatonin supplements have been shown to restore regular ovulation in women with PCOS.[205]

> **How it works:** It protects the ovarian follicle from oxidative stress and promotes ovulation.

> **What else you need to know:** I recommend 0.5 to 3 mg at bedtime. It can also be used topically for hair loss, as described in the androgenetic alopecia section below.

Checklist for inflammatory PCOS

- Avoid wheat and cow's dairy.
- Identify and avoid other food sensitivities.
- Fix any digestive problems.
- Consider taking a zinc supplement.
- Consider an additional anti-androgen supplement, as discussed later in the chapter.

Adrenal PCOS

Hopefully, you have by now identified your type of PCOS. Chances are it is the first type, insulin-resistant PCOS, but if not, here's one more to consider.

Your PCOS is adrenal PCOS if you:

- meet all the criteria for PCOS
- do *not* have insulin resistance
- were *not* negatively affected by coming off the pill
- have *no* signs and symptoms of inflammation
- have *normal* ovarian androgens (testosterone and androstenedione) but elevated *adrenal androgens* (DHEAS).

If you need a visual of these criteria, please refer again to the PCOS flow-chart above (*image 9*).

Most women with PCOS have an elevation of one or *all* types of androgens:

- testosterone from the ovaries
- androstenedione from the ovaries and adrenal glands
- DHEAS (dehydroepiandrosterone sulfate) from the adrenal glands.

If you have elevated ovarian androgens, then you have one of the earlier types of PCOS. This is the section for when you have *only* elevated DHEAS, but normal testosterone and androstenedione.

If you have elevated DHEAS, your doctor should first rule out other reasons for it, such as high prolactin or nonclassic congenital adrenal hyperplasia (NCAH), discussed earlier in the chapter. Once those conditions have been ruled out, you're left with the diagnosis of adrenal PCOS,[206] which accounts for about 10 percent of PCOS,[207] and is different from the classic ovarian PCOS discussed so far. For example, you can ovulate regularly with adrenal PCOS.

Like ovarian androgen PCOS, adrenal PCOS is associated with endocrine disrupting chemicals[208] and an underlying genetic susceptibility.

Unlike ovarian androgen PCOS, adrenal PCOS is *not* driven by insulin resistance or impaired ovulation. Instead, it's driven by an abnormal stress response system[209] or HPA (adrenal) axis, which may be the result of stress around the time of puberty.[210]

There is no conventional treatment for adrenal PCOS, although some doctors used to prescribe low-dose hydrocortisone,[211] which worked by reducing the production of DHEAS.

Diet and Lifestyle for Adrenal PCOS

Your first step is to reduce stress to lower the DHEAS made by your adrenal glands. Helpful stress-busting strategies include those discussed in Chapter 6 such as making time for rest and joy; engaging in relaxation techniques such as meditation, massage, and yoga; and, finally, maintaining a stable blood sugar.

Supplements and Herbal Medicines for Adrenal PCOS

Both zinc and magnesium are once again helpful here. As described in previous sections, they help to regulate the HPA axis.

B vitamins reduce stress and help to regulate the HPA axis.

How they work: B vitamins boost levels of the calming neurotransmitters serotonin and GABA.

What else you need to know: For stress and HPA axis dysfunction, I recommend a B-complex that contains choline and vitamin B5, the "anti-stress factor."

Licorice (*Glycyrrhiza glabra*) is great for adrenal PCOS. It is, of course, the same herb used in the peony and licorice formula discussed earlier.

> **How they work:** Like hydrocortisone, licorice can downregulate the production of the adrenal androgen DHEAS.

> **What else you need to know:** The exact quantity of the herb depends on the concentration of the formula, so please take as directed on the bottle. And as previously mentioned, watch your blood pressure, because licorice raises blood pressure!

Rhodiola (*Rhodiola rosea*) is the adaptogen herbal medicine we met in Chapter 6. Together with licorice, it can help to reduce DHEAS.

> **How they work:** It calms the brain and the HPA axis.

> **What else you need to know:** The exact quantity of the herb depends on the concentration of the formula, so please take as directed on the bottle. You can take Rhodiola on its own or as part of a combination formula with other adaptogen herbs like Siberian ginseng and ashwagandha.

If you have adrenal PCOS, you are probably going to have an ongoing struggle with androgen symptoms such as hirsutism. So, in addition to the treatments discussed in this section, you may require long-term treatment with a natural androgen blocker. Refer to the Anti-Androgen Treatments section later in this chapter.

Checklist for adrenal PCOS

- Reduce stress.
- Consider supplements such as magnesium and B vitamins to regulate the HPA axis.
- Consider the long-term use of an anti-androgen supplement discussed later in the chapter.

There is a degree of overlap between the different PCOS types. For example, inflammation is also a factor in both the insulin-resistant and adrenal types of PCOS.

Still Confused?

What if you've been told you have PCOS, but you do not seem to meet any of the criteria discussed above? You do not have insulin resistance. You did not develop PCOS after the pill. You have no obvious signs of inflammation or exposure to environmental toxins.

Go back to the drawing board. First, do you truly have PCOS? Do you have either high androgens on a blood test or clear physical signs of androgen excess?

If you do *not* have androgen excess, and your *only* symptom is a lack of periods (and maybe acne), then you could have hypothalamic amenorrhea, which we'll discuss soon. Remember, an ultrasound finding of polycystic ovaries is not enough to diagnose PCOS.

If you *do* have PCOS, but meet none of the above criteria, then your problems may stem from something a bit less obvious. Before we leave the topic of PCOS, let me share some *hidden drivers* of PCOS that I've observed with my patients. Hidden drivers are things that—once corrected—can improve or reverse androgen excess.

Hidden Drivers of PCOS

Many things can impair ovulation and promote excess androgens. They include:

Thyroid disease, because hypothyroidism impedes ovulation and worsens insulin resistance.[212]

Vitamin D deficiency, because your ovaries need vitamin D.

Zinc deficiency, because your ovaries need zinc.

Iodine deficiency, because your ovaries need iodine.

Elevated prolactin, because it increases DHEA.

Too little food or too few carbs, because you need carbs to ovulate. If you're undereating, then you've slipped into HA.

The great thing about identifying a *hidden* driver of PCOS is that once you correct it, your symptoms should improve fairly quickly.

Treatment of Facial Hair, Acne, and Female Pattern Hair Loss

Facial hair, acne, and androgenetic alopecia (female pattern hair loss) are all common symptoms of PCOS, but they can also occur for other reasons. This is the treatment section for those symptoms whether or not you have PCOS.

Treatment of Facial Hair (Hirsutism)

Conventional treatment includes the pill or the anti-androgen drugs cyproterone (Androcur®) and spironolactone (Aldactone®).

Natural treatment is to treat PCOS (if you have PCOS) and also to choose one of the supplements listed later in the chapter in the Natural Anti-Androgen section.

You will also require mechanical hair removal such as tweezing, waxing, laser, or electrolysis.

Facial hair is a frustrating symptom because even with the best treatment, it can take at least twelve months to start to improve.

Treatment of Acne

Conventional treatment includes the pill, spironolactone (Aldactone®), and isotretinoin (Accutane®). Isotretinoin's mechanism of action is to alter DNA expression, and studies have associated it with serious side effects such as depression,[213] inflammatory bowel disease, and osteoporosis.[214] I beg you not to take it.

Natural treatment includes the following:

- Treat PCOS, if you have PCOS.
- Choose one of the supplements listed later in the chapter in the Anti-Androgen Treatments section.
- Choose one or more of the following acne treatments.

Acne treatments

The following treatments are effective for acne regardless of the underlying cause of PCOS, post-pill, or otherwise.

Quit sugar to reduce a hormone called insulin growth factor or IGF-1. IGF-1 is the perfect storm for acne because it increases sebum, keratin, and inflammation.[215]

Avoid cow's dairy to reduce inflammation and IGF-1 hormone. According to the 2005 Nurses' Health Study, women who drink less milk are less likely to suffer acne.[216] You can still have non-inflammatory dairies, such as goat, sheep, and Jersey milk. See the Dairy Products section in Chapter 6.

Address digestive problems because acne can be caused by stomach acid deficiency and SIBO and other digestive problems. That may mean avoiding common food sensitivities such as gluten and eggs. Refer to the Digestive Health section in Chapter 11.

Address histamine intolerance, which is the condition of excess histamine we discussed in the last chapter. High histamine foods include fermented foods and cheese. They can worsen acne.

Zinc is a great treatment for acne. It works by reducing keratin and therefore keeping pores open. Zinc also kills bacteria, reduces inflammation, and lowers androgens. It has done well in several clinical trials.[217]

Berberine is a natural antibiotic, and so it kills the bacteria that cause acne. It also reduces inflammation and IGF-1. In one clinical trial, acne improved by 45 percent after just four weeks on berberine.[218] Berberine may not be safe for long-term use. Please refer to the full discussion of berberine earlier in this chapter.

DIM (diindolylmethane) is a phytonutrient derived from vegetables such as broccoli. It's discussed in the Anti-Androgen section below.

Even with the best treatment, acne can take six months to improve. And remember, coming off a pill like Yasmin® can cause a post-pill type of acne that worsens for six months before it starts to get better.

Treatment of Female Pattern Hair Loss

Female pattern hair loss or androgenetic alopecia is the long-term thinning type of hair loss caused by male hormones. It's different from the temporary hair loss caused by thyroid or iron deficiency. For a full discussion of all the types of hair loss, see the Hair Loss section in Chapter 11.

Conventional treatment includes the pill, cyproterone (Androcur®), spironolactone (Aldactone®), and the topical drug minoxidil or Rogaine®.

Natural treatment includes the following:
- Treat PCOS if you have PCOS.
- Choose one of the supplements listed later in the chapter in the Anti-Androgen Treatments section.
- Choose one of the following topical treatments.

Topical treatments for androgenetic alopecia

Rosemary inhibits 5-alpha reductase which is the enzyme that converts testosterone to the more potent hormone dihydrotestosterone (DHT).[219] For topical use, put four drops of rosemary essential oil into a tablespoon of a carrier oil like jojoba oil. Massage gently into the scalp for 30 minutes before washing your hair. Use three times per week.

Melatonin reduces oxidative stress at the hair follicle and promotes hair growth.[220] One study used a 0.1 percent solution applied once daily at bedtime.

Even with the best treatment, androgenetic alopecia can take months or even years to improve.

Anti-Androgen Treatments

You need this section if you:

- have PCOS and have already put in place the *core treatment* for your type of PCOS
- have androgen symptoms for another reason such as from a post-pill androgen surge.

---

 anti-androgen

Anti-androgens (also known as androgen antagonists, androgen blockers, or testosterone blockers) are drugs or supplements that reduce androgens or block their effects.

(tip) **Anti-androgen supplements** are not a *stand-alone* treatment for PCOS. They're to be used as adjuncts to the other core treatments discussed earlier in this chapter.

Conventional anti-androgen treatment includes the drugs cyproterone (Androcur®) and spironolactone (Aldactone®).

Natural anti-androgen treatment includes the following:

Zinc, which did well in a recent clinical trial where it significantly improved hirsutism in just eight weeks.[221] Zinc works by normalizing hormones. It will not push testosterone below normal.

Peony and licorice combination reduces serum testosterone. I prescribe it primarily for PCOS. Refer to the peony and licorice section earlier in this chapter.

DIM (diindolylmethane) is a phytonutrient derived from vegetables such as broccoli, brussels sprouts, cabbage, and kale. It blocks androgen receptors.[222] It also inhibits the aromatase enzyme, and so could have the unwanted effect of decreasing estrogen. I prescribe 100 mg DIM per day for both acne and hirsutism.

Micronized or natural progesterone inhibits 5-alpha reductase and blocks androgen receptors. The best way to obtain progesterone is to ovulate and *make your own*. You can also supplement it.

Reishi mushroom (*Ganoderma lucidum*) inhibits 5-alpha reductase.[223] Reishi has several other health benefits including support of the immune system and stabilization of the HPA (adrenal) axis.

Vitex agnus-castus lowers prolactin, thereby improving prolactin-induced androgen excess and hirsutism. High prolactin is not typical of PCOS, which is why I usually don't prescribe Vitex for PCOS. I do prescribe it for hypothalamic amenorrhea, discussed below.

Saw palmetto (*Serenoa repens*) inhibits 5-alpha reductase and did well in a recent clinical trial where it was combined with green tea, vitamin D, melatonin, and soy.[224] Like DIM, saw palmetto might have the unwanted effect of decreasing estrogen. I never prescribe saw palmetto, primarily because I prefer other treatments such as zinc, and peony and licorice combination.

> (tip) **You don't need *all* the supplements** discussed in this chapter. Start with your core PCOS treatment such as quitting sugar and taking magnesium, and then choose one additional anti-androgen treatment such as zinc.

Hypothalamic Amenorrhea (HA)

Hypothalamic amenorrhea is defined as the lack of a menstrual period for more than six months when *no medical diagnosis can be found.*

The "no medical diagnosis" part is important. It means your doctor should have ruled out other conditions such as thyroid disease, celiac disease, PCOS, high prolactin, and others.

Before we move on to discussing hypothalamic amenorrhea, there are two more possibilities to consider.

First, is your lack of periods due to too much soy in your diet? As we saw in Chapter 6, too many phytoestrogens can stop periods.[225] If soy is the problem, then please reduce your intake and your periods should return.

Next, is your lack of periods due to recently coming off the pill? If so, then you may just need a bit more time, as did Christine in Chapter 1. Or you may benefit from the treatments discussed in this section. Please also refer to the How to Come Off Hormonal Birth Control section in Chapter 11.

The wisdom of the hypothalamus

If there is no medical reason for your lack of periods, then it's because your hypothalamus (your master hormonal command center) has decided you should not ovulate. Why would it make such a decision? Your hypothalamus is not trying to be mean. It's trying to *help* you because it perceives that something is not right in your world. You are either stressed or not getting enough to eat, so your hypothalamus does not want you to attempt the difficult business of bringing a baby into the world. It temporarily dials back reproduction—just until things get better.

But wait—what if you don't actually want to make a baby? You just want periods. From the perspective of your hypothalamus, it's the same thing. Being healthy enough to make a baby is how you are healthy enough to have a period.

Hypothalamic amenorrhea is not a disorder. It's a *normal* response to undereating or stress.

Let's now look at the two main causes of hypothalamic amenorrhea: undereating and stress.

Eat More

If you were my patient, I would start with one simple question: Do you feel like you're getting enough to eat? For example, yesterday—did you feel *satisfied* with your food?

I like this question because it sends the message that you *deserve* to feel satisfied and be fully nourished. As a woman, you need more food than you've been led to believe.

Undereating can cause you to lose your periods, and, as we saw in Chapter 5, you don't have to be underweight. Undereating can be a problem when you are normal weight or even *over*weight. Your hypothalamus cares less about body weight and more about whether you eat enough to keep up with your activity level.

 You can exercise as long as you eat enough.

To get a period, you need to be fully nourished in every respect. That means enough calories and enough micronutrients such as zinc and iodine. It also means enough of *all* of the macronutrients including protein, fat, and carbohydrate.

Undereating carbohydrate can impair hypothalamic signaling and cause amenorrhea—even if you eat enough calories.[226]

If you feel better on a low-carb diet, then ask yourself:

- Is it because you stopped having wheat? If so, your better strategy is to avoid wheat, but continue to have rice, potatoes, and oats.
- Is it because you've relieved a digestive problem? If so,

your better strategy is to fix your digestion (see Chapter 11).

Eating disorder

If you think you might have an eating disorder, then please know you're not alone. One study showed that the majority (63 percent) of young women with amenorrhea go on to be diagnosed with an eating disorder.[227]

Be gentle with yourself and *reach out for professional help*. I've provided the names of reputable organizations in the Resources section.

In addition to seeking help from a professional psychologist, here are some simple ideas:

- Unfollow any social media accounts that glorify undereating or skinny bodies.
- Hang out with friends who enjoy eating and are comfortable with food.
- Never use the word "bad" or "clean" to refer to food or eating.
- Let go of being perfect at anything—including your diet.

Even once you start eating more, you'll still have to wait at least four months to get a period. Why? Because that's how long it takes your ovarian follicles to travel all the way to ovulation.

 If you cannot gain weight no matter how much you eat, you might have a medical condition such as celiac disease. Speak to your doctor.

Stress Less

The best way to reduce stress is to follow all the guidelines described in the HPA axis dysfunction section in Chapter 6.

Conventional Treatment of Hypothalamic Amenorrhea

Hypothalamic amenorrhea is one condition where the conventional and natural treatment recommendations are the same: Eat more and stress less.

Your doctor may also recommend the pill, but remember, pill bleeds are not periods. The pill does not protect against osteoporosis[228] and can actually impair recovery from hypothalamic amenorrhea.[229]

Supplements and Herbal Medicines for Hypothalamic Amenorrhea

The most important strategy for hypothalamic amenorrhea is to *eat more*. Unless you also do that for at least four months, none of the following supplements can do anything to help you.

Magnesium is The Miracle Mineral for Periods, and is helpful here again. It helps you cope with stress and regulates your hypothalamus.

Ashwagandha (*Withania somnifera*) is a herbal medicine that's been used for thousands of years in the Ayurvedic medical tradition of India. It was traditionally given as an energy and reproductive tonic.

> **How it works:** It reduces anxiety and counters the long-term effects of stress such as blood sugar instability, insomnia, depression, and suppression of the hypothalamus.

> **What else you need to know:** The exact quantity of the herb depends on the concentration in the formula, so please use as directed on the bottle. Ashwagandha can be taken as tea, liquid, or tablet. For full benefit, I recommend taking it twice daily for at least three months.

Vitex agnus-castus (chaste tree or chasteberry) is a medicine prepared from the berries of a large Mediterranean tree. In ancient times, it was purportedly used to suppress the libido of monks, hence its name. Fortunately, it does not have that effect in women.

How it works: It promotes ovulation by protecting your hypothalamus from chronic stress and by preventing your pituitary gland from making too much prolactin. Vitex also contains opiate-like constituents, which calm your nervous system.[230] That's why Vitex is also a great treatment for premenstrual syndrome, as we'll see in Chapter 8.

What else you need to know: The exact quantity of the herb depends on the concentration in the formula. One tablet can contain anywhere from 200 to 1000 mg. For best effect, take the herb first thing in the morning before breakfast, because that's when your pituitary is most receptive. I recommend pulsing the dose by stopping it for five days each month. Not all clinicians dose it this way, but I think it prevents attenuation of its effect over time. If you have periods (but are using it for PMS),stop the herb for five days from the start of each period. If you don't have periods, take it for 25 days on and then five days off.

Vitex is a powerful medicine, so you need to be careful about how you take it. For example, do not take it if you are also taking a fertility drug. Do not take it if you are younger than 18, because your pituitary-ovarian communication is still developing. Do not take it for more than six months continuously, except under professional guidance. If you are using Vitex to get your periods going, you should not need it for longer than that because it should have worked within that time. You should then be able to stop it and your periods remain regular. Finally, be careful with Vitex if you have PCOS, because it can increase LH and worsen the condition. If in doubt, speak to your doctor.

High Prolactin

Prolactin is a pituitary hormone that promotes lactation and regulates hormones. Too much prolactin inhibits ovulation.

Severely elevated prolactin is a serious medical problem that can stop periods completely.

Mildly elevated prolactin can cause irregular periods, breast pain, and loss of libido. It can also cause androgen excess by two different mechanisms.

- Prolactin increases the adrenal androgen DHEA.[231]
- Prolactin up-regulates 5-alpha reductase leading to more dihydrotestosterone (DHT).[232]

High prolactin can be identified with a simple blood test.

What Causes High Prolactin?

Very high prolactin (greater than 1000 mIU/L or 50 ng/mL) is usually the result of a benign pituitary tumor called a prolactinoma, which requires medical diagnosis and management. Your doctor will probably order an imaging study such as an MRI (magnetic resonance imaging study) and treat you with the drug bromocriptine, which reduces prolactin. There is no natural treatment for an active prolactinoma.

Moderately high prolactin (greater than 480 mIU/L or 23 ng/mL) can be caused by prolactinoma, thyroid disease, alcohol, or medications such as hormonal birth control, stomach acid tablets, and some types of psychiatric and blood pressure medications. It requires medical diagnosis and management.

Mildly high prolactin (around 480 mIU/L or 23 ng/mL) is common, and cannot be diagnosed by a single result. Why? Because your prolactin might have been temporarily elevated by any of the following:

- sex
- exercise
- alcohol
- eating
- sleep
- dehydration
- stress
- luteal phase (post-ovulation)
- mild thyroid disease

- hormonal birth control.

For accuracy, you'll want to recheck your prolactin under the following conditions:

- during the follicular phase
- between 8 a.m. and 12 p.m.
- fasting
- hydrated
- not directly after exercise or sex
- relaxed
- not on hormonal birth control.

 Mildly elevated prolactin can be a feature of both hypothalamic amenorrhea and PCOS.

Once your doctor has ruled out a medical explanation for your high prolactin, you can consider using natural treatments

Diet and Lifestyle to Lower Prolactin

Reduce alcohol, especially beer, because barley stimulates prolactin. That's why beer was traditionally prescribed to increase milk supply. Do not exceed four alcoholic drinks per week.

Reduce stress with yoga, meditation, and long slow walks.

Herbal Medicine to Lower Prolactin

Vitex is the best natural treatment to lower prolactin. For dosing instructions, refer to the section dealing with Vitex earlier in the chapter.

A Final Word About Irregular Periods

Irregular periods can be frustrating. It's difficult to obtain an accurate diagnosis, and even once you do, there are so many different natural treatments to choose from.

My experience with thousands of patients is that the mystery of irregular periods can eventually be solved. Go deeper with your diagnosis. Try to figure out *why* you do not ovulate. Recruit your doctor to help you, using the list of questions in the How to Talk to Your Doctor section in Chapter 11.

Once you select a treatment, please commit to it for *at least three months*. You need to wait at least that long because that's how long it takes your ovarian follicles to journey all the way to ovulation.

Take heart. Keep going, and remember: Your body *wants* to have regular periods.

Chapter 8

➤————————➤

The PMS Solution: 3 Steps to Hormonal Resilience

This is the chapter that many of you have been waiting for. What, for goodness sake, can be done to relieve premenstrual irritability, breast pain, acne, headaches, and other symptoms?

Let me start by saying flat out that for most of you, premenstrual syndrome (PMS) can become a thing of the past. I am serious. PMS responds well to natural treatment, and it responds quickly. It will be the first thing to change on your monthly report card.

I love to hear patients say: "I was surprised when my period just arrived. I didn't even feel it coming."

No irritability. No headache. No food cravings. It *is* possible.

Does that surprise you? The majority of women report some physical or emotional changes in the second half of their cycle. About twenty percent of women experience symptoms severe enough to seek medical help.

No wonder PMS is widely portrayed as something universal and inevitable. Yet here I am, telling you it does not need to be that way. I stand by what I say. PMS is common, but it's not inevitable. In fact, PMS is curable. That's why I've dedicated a full chapter of this book to a PMS solution.

A Controversial Diagnosis

PMS was first described in the early 1980s and has been controversial ever since. It's controversial for a couple of reasons.

First, the term PMS is subject to misuse. Too often, it's used to trivialize any and all of women's emotions, which is a problem. As a woman (and a human being), you have the *right* to emotions. Your emotions should not be dismissed by your partner or family member as simply "hormonal." In fact, I reject the very word when used as an adjective to describe a woman. It's crazy to me that *hormonal* has come to be an insult. It implies that female hormones themselves are negative for mood, which, as we'll discover later in the chapter, is simply not true.

The second reason PMS is controversial is that it refers not to one thing, but rather to a large and varying set of symptoms. In its broadest interpretation, PMS can refer to virtually *any* symptom you experience two out of every four weeks.

PMS Symptoms

Despite the controversy, I am convinced that PMS is real.

The most commonly reported emotional symptoms are irritability, anxiety, depression, and weepiness. The most commonly reported physical symptoms are sleep disturbance, fluid retention, abdominal bloating, palpitations, joint pain, headaches, brain fog, food cravings, breast pain, and pimples. To qualify as PMS, symptoms must occur during the ten days *before* your period and then disappear during or shortly after your bleed.

Premenstrual magnification

If your PMS symptoms are a temporary *worsening* of symptoms you tend to experience anyway (e.g., headaches, digestive problems, acne, and sugar cravings), then it is not PMS. It's *premenstrual magnification.*

Premenstrual magnification is different from premenstrual syndrome in that your best strategy is to treat your *underlying* condition. That way, it will not be aggravated by the natural shift to inflammation that occurs at the end of your luteal phase. You may also benefit from some of the strategies discussed in this chapter.

What Causes PMS?

Your hormones themselves are *not to blame for PMS*. Neither estrogen nor progesterone is inherently negative for mood or any other thing—far from it. Your hormones are *beneficial.*

Remember from previous chapters that both estrogen and progesterone are powerful enhancers of mood and metabolism.

For example, when estrogen rises in your follicular phase, you will feel great because estrogen boosts serotonin and gives you stronger muscles and better insulin sensitivity. Wonderful, to a point. If your estrogen goes too high, you will feel less than wonderful.

The Ups and Downs of Estrogen

Estrogen is like an interesting and charismatic friend: she's great to have around, but she can become a bit overwhelming after a while. Some estrogen is great. Too much estrogen is overstimulating and can cause breast pain, fluid retention, irritability, and headaches.

The departure of estrogen can also cause symptoms. Your estrogen cannot stay high forever, and you wouldn't want it to. Estrogen has to drop at the end of your cycle, and when it does, it brings serotonin and dopamine down with it. The higher your estrogen, the further your fall. The withdrawal from estrogen can cause fatigue, night sweats, and migraines.

Progesterone to the Rescue

At the same time that estrogen is going up and down, progesterone should be coming to your rescue. If you can make enough progesterone, it will soothe you and shelter you from the ups and downs of estrogen.

Recall from Chapter 4 that progesterone counterbalances estrogen. Progesterone has other superpowers such as converting to the neurosteroid allopregnanolone which calms your brain just like the neurotransmitter GABA. It stabilizes your HPA (adrenal) axis.

If you can make enough progesterone, and if you are sufficiently sensitive to it, then you will be soothed by allopregnanolone all the way to your period. If, on the other hand, you don't make enough progesterone, or if progesterone drops away too quickly, [233] or if you have altered sensitivity to progesterone[234]—then you may experience mood symptoms.

The conventional approach to PMS and hormonal fluctuation is to flat-line your hormones with hormonal birth control. Yes, that stabilizes things, but not in a good way. You will no longer have hormonal fluctuation, but that's because you will no longer have hormones. You throw the baby out with the bathwater.

 Hormonal birth control can also cause symptoms, but they're *drug side effects*—not PMS.[235]

Hormonal Resilience

The natural approach to hormonal fluctuation is different. It does not switch off hormonal fluctuation. Instead, it embraces the shift as a normal and beneficial process. Your hormones fluctuate because you make them in a cyclical pattern with ovulation. That is the only way you *can* make them.

Put it this way: if you're going to have hormones, they're going to fluctuate.

You don't need to flat-line your hormones. You need only be able to *adapt* to their ups and downs. That ability to adapt to hormonal fluctuation is what I call *hormonal resilience*.

New research supports the idea of hormonal resilience and suggests there's a genetic component. The cells of women with premenstrual dysphoric disorder (PMDD) respond differently to hormones compared to women without the condition.[236]

PMDD

Premenstrual dysphoric disorder is a condition of severe premenstrual depression, irritability, or anxiety. It affects about one in twenty women.

So, you may have been lucky enough to be born with genes that protect you from premenstrual symptoms. If not, you can protect yourself by *cultivating hormonal resilience* in three easy steps:

- Enhance progesterone and GABA.
- Stabilize estrogen and metabolize it properly.
- Reduce inflammation to calm your hormone and neurotransmitter receptors.

Did you notice the third point? *Reduce inflammation.* Why is that important for PMS?

The Role of Inflammation

Inflammatory cytokines put you at greater risk of PMS.[237] Why? Because, as we saw in Chapter 6, chronic inflammation distorts hormonal communication.

More precisely, inflammation impairs both the manufacture of progesterone and the responsiveness of progesterone receptors. So, you end up needing *more* progesterone just to be able to feel its soothing effect.

Inflammation also downregulates GABA receptors, which further impairs your response to progesterone and worsens PMS.

Finally, inflammation interferes with estrogen detoxification and hyper-sensitizes you to estrogen.

In summary, inflammation can cause 1) less progesterone and GABA, and 2) more estrogen.

Inflammation is the perfect storm for PMS.

Fortunately, you can reduce inflammation with the anti-inflammatory strategies we discussed in Chapter 6. You can also harness the natural anti-inflammatory effects of progesterone.[238]

Let's start with progesterone.

Enhance Progesterone and GABA

Progesterone is central to the PMS story because it shelters you from the ups and downs of estrogen. It also reduces inflammation and calms your mood by enhancing the neurotransmitter GABA.

You want more progesterone *and* more GABA so you can experience a greater benefit from progesterone. This section will give you strategies for both progesterone and GABA.

 More progesterone and more GABA can result in less PMS.[239]

How do you know if you have enough progesterone?

Symptoms of low progesterone include PMS, fertile mucus during the premenstrual phase, premenstrual bleeding or spotting, and prolonged or heavy menstrual bleeding.

You can measure progesterone with a mid-luteal blood test or by tracking your temperatures. Remember, you're looking for a consistent rise in temperature in your luteal phase. See the Progesterone Deficiency section in Chapter 5.

As we've seen in previous chapters, progesterone is difficult to make and difficult to hold on to. No wonder premenstrual symptoms are so common!

Diet and Lifestyle to Enhance Progesterone and GABA

As we saw in the Roadmap to Progesterone section in chapter 4, your progesterone in any given cycle is the result of the health of your corpus luteum which is the result of the health of your ovarian follicle during all its 100-day journey to ovulation.

Boosting progesterone is a long-term project.

Reduce inflammatory foods

By reducing inflammatory foods such as sugar, wheat, and cow's dairy, you can support progesterone in two ways:

- Less inflammation leads to better ovulation, and therefore *more* progesterone.
- Less inflammation enhances the sensitivity of both progesterone and GABA receptors.

Of all the inflammatory foods, cow's dairy seems to be the most significant for PMS, probably because it can trigger the release of histamine.

Special Topic: The Curious Link Between PMS and Histamine

If your PMS symptoms include headaches, anxiety, or brain fog, then you might be suffering *histamine intolerance*. As you may recall from the Histamine Intolerance section in Chapter 6, histamine is a normal part of your immune system, but too much histamine can cause symptoms.

Histamine intolerance is often worse just before the period

because estrogen increases histamine and vice versa. Progesterone, on the other hand, decreases histamine, which is one way that progesterone relieves PMS.

Treatment for histamine intolerance can include:

- enhancing progesterone or taking progesterone

- reducing *histamine-stimulating* foods such as dairy and alcohol[240]

- reducing *histamine-containing* foods such as red wine, cheese, bone broth, and fermented foods

- Taking vitamin B6, which upregulates the DAO enzyme that breaks down histamine.[241]

Histamine intolerance can also be a factor in period pain and ovarian cysts, which we'll discuss in Chapter 9.

 Histamine reduction is a big part of why vitamin B6 and natural progesterone work so well for PMS and other conditions.

Reduce alcohol

Alcohol lowers allopregnanolone[242] and interferes with progesterone's soothing effect. Alcohol can also worsen histamine intolerance. You can probably enjoy the occasional wine or beer, but for the sake of your progesterone and PMS, please do not exceed four drinks per week.

Reduce stress

A high level of perceived stress doubles the risk of severe PMS. [243] There are a few things going on. First, adrenaline directly blocks progesterone receptors and depletes GABA. That alone can cause PMS.

In the longer term, stress also impairs ovulation and depletes progesterone. Finally, low progesterone can further destabilize your stress response or HPA (adrenal) axis.[244] That's why you may notice a delayed effect with stress. Stress *now* can lead to PMS weeks in the future.

Stress-reduction is critical for hormonal resilience. If you suffer PMS, you now have an excuse to say: "To balance my hormones, I need to go for that walk, or book a massage, or spend the entire afternoon reading a novel."

Exercise

Exercise helps PMS[245] because it reduces both stress and inflammation.

Supplements and Herbal Medicines to Enhance Progesterone and GABA

Magnesium is my front-line treatment for PMS. It improves premenstrual symptoms so dramatically[246] that some scientists have suggested that magnesium deficiency is the main *cause* of PMS.[247]

> **How it works:** It aids in the manufacture of steroid hormones, including progesterone. It also normalise the action of progesterone on the central nervous system. But magnesium's benefits don't stop there. It also reduces inflammation, regulates the stress response, and enhances GABA activity.

> **What else you need to know:** Food sources of magnesium include nuts and seeds and dark leafy vegetables, but food sources of magnesium are often not enough. I recommend a supplement of 300 mg magnesium glycinate per day. See the Magnesium section in Chapter 6.

Vitamin B6 is the next strongest treatment for PMS. It is effective for both PMS and the more severe condition of PMDD. [248]

> **How it works**: Vitamin B6 (also called pyridoxal-5-phosphate or P5P) works on almost every aspect of the PMS story. It's essential for the synthesis of both progesterone and GABA. It

reduces inflammation and assists with the healthy detoxification of estrogen. Finally, vitamin B6 is a natural diuretic and relieves histamine intolerance.

What else you need to know: I generally recommend between 20 and 150 mg per day of vitamin B6 in divided doses spaced out during the day (e.g. 50 mg twice daily). You can expect to feel its benefits within one hour. Vitamin B6 works well in combination with magnesium as we saw in Amy's story in Chapter 6. Note that long-term supplementation of more than 200 mg can cause nerve damage.

 Magnesium plus vitamin B6 is my favorite treatment for PMS.

Vitex agnus-castus (chaste tree or chasteberry). We met the herbal medicine Vitex in the last chapter as a treatment for hypothalamic amenorrhea. Vitex is also great for PMS. It was recently evaluated by a large systematic review of seventeen randomised controlled trials and was determined to be safe and effective for the treatment of PMS and PMDD.[249]

Vitex relieves mood, fluid retention, and breast tenderness. We'll look at breast tenderness later in the chapter.

How it works: By inhibiting the pituitary hormone prolactin, it enhances ovulation and progesterone. Vitex also contains opiate-like constituents, which calm the nervous system.[250]

What else you need to know: The exact quantity of the herb depends on the concentration of the formula. One tablet can contain anywhere from 200 to 1000 mg.

For best effect, take the herb in the morning before breakfast, because that's when your pituitary is most responsive. Stop it for five days from the start of each period. For detailed instructions, refer to the Vitex section in Chapter 7.

Selenium is a key nutrient for progesterone production.

How it works: it's essential for the formation and integrity of the corpus luteum.

What else you need to know: Food sources of selenium include seafood, organ meats, and brazil nuts. One serving of salmon, for example, provides 40 mcg of selenium. If you decide to supplement, take only 100 to 150 mcg per day to allow for the amount you're getting from food. The safe upper limit for selenium from all sources is 200 mcg per day.

Micronized progesterone or natural progesterone is something to consider after you have tried the other treatments.

How it works: It is the hormone progesterone, so is a type of hormone replacement. Progesterone relieves PMS because it converts to the calming neurosteroid allopregnanolone and because it assists with the healthy removal of histamine.

What else you need to know: Take during your luteal phase as a topical cream or capsule. For more information about natural progesterone and bioidentical hormones, see the Bioidentical Hormones section in Chapter 10.

Checklist to enhance progesterone and GABA:
- Maintain healthy ovarian follicles for all of their 100-day journey to ovulation.
- Reduce stress.
- Consider taking magnesium, vitamin B6, and Vitex.

 Natural treatment works best to prevent PMS. Follow the guidelines during *all* the days of your cycle—not just when you're premenstrual.

Stabilize and Metabolize Estrogen

As we saw earlier in the chapter, estrogen is a beneficial and charismatic friend, but you do need to rein her in a little. By keeping estrogen in check, you will prevent symptoms of *estrogen excess* such as premenstrual irritability and breast tenderness. You will also prevent the depression that can occur when estrogen crashes from high to low.

Diet and Lifestyle to Metabolize Estrogen

Reduce alcohol

Reduce alcohol to improve estrogen metabolism or detoxification. Just two drinks per day can *double* your exposure to estrogen.[251]

Maintain healthy gut bacteria

Healthy gut bacteria escort estrogen safely out of your body. Unhealthy gut bacteria do the opposite. They impair estrogen metabolism and cause estrogen to be reabsorbed into your body. One of the best ways to maintain a healthy microbiome is to avoid as much as possible drugs such as antibiotics that damage gut bacteria.

Maintain a healthy body weight

Maintain a healthy body weight, because body fat makes a type of estrogen called *estrone*.

Avoid endocrine disrupting chemicals

Endocrine disrupting chemicals such as plastics and pesticides impair your ability to metabolize estrogen. They can also hyperstimulate your estrogen receptors. See the Environmental Toxins section in Chapter 11.

Reduce inflammatory foods

By reducing inflammatory foods such as sugar, wheat, and cow's milk, you support the healthy detoxification of estrogen. You also reduce histamine, which in turn can reduce estrogen excess, and thus relieve PMS symptoms.

Eat phytoestrogens

Phytoestrogens are natural estrogen-like substances from legumes, flaxseed, grains, and vegetables. They're beneficial for PMS because they bind weakly to your estrogen receptors and buffer you from the ups and downs of your stronger estrogen estradiol.

 Phytoestrogens reduce estrogen because they block estrogen receptors and speed up estrogen metabolism. [252]

Supplements and Herbal Medicines to Stabilize and Metabolize Estrogen

Iodine is helpful for PMS and especially for breast pain, which we'll discuss later in the chapter.

How it works: It stabilizes and downregulates your estrogen receptors.

What else you need to know: Please be careful with iodine if you have thyroid disease. See the Iodine section in Chapter 6.

Calcium d-glucarate is an effective phytonutrient for PMS. The active part is the *glucarate* (not the calcium). Glucarate is normally made by your body in small amounts. It's also found in foods such as oranges and broccoli.

How it works: Glucarate assists with estrogen detoxification in two ways. First, it binds to estrogen in the liver and deactivates it. Second, it inhibits *beta-glucuronidase*, which is an enzyme made by gut bacteria that causes estrogen to be reabsorbed.

What else you need to know: I recommend taking 1000 to 1500 mg per day. It may also help to prevent breast cancer.[253]

A **Probiotic supplement** promotes healthy gut bacteria.

How it works: Healthy gut bacteria escort estrogen out of your body.

What else you need to know: The best probiotic to promote healthy estrogen metabolism is one that inhibits the enzyme beta-glucuronidase. The bacteria strain *Lactobacillus casei* has shown promising results in this regard, but the research is still in its infancy. For a full discussion of the rapidly changing field of probiotic research, refer to the Digestive Health section in Chapter 11.

Checklist to stabilize and metabolize estrogen:
- Reduce alcohol.
- Maintain healthy gut bacteria.
- Identify and treat histamine intolerance.
- Consider taking calcium-d-glucarate and low-dose iodine.

Reduce Inflammation

As we saw earlier in the chapter, chronic inflammation distorts hormonal communication. By interfering with hormone production and hormone receptors, inflammation is a major cause of PMS.

How can you reduce inflammation?

Diet and Lifestyle to Reduce Inflammation

Reduce inflammatory foods
Removing dairy from your diet can dramatically improve PMS as we saw with Nina in Chapter 6. Other potentially PMS-causing foods include wheat, sugar, vegetable oil, and high histamine foods (discussed above).

 Food sensitivities can cause PMS.

Supplements and Herbal Medicines to Reduce Inflammation

As we saw a few pages ago, **magnesium** plus **vitamin B6** is my front-line treatment for PMS. Both nutrients help with the formation of progesterone, but they also have a powerful anti-inflammatory effect. For dosing instructions, refer to the progesterone section above.

Beyond magnesium and vitamin B6, you can look at zinc.

Zinc is one of the strongest anti-inflammatory supplements and did well in a recent clinical trial for PMS.[254]

> **How it works:** It decreases inflammation and histamine, and it increases progesterone and GABA. If you're deficient in zinc, you're more likely to suffer PMS.[255]

> **What else you need to know:** I recommend 30 mg per day to be taken directly after dinner, as dinner is usually the biggest meal. Avoid taking zinc on an empty stomach or it may cause nausea.

Advanced Treatment of PMS

So far, we've discussed a general PMS treatment plan which should be effective for most premenstrual symptoms including those discussed in this section.

As a review, the most effective treatments for PMS are:

- magnesium
- vitamin B6
- Zinc
- avoid inflammatory or histamine-inducing foods (usually dairy).

With these treatments, you could see results within the very first month, but it could take longer. Allow at least three months before you try something different.

Here are some additional treatment ideas to try *together with* those core treatments.

PMS with Depression and Anxiety

Mood symptoms are common with PMS. If they're severe enough, they can qualify you for the medical diagnosis of *premenstrual dysphoric disorder* (PMDD). The conventional treatment for PMDD is an antidepressant, for which you will need to consult your doctor.

Premenstrual mood symptoms should improve with the treatments offered earlier in the chapter, particularly magnesium, vitamin B6, and Vitex. All of those supplements can be used safely in combination with a conventional antidepressant.

 Vitex outperforms antidepressants for premenstrual dysphoric disorder. (PMDD)[256]

You can also consider one of the following treatments.

SAM-e (S-adenosylmethionine) is a strong mood enhancer. It works quickly over just a few days so that you can use it in the short-term, on an as-needed basis.

> **How it works:** SAMe is a derivative of the amino acid methionine. It occurs naturally in your body and has many different functions, including the manufacture of serotonin and dopamine. It also reduces histamine.

> **What else you need to know:** I recommend 100 to 200 mg per day. A higher dose can cause anxiety. Do not combine with other antidepressants except under medical advice.

St John's wort (*Hypericum perforatum*) is a herbal medicine with a long tradition of use for depression and anxiety. In recent years, it has undergone several clinical trials for PMS. In one study, a group of 35 PMS sufferers took St John's wort for two cycles and reported a significant reduction in all emotional and physical symptoms including anxiety.[257]

How it works: St John's wort boosts serotonin, dopamine, and GABA. It also reduces inflammation. Scientists are still working to discover the full mechanism for the benefits of St John's wort.

What else you need to know: I recommend 300 mg of a standardized extract. For best results, take twice daily for at least two months. Do not combine with other antidepressants except under medical advice. Do not combine with the birth control pill because it can reduce the pill's contraceptive efficacy.[258]

Rhodiola rosea is the herbal medicine we met in Chapter 6 for regulating the stress response.

How it works: Rhodiola calms anxiety and regulates the HPA (adrenal) axis.

What else you need to know: The exact quantity of the herb depends on the concentration of the formula, so take as directed on the bottle. For more information about Rhodiola, refer to Chapter 6.

PMS with Breast Pain

Cyclic breast pain (also called *cyclic mastalgia* or *fibrocystic breast pain*) is common with PMS. Symptoms include breast enlargement, pain, lumpiness, cysts, warmth, nipple soreness, and sometimes nipple discharge. Fibrocystic lumpiness of the breasts can be frightening, but it does not directly lead to breast cancer. The biggest concern is that it can mask the presence of other types of lumps, so it should be assessed by your doctor.

Iodine is the best treatment for breast pain.

How it works: As we saw in Chapter 6, iodine stabilizes and downregulates estrogen receptors. Breast tissue has a lot of estrogen receptors, so breasts need a lot of iodine. Iodine supplementation has been demonstrated to improve fibrocystic breast lumpiness[259] and to reduce the risk of breast cancer.[260] It also has a nice diuretic effect and so can relieve premenstrual fluid retention.

What else you need to know: The best type of iodine for breasts is *molecular iodine* (I2). Compared to iodide, I2 is absorbed more *slowly* into the thyroid and more *quickly* into the breasts.[261] That makes I2 safer for thyroid and better for breast pain. That said, any type of iodine can be harmful to your thyroid, so please do not take more than 500 mcg (0.5 mg) except under professional supervision. Too much iodine can worsen acne.

June: Iodine for breast pain

June told me that when she was coming up to her period her breasts were so painful, it hurt to walk downstairs. Her breasts were also lumpy, which her doctor said was benign breast disease and told her not to worry.

June wasn't *worried*, but she was in pain. She needed help.

"Let's check your thyroid," I said. "So we can decide if it's safe for you to take iodine."

June had a normal thyroid function test (TSH) and was negative for *thyroid antibodies*, which to me, is the single most important test before giving iodine. If she had tested positive for thyroid antibodies, then I would have been reluctant to prescribe any amount of iodine in supplement form.

I didn't test June for iodine because as we saw in Chapter 6, iodine is not easy to test. For me, as a clinician, the symptom of breast pain is enough to demonstrate iodine deficiency.

I asked June to take one tablet per day of the Violet® brand of iodine which provides 3000 mcg (3 mg) of molecular iodine. She also took magnesium plus vitamin B6, which I recommend for almost every PMS patient.

Three months later, June had almost no breast pain.

I then asked June to reduce her iodine to one tablet every

second day, because I expected she had replenished her body's iodine, and so would need less over time. Eventually, we dropped her to a maintenance dose of one tablet per week, which equates to 428 mcg per day.

Vitex is another reliable treatment for premenstrual breast pain. It can reduce lumps and pain within just two cycles[262]. For further instruction, refer to the Vitex section earlier in the chapter.

PMS with Acne

Both estrogen and progesterone are generally good for skin. That's why you have clearer skin during the middle of your cycle when those hormones are high. You may then notice more acne during your premenstrual time when those hormones drop. You can *somewhat* improve acne by supporting progesterone, and by stabilizing estrogen with the treatments discussed in this chapter.

I say "somewhat" because acne is almost never about estrogen or progesterone. Instead, acne is almost always about other underlying issues such as insulin resistance and inflammation. The best treatments are those that address those issues, such as removing both dairy and sugar from your diet, and taking zinc. I provide other acne treatment ideas in the Acne Treatment section in Chapter 7.

PMS with Migraines or Headaches

Migraines are triggered by a drop in estrogen,[263] which is why the premenstrual phase is a dangerous time for migraines. Seventy percent of female migraine sufferers report a worsening of migraines just before or during their period. Melatonin insufficiency during menstruation may also play a role.[264]

Conventional treatment is hormonal birth control, but it's not

effective because most types of hormonal birth control make migraines worse. Also, hormonal birth control carries a higher stroke risk for migraine-sufferers than it does for other women.
[265]

Natural treatments are a good solution.

Avoid wheat, because it's a common migraine trigger. One study found that avoiding wheat eliminated migraines in 89 percent of patients.[266]

Magnesium is highly effective for migraine prevention, which makes sense since 50 percent of migraine sufferers are deficient in the mineral. Neurologist Dr Alexander Mauskop from the New York Headache Center recommends that *all migraine patients be treated with magnesium*.[267] A 2016 meta-analysis further supports the use of magnesium for migraine prevention.[268]

> **How it works:** It calms your nervous system, reduces inflammation, and stabilizes serotonin receptors. Magnesium also prevents the release of *substance-P*, which is a pain-promoting neurotransmitter involved in migraines.

> **What else you need to know:** I recommend 300 mg of magnesium glycinate per day. You can take an extra dose if you feel a migraine coming on. It works well in combination with 100 mg of vitamin B6.

Melatonin supplements reduce the frequency of menstrual migraines and have outperformed conventional migraine medication in at least one clinical trial.[269]

> **How it works:** It reduces inflammation, and stabilizes the neurotransmitters serotonin and GABA.

> **What else you need to know:** It works as prevention, so should be taken every night throughout the luteal phase. I recommend 0.5 to 3 mg at bedtime.

Vitamin B2 (riboflavin) has been shown to reduce the frequency of migraines by 50 percent.[270]

> **How it works:** It normalizes the production of serotonin and improves the function of a gene called MTHFR that has been

linked to migraines.

What else you need to know: The dose used in the clinical trials was 200 mg twice daily, which is the dose I prescribe for my migraine patients.

MTHFR

MTHFR (methylenetetrahydrofolate reductase) is an enzyme that transforms folate (folic acid) to its active form. About one in three people have a variant of the gene that makes the enzyme. The MTHFR gene mutation can be assessed with a simple blood test. If you have the variant gene, then you may need a higher dose of B vitamins.

Micronized progesterone or natural progesterone is highly effective for premenstrual migraines. I said earlier that I recommend trying other treatments before trying progesterone. Premenstrual migraines are the exception. When a patient comes to me for help with migraines, I often recommend progesterone on the first visit.

How it works: Progesterone calms your nervous system and brain.

What else you need to know: I recommend a cream or capsule. Take at bedtime throughout your migraine "danger window" (from five days before your period until two days into your period). If you feel a migraine coming on, take a second daytime dose. See the Natural Progesterone section in Chapter 10.

And just a reminder: There is *no* progesterone in hormonal birth control.

Postmenstrual or end-menstrual migraines

End-menstrual migraines are not triggered by hormones as are premenstrual migraines. Instead, end-menstrual migraines are triggered by a brief iron-deficiency anemia due to menstrual blood loss.[271] The best treatment is to take iron.

PMS with Fatigue

To treat premenstrual fatigue, you must first figure out *why* it's happening.

Inflammatory fatigue

A common reason for premenstrual fatigue is the inflammation as progesterone drops away (remember, progesterone is anti-inflammatory). With this type of fatigue, you feel a bit like you have the flu, with achy muscles and a sore throat. Histamine intolerance may also play a role in this type of premenstrual fatigue. The best treatment is to remove cow's dairy from your diet, and to take the anti-inflammatory nutrients magnesium, vitamin B6, and zinc.

HPA (adrenal) axis fatigue

Another reason for premenstrual fatigue is HPA axis dysfunction or a problem with your stress response system. Losing progesterone at the end of your cycle can destabilize your HPA axis and worsen symptoms of "adrenal fatigue." With this type of fatigue, you feel agitated or stressed before your period. The best treatments are magnesium plus vitamin B6 plus an *adaptogen* herb such as Rhodiola or ashwagandha.

Sleep problems

Yet another reason for premenstrual fatigue is the insomnia you might experience as your estrogen and progesterone drop away. Both hormones have direct sleep-enhancing effects[272] and so losing them can disrupt sleep.

Special Topic: The Sleep-Enhancing Effect of Progesterone

Progesterone enhances sleep so profoundly that it can be detected on EEG or brainwave studies. For example, in the days immediately after ovulation (when progesterone is highest), women exhibit more sleep spindles, which are brainwaves that indicate the onset of deep sleep.[273] Conversely, women on the Pill (who have no progesterone) exhibit fewer sleep spindles and fewer restorative sleep cycles.[274]

The best treatment for premenstrual insomnia is magnesium, and the other progesterone-enhancing treatments discussed earlier in the chapter. Micronized progesterone capsules can also give great relief.[275]

Iron deficiency

A final consideration for premenstrual fatigue is iron deficiency, which is common in women with PMS.[276] You are particularly at risk of deficiency if you suffer heavy periods.

If you suspect iron deficiency, look for symptoms such as breathlessness and easy bruising. Ask your doctor to test your *serum ferritin.*

 ferritin

Serum ferritin is the blood test for stored iron.

Your doctor needs to test your *actual* iron or ferritin levels. It's not enough to just order a blood count, and then say your hemoglobin is okay, so your iron must be okay. Your serum ferritin should be between 50 and 200 ng/mL.

> 📖 *blood count*
>
> Blood count is a blood test to determine the number of blood cells and hemoglobin.

> 📖 *hemoglobin*
>
> Hemoglobin is the iron-containing protein found in red blood cells.

Iron is a key energy nutrient.

How it works: It transports oxygen in your blood and supports the production of thyroid hormone.

What else you need to know: If you are deficient, take 15 to 50 mg of iron bisglycinate (a gentle and highly absorbable form of iron) directly after food. Food sources of iron include red meat, eggs, lentils, and leafy green vegetables.

PMS with Sugar Cravings

Premenstrual cravings are so common they've become a kind of joke in popular culture. And yet, like all things premenstrual, you do not have to put up with them.

The first thing to understand is that it's *normal* to be hungrier before your period. It happens because both estrogen and serotonin drop away and they were your natural appetite suppressants. So, you're left with relatively more progesterone, which is an appetite stimulant. Progesterone's appetite-enhancing effect is nothing to worry about because progesterone also increases your metabolic rate, so you burn more calories.

If you're hungrier during your premenstrual time, then please *eat more*. It's fine and normal. Have that second serving of your meal if you need it. Snack on satisfying high-calorie foods like nuts or boiled eggs. But *please avoid sugar,* because sugar is inflammatory and that will only worsen your PMS.

Here are a few tricks to get rid of sugar cravings.

Get enough sleep

Sleep normalizes appetite, and so adequate sleep is one of the single best ways to prevent premenstrual sugar cravings.

Eat protein

Protein promotes satiety. In other words, protein makes you feel full, which will make you far less likely to crave sugar.

Quit sugar

As we saw in the Sugar section of Chapter 7, sugar can be addictive. Yes, you crave it more intensely during PMS, but if you crave it all the time, then your sugar cravings are only a *premenstrual magnification* of a bigger problem.

It's time to break up with sugar. I assure you: You cannot just "cut back." Quitting all dessert type foods is the only way to permanently escape your cravings.

The best supplements to relieve sugar cravings are the core PMS supplements of magnesium plus vitamin B6. Together, they calm your nervous system, reduce inflammation, and improve insulin resistance.

Other helpful supplements for sugar cravings include SAMe and St John's wort.

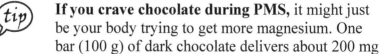 **If you crave chocolate during PMS,** it might just be your body trying to get more magnesium. One bar (100 g) of dark chocolate delivers about 200 mg of magnesium. Supplementing magnesium is an easy way to relieve chocolate cravings.

Occasional PMS Is a Useful Part of Your Monthly Report Card

With the help of the treatments we've just discussed, your PMS should improve rapidly, and you can expect months of little or no symptoms. Every once in a while, your PMS will return. It's not because the treatments have stopped working. It's because something has changed with *you*.

For example, you may have encountered some work stress. Or overseas travel. Perhaps you suffered an infection and had to take antibiotics. Or perhaps desserts crept back into your diet.

Any and all of those things can bring back your old PMS.

Remember, your period is your monthly report card. Your premenstrual time is an exquisitely sensitive part of that report card. It reports on things that have happened that month. Maybe those 50 hours of work per week were just too much for you. Maybe you need to quit sugar again.

You can thank your PMS for telling you so.

Chapter 9

Easy Flow: No More Pain and Suffering

We've talked about irregular periods, and also the difficult premenstrual build-up to periods. We now come to the all-important bleed itself.

Let's review what is normal. Your menstrual fluid should be mostly liquid, with no large clots. It should be bright red. Your period should not be painful.

You should lose anywhere from 25 to 80 mL over all the days of your period. That allows for a significant amount of variation. For example, it's normal to have a scanty little bleed that lasts only two days. It's normal to have a longer, heavier bleed that goes on for seven days. As we saw in Chapter 5, the average blood loss is 50 mL, which equates to ten fully soaked regular tampons or five fully soaked super-tampons over all the days of your period. Remember, one soaked regular pad or tampon holds 5 mL. A half-soaked tampon holds 2.5 mL, and a fully soaked super-tampon holds 10 mL.

Heavy Periods

Heavy menstrual bleeding affects about 25 percent of women. The medical term is *menorrhagia* (meaning "menstrual burst") and is defined as blood loss of greater than 80 mL, or lasting longer than seven days. To visualize this, 80 mL equates to sixteen fully soaked regular tampons, or eight fully soaked super-tampons over all the days of your period.

It's possible you lose far, far more than 80 mL. That kind of scary period is called *menstrual flooding* and can happen during perimenopause when you may lose more than 500 mL (two cups) in a single period.

Prolonged bleeding

If you flow for more than seven days, you almost certainly had an *anovulatory cycle.* That can occur with PCOS (Chapter 7) or perimenopause (Chapter 10). If you have PCOS, your strategy is to figure out your type of PCOS and treat it. See Chapter 7. You may also want to consider micronized or natural progesterone.

Get a Diagnosis

If you have not already done so, please see your doctor about your heavy periods. She will likely do a pelvic exam, as well as order blood tests and a pelvic ultrasound. She will probably find that your heavy periods are the result of a *hormone imbalance*, by which she means too much estrogen and not enough progesterone.

 Progesterone lightens periods.

Your doctor could also discover a *medical reason* for heavy menstrual bleeding. The two most common are coagulation disorders and thyroid disease. Let's look at each.

Coagulation disorders

A coagulation disorder is an impairment of your body's ability to clot blood. It can happen for different reasons, the most common being that you have a genetic variant of one of the many clotting factors. You've probably heard of the coagulation disorder *hemophilia*, but there are several others including the common *von Willebrand disease.*

If you've suffered heavy periods all your life, please ask your doctor to test you for von Willebrand disease. The condition accounts for at least 20 percent of all cases of heavy menstrual bleeding,[277] which is sometimes the only symptom.

Your doctor can rule out a coagulation disorder with a simple screening blood test. If you test positive, she will then refer you to a hematologist or blood specialist.

Thyroid disease

Underactive thyroid or hypothyroidism is a common cause of heavy menstrual bleeding and has been recognized as such since 1840. Oddly, your doctor may not consider it. According to Dr Andrew Weeks, a senior doctor writing in the BMJ: "Hypothyroidism may be greatly underdiagnosed as a cause of menorrhagia...and all women with unexplained menorrhagia should be tested for thyroid."[278]

How does hypothyroidism cause heavy periods? For one thing, it deprives your ovarian follicles of the thyroid hormone they need to ovulate and make progesterone. And remember, progesterone is your "period-lightening" hormone.

Hypothyroidism also decreases coagulation factors,[279] which impairs your ability to clot blood. And finally, hypothyroidism increases your exposure to estrogen by slowing estrogen metabolism and reducing the "estrogen-binding protein" SHBG.

If you have thyroid disease, then thyroid hormone is the best treatment for your heavy menstrual bleeding. Read more in the Thyroid Disease section in Chapter 11.

Other medical reasons for heavy periods

Other medical reasons for heavy menstrual bleeding include liver disease, pelvic infection, miscarriage, uterine polyps, fibroids, copper IUD, adenomyosis, and endometriosis. Of these possibilities, adenomyosis and endometriosis are the most common. We'll discuss those two important conditions later in this chapter.

When Are You Most at Risk?

You can suffer heavy menstrual bleeding at any age, but you're most at risk when you're a teenager and again when you're in your forties (perimenopause). This section is about heavy periods in your teens, twenties, and thirties. If you're in your forties, please first read this section and then go on to the Heavy Menstrual Bleeding of Perimenopause section in Chapter 10.

The heavy periods of teenagers

Why might you suffer heavy periods as a teen? Two reasons.

- Your estrogen receptors are still getting used to estrogen, so they react more strongly. That estrogen sensitivity will persist for a year or two while you form your "hormonal river system," described in Chapter 1.
- You don't yet make enough progesterone because you don't yet ovulate regularly.

With time, your estrogen receptors will adjust to estrogen and become less sensitive. You will also start to ovulate and make progesterone—so your periods should lighten.

If you're a teenager, your heavy periods are probably a temporary thing. You don't need the pill. Instead, you can use natural treatments such as iron, turmeric, and a dairy-free diet, as we'll see below. While you're waiting for the natural treatments to take effect, you can manage the flow with ibuprofen.

Conventional Treatment of Heavy Periods

Ibuprofen

The conventional anti-inflammatory medication ibuprofen (Advil® or Nurofen®) reduces menstrual flow *by half*.[280] It works by lowering the prostaglandins that contribute to heavy flow. Take 200 mg every six hours during your first one or two days of bleeding.

Ibuprofen is a simple and practical solution for heavy bleeding. Yes, it's a pharmaceutical drug, but you take it for only a couple of days per month. In my view, it's a far better option than hormonal birth control.

Hormonal birth control

Hormonal birth control is the standard prescription for heavy periods, but for reasons I explained in Chapter 2, it's not a great solution.

Mirena® IUD

Mirena® is a better option than other types of hormonal birth control. It delivers a smaller dose of progestin than the pill and so does not completely suppress ovulation. Plus Mirena® reduces flow by *90 percent*, thereby offering great relief for heavy periods. Unfortunately, once you remove Mirena®, your heavy bleeding will return.

Of course, I hope the natural treatments will work for you, so that you won't need a hormonal IUD. If you're stuck and *have to* choose a conventional treatment such as the pill or Mirena®, I recommend Mirena®.

Diet and Lifestyle to Prevent Heavy Periods

Natural treatments work to *prevent* heavy periods. They cannot stop a heavy period once it's underway.

Avoid cow's dairy

My clinical observation is that dairy makes periods heavier. That's consistent with a recent research finding that dairy may alter hormones and impair ovulation.[281]

Avoiding dairy is a safe and simple solution to try for a few months. And remember, you can still have goat and sheep milk products.

A dairy-free diet can work particularly well for the heavy periods of teenagers.

Keep insulin low

Insulin is a growth hormone and thickens your uterine lining. And as we saw in Chapter 7, too much insulin can impair ovulation and cause progesterone deficiency. You're more at risk for heavy periods if you have insulin resistance and insulin-resistant PCOS. For treatment ideas, refer to the insulin resistance sections in Chapters 7 and 11.

Exercise

Exercise improves insulin sensitivity, reduces inflammation, and promotes the healthy removal of estrogen through perspiration.

Maintain healthy gut bacteria

Healthy gut bacteria escort estrogen safely out of your body. Unhealthy gut bacteria do the opposite. They impair estrogen metabolism and cause estrogen to be reabsorbed into your body. One of the best ways to maintain a healthy microbiome is to avoid as much as possible drugs such as antibiotics that damage gut bacteria.

Eat phytoestrogens

Phytoestrogens are found in plant food such as nuts, legumes, and flax seeds. They reduce your exposure to estrogen by blocking estrogen receptors and promoting the healthy metabolism of estrogen.

Supplements and Herbal Medicines to Prevent Heavy Periods

Iron is a critical nutrient for heavy periods.

How it works: Iron corrects the iron deficiency caused by your heavy periods, but it can also lighten your period. That's because iron deficiency is both a cause and effect of heavy periods.[282]

What else you need to know: Ask your doctor to test serum ferritin (see the Iron Testing section in Chapter 8). If you're deficient, take 15 to 50 mg of a gentle and absorbable form of iron called iron bisglycinate. The best food sources of iron are animal products including red meat and eggs.

 Can't get your iron up? It could be because you're consuming too much dairy. Dairy inhibits the absorption of iron.

Turmeric is the yellow spice commonly used in Indian curries. It contains the active ingredient *curcumin*. Both turmeric and curcumin are available in the form of a concentrated capsule.

How it works: It reduces inflammation and prostaglandins, thereby reducing menstrual flow in a way similar to ibuprofen. Turmeric also lowers estrogen by blocking an enzyme called aromatase.

What else you need to know: Unlike ibuprofen (which you take only during your period), you take turmeric every day of your cycle and then increase the dose during your period. It can also relieve period pain.

Take turmeric after a meal for better absorption. The exact quantity depends on the concentration of the formula, so please take as directed on the bottle. Turmeric is generally safe and non-toxic even at high dose. That makes it an excellent treatment choice for teenagers. The only precaution is that it can interact with anticoagulant medication.

Other supplements for heavy periods include calcium-d-glucarate and micronized progesterone. We'll discuss those treatments in Chapter 10.

Checklist for heavy periods

- Rule out a medical cause such as thyroid disease.
- Consider taking ibuprofen on your heavy days.
- Avoid cow's dairy.
- Consider taking iron and turmeric.
- If you're over 40, then also refer to the section on heavy periods in Chapter 10.

Light Periods

You can lose as little as 25 mL of menstrual fluid, and that is still normal. This equates to five fully soaked regular tampons, spread over all the days of your period.

If you see less than 25 mL of menstrual fluid, then ask yourself: is it a true period or is it an anovulatory bleed?

Remember, a true period is one that follows a follicular phase, ovulation, and a luteal phase. An anovulatory bleed is one that follows a cycle in which you did not ovulate. It's not a real period and is better described as breakthrough bleeding.

If you're having anovulatory cycles, then your best strategy is to find a way to ovulate. Please see Chapter 7 for guidance.

If you're certain you *do* ovulate, then your next question is: is it a true period or is it another type of bleeding like mid-cycle spotting?

That's what happened to my patient Sam.

Sam: A short light cycle

Sam was pretty worried about what she described as very light periods coming every two to three weeks.

"Do you know if you ovulate?" I asked.

With a two-week cycle, Sam was either not ovulating, or seeing mid-cycle spotting and mistaking it for a period.

Sam had no idea if or when she ovulated, so I asked her to track her fertile mucus and temperatures for a couple of months. (See the Physical Signs of Ovulation section in Chapter 3.)

We were happy to discover that Sam did ovulate. When she knew what to look for, Sam noticed fertile mucus just before her first "period," which was really just half a day of light ovulation bleeding. After that, her temperatures went up for an eleven-day luteal phase and then dropped for her real period of two more days of light bleeding.

"The first bleed is ovulation," I said. "The second bleed after your temperature drop is your period. Count the first day of that bleed as your 'day 1.'"

Counting properly from "day 1" to "day 1" Sam had about a 37-day cycle. Yes, her period was light, but that was because she was vegetarian and ate a lot of phytoestrogens in beans and grains.

"The phytoestrogens in your diet are blocking estrogen and making your period lighter," I explained. "I'm not worried about the light period, but I'm concerned your cycle is a little long at 37 days. It would be nice to get you to ovulate earlier in your follicular phase. One way is to cut back the phytoestrogens. The other is to look at supplementing zinc and iodine—two nutrients that are essential for ovulation and are probably deficient with your vegetarian diet."

I ordered a blood test for zinc, which came back low, so I prescribed my "ovulation cocktail for vegetarians," which is

30 mg zinc plus 200 mcg iodine.

Sam also diversified her protein to include eggs and goat cheese, which do not contain phytoestrogens.

A few months later, Sam's cycle shortened to 32 days, and she stopped seeing the mid-cycle spotting.

A light period is a sign of *lower than average* estrogen, but as long as you ovulate, you probably do not need treatment. You have enough estrogen, or you could not reach ovulation. You just don't have as much estrogen as other women. In other words, your estrogen is *relatively* low. It's not truly low—like it would be if you did not ovulate, or if you were in menopause.

The relatively low estrogen of ovulatory cycles generally does not require treatment.

Checklist for light periods
- Are they real periods or anovulatory cycles?
- If they're anovulatory cycles, then find a way to ovulate. Refer to Chapter 7 for strategies.

Uterine Fibroids

If your doctor ordered a pelvic ultrasound to investigate heavy menstrual bleeding or pain, she might have discovered a fibroid or fibroids. What does that mean?

A uterine fibroid (also called leiomyoma or myoma) is a benign growth of your uterine muscle. Fibroids are common after age 35, and most of us have at least one or two small fibroids. In the majority of cases, they don't cause symptoms and may simply be an *incidental finding* that does not require treatment.

Fibroids and heavy bleeding often occur together because both conditions are caused by estrogen excess. But fibroids themselves are rarely the *cause* of heavy bleeding because most fibroids are located inside the muscle or on the outside of the uterus where they do not affect flow. Only ten percent of fibroids grow into the uterine cavity where they can cause heavy bleeding.[283]

Fibroids can, however, cause other symptoms, such as pain or other pelvic discomfort, and frequent urination because of your uterus pressing on your bladder.

Risk factors for uterine fibroids include anything that increases your lifetime exposure to estrogen. For example, taking the pill at a young age increases your risk of fibroids.[284] So does chronic alcohol use because it increases estrogen. Finally, exposure to endocrine disrupting chemicals increases the likelihood that you'll eventually be diagnosed with a fibroid.[285]

Fibroids grow slowly over many years and tend to run in families, which means they also have a genetic component.[286]

 Fibroids are easier to prevent than they are to treat.

Conventional Treatment of Uterine Fibroids

Unless it's particularly large or growing inside your uterus, a fibroid usually does not require medical treatment. The standard medical approach is to watch and wait. Fibroids will naturally reduce in size with menopause.

If your fibroids do require treatment, then you will be offered a procedure such as a hysterectomy, myomectomy, or uterine artery embolization.

Myomectomy

Myomectomy is the surgical removal of the fibroid but leaving the uterus.

Myomectomy carries a risk of bleeding, which is why some doctors are reluctant to attempt it. The bleeding risk depends on the size and location of your fibroid. Fibroids on the outside of the uterus are easier to remove.

Uterine artery embolization

Uterine artery embolization is a non-surgical treatment option for fibroids. It's done under local anesthetic in an outpatient setting. Guided by an X-ray image, a radiologist inserts a catheter into your leg and injects small beads or particles into your uterine artery to block the fibroid's blood supply. With time, the fibroid will then shrink.

Uterine artery embolization carries a small risk of infection and pain. It is a safer procedure than hysterectomy or myomectomy.

Diet and Lifestyle for Uterine Fibroids

Natural treatment *cannot* substantially shrink fibroids, but it can prevent further growth. That may be enough to get you through to menopause when your fibroids will naturally shrink anyway.

Reduce alcohol

Alcohol impairs your liver's ability to metabolize or detoxify estrogen. There's a strong association between alcohol consumption and fibroids.[287]

Maintain healthy gut bacteria

As discussed in the heavy period section, healthy gut bacteria escort estrogen safely out of your body.

Maintain a healthy body weight

Maintain a healthy body weight, because body fat makes a type of estrogen called estrone.

Avoid endocrine disrupting chemicals

Endocrine disrupting chemicals such as plastics and pesticides impair your ability to metabolize estrogen. They can also hyperstimulate your estrogen receptors. See the Environmental Toxins section in Chapter 11.

Supplements and Herbal Medicines for Uterine Fibroids

Iodine may help to slow the growth of fibroids.

How it works: It downregulates estrogen receptors, thereby reducing estrogen stimulation.

What else you need to know: Iodine can harm your thyroid gland. Do not exceed 500 mcg (0.5 mg) daily except under professional advice. See the Iodine section in Chapter 6.

Calcium d-glucarate assists with the healthy metabolism or detoxification of estrogen.

How it works: Glucarate assists with estrogen detoxification in two ways. First, it binds to estrogen in the liver and deactivates it. Second, it inhibits *beta-glucuronidase*, which is the enzyme made by gut bacteria that causes estrogen to be reabsorbed.

What else you need to know: Take 1000 to 1500 mg per day. It may also help to prevent breast cancer.[288]

Cinnamon and hoelen combination is a traditional Chinese herbal medicine that contains *Peonia lactiflora, Cinnamomum cassia*, and other herbs. Regular use has been shown to prevent fibroid growth.[289]

I like Cinnamon and hoelen combination, but I prefer to start with less expensive lifestyle changes, low-dose iodine, and calcium-d-glucarate.

Checklist for fibroids

- Keep estrogen low by reducing alcohol and maintaining healthy gut bacteria.
- Consider taking calcium d-glucarate and low-dose iodine.
- Know that fibroids naturally shrink with menopause.

Adenomyosis

Adenomyosis is a different kind of abnormal growth in your uterine wall. It's similar to uterine fibroids, and until recently, was often mistaken for fibroids.

According to Professor Edward Lyons of the University of Manitoba, adenomyosis is under-diagnosed. He says that the majority of women with lumpy or enlarged uteruses have adenomyosis—not fibroids.[290]

Please seek an accurate diagnosis. The treatment of adenomyosis is different from the treatment of fibroids.

With adenomyosis, the uterine growths are not muscle like they are with fibroids. Instead, they are bits of uterine lining that have grown into the uterine muscle. It is similar to another condition called endometriosis, which we'll come to next.

Symptoms of adenomyosis include abdominal distension, pelvic pain, and very heavy periods. Adenomyosis is more common after 35, but it can occur at any age. Diagnosis is by pelvic ultrasound or MRI.

Conventional Treatment of Adenomyosis

Conventional treatment is hysterectomy, oral contraceptives, or the Mirena® IUD.

The hormonal IUD reduces blood flow by 90 percent, which can be pretty helpful for a condition like adenomyosis. I sometimes recommend that my patients with severe adenomyosis resort to an IUD.

Myomectomy or uterine artery embolization can be attempted for adenomyosis but carries a higher risk of complications compared with uterine fibroids. Many women who undergo embolization ultimately end up requiring a hysterectomy anyway.[291]

Like fibroids, adenomyosis will shrink somewhat with menopause.

238 — Period Repair Manual

Diet and Lifestyle for Adenomyosis

The natural approach to adenomyosis is a combination of the treatment of endometriosis (discussed below) and the treatment of the very heavy periods of perimenopause (discussed in Chapter 10). Please read those sections for additional treatment ideas.

Natural treatment can help the condition, but it cannot cure it.

Avoid cow's dairy

Dairy makes periods heavier and may also worsen the underlying inflammation or immune dysfunction that drives both adenomyosis and endometriosis.

Consider avoiding gluten

Like dairy, gluten worsens the immune dysfunction that lies at the heart of both adenomyosis and endometriosis.

Reduce alcohol

Alcohol impairs your liver's ability to metabolize or detoxify estrogen.

Maintain healthy gut bacteria

As discussed earlier in the chapter, healthy gut bacteria escort estrogen safely out of your body.

Supplements and Herbal Medicines for Adenomyosis

Turmeric lightens periods and reduces estrogen, pain, and inflammation. For dosing instructions, refer to the Heavy Period section earlier in this chapter.

Zinc is helpful for adenomyosis and endometriosis and period pain. It reduces both pain and inflammation.[292] I recommend 30 mg per day taken after dinner. Do not take zinc on an empty stomach or it may cause nausea.

Cinnamon and hoelen combination is helpful for adenomyosis as well as fibroids (see above).

Micronized progesterone or **natural progesterone** makes periods lighter. It's as effective as a synthetic progestin, but without the side effects. Please see the Heavy Period section in the next chapter.

How it works: It thins the uterine lining and reduces inflammation.

What else you need to know: A progesterone capsule works better than a topical cream for adenomyosis. See Chapter 10.

Checklist for adenomyosis

* Avoid cow's dairy.
* Consider taking turmeric, zinc, and micronized progesterone.
* Refer to the sections about endometriosis and the heavy periods of perimenopause.

Endometriosis

Endometriosis is a common condition that affects at least one in ten women. Its main symptom is *pain*, which can be severe. Remember from the Period Pain section in Chapter 5 that there's a big difference between *normal* period pain and the *severe* period pain of endometriosis or adenomyosis.

Normal period pain is a bit of cramping in your pelvis or lower back. It occurs just before or during your period. It improves with ibuprofen, and does not interfere with your daily activities. We'll discuss natural treatment for normal period pain later in the chapter.

Severe period pain is throbbing, burning, searing, or stabbing pain that lasts for many days and can occur between periods. It doesn't improve with ibuprofen, and can be so bad you vomit or miss work.

Endometriosis pain can occur in your uterus during your period. Or it can occur in other *places* such as your rectum, bladder, legs, or throughout your pelvis. Or it can occur at other *times* such as ovulation and during sex. With endometriosis, you could have pain *all the time*, or, oddly, you could have no pain at all.

Other symptoms of endometriosis:

- bladder problems such as urgency, frequency, and painful voiding
- bowel problems such as diarrhea and constipation
- abdominal bloating
- nausea and vomiting
- headaches
- fatigue
- low-grade fever
- bleeding between periods
- infertility and recurrent miscarriage.

As you can see, endometriosis is not just a period problem. It is a *whole body inflammatory disease*, and your doctor may have missed it. Endometriosis typically takes up to ten years to diagnose.

 One review concluded that 70 percent of teens reporting chronic pelvic pain will eventually go on to be diagnosed with endometriosis.[293]

What Is Endometriosis?

Endometriosis is a condition in which bits of tissue that are *similar to the endometrium* (uterine lining) grow in places other than inside your uterus. The bits of tissue are called *endometriosis lesions* and can occur anywhere in the body, including the bowel and bladder. The most common sites for endometriosis are around the uterus and ovaries and on the Fallopian tubes. When endometriosis occurs on the ovaries, the lesion is called an *endometrioma* or chocolate cyst.

Researchers don't yet know what causes endometriosis. The most widely accepted theory is *retrograde menstruation,* which means that menstrual fluid flowed back through your Fallopian tubes and entered your pelvic cavity. This old theory is falling out of favor because retrograde menstruation occurs in most women, yet only ten percent develop endometriosis. Instead, some researchers think that endometrial tissue is laid down before birth and lies dormant until it's activated by hormones at puberty.

Whatever the origin of the endometriosis lesions, your immune system plays a big part in what happens next. It produces inflammatory cytokines and other immune factors that inflame the endometriosis lesions and promote their growth.

The growing consensus is that endometriosis is caused by *immune dysfunction.*[294] For example, endometriosis shares many features with other immune diseases such as lupus and rheumatoid arthritis, including *angiogenesis*, which is the ability of the lesions to establish a blood supply.[295]

There is also a strong genetic component to endometriosis. If you have a sister or mother with the disease, then you are more likely to develop it yourself.[296]

Finally, endometriosis has been linked to dioxin exposure in the womb,[297] which means you may have been predisposed to the disease before you were even born. On the one hand, that's frustrating because the cause was out of your control. On the other hand, it means you did not cause the disease by something you did or something you ate. Endometriosis is *not* a lifestyle disease.

Other endocrine disrupting chemicals may play a role in endometriosis.[298] We'll talk more about environmental toxins in the Environmental Toxins section in Chapter 11.

The link with digestive problems

Endometriosis and digestive problems go hand in hand. For one thing, endometriosis lesions and adhesions can occur on the bowel and directly cause digestive problems. Up to 90 percent of women with endometriosis also experience bowel symptoms.[299]

adhesions

Adhesions are bands of connective tissue or scar tissue that bind together pelvic structures and cause pain. They are the result of both the disease process of endometriosis and the surgery used to treat it.

So, endometriosis can cause digestive symptoms but, at the same time, digestive problems can worsen endometriosis. Why? Because digestive problems can affect the immune system and endometriosis is primarily a disease of immune dysfunction.

As we saw in Chapter 6, your digestion and your immune system are, in a sense, one continuous entity. Anything that upsets your digestion will upset your immune system and cause it to make more inflammatory cytokines. One example is the presence of too many of the wrong kind of bacteria in your digestion. They produce a toxin called LPS (lipopolysaccharide) which promotes both inflammatory disease[300] and endometriosis.[301][302]

> **Endometriosis can also be promoted** by LPS-producing bacteria in the uterine lining and pelvic cavity.[303]

Digestive problems can also lead to intestinal permeability which we discussed in Chapter 6. It occurs when the intestinal wall becomes too permeable and permits bacterial toxins and other proteins to enter your body and activate your immune system. Intestinal permeability can worsen inflammatory disease, and I argue that it plays a role in endometriosis. We'll discuss Intestinal Permeability in more detail in Chapter 11.

Since digestion plays a role in promoting endometriosis, fixing digestion can go a long way to relieving endometriosis, as we'll see.

The role of estrogen and progesterone

Endometriosis is fundamentally an inflammatory disease—not a hormonal condition. That said, hormones do play a role.

Estrogen strongly stimulates the growth of endometriosis lesions, which is why the current conventional approach is to shut down estrogen. Shutting down estrogen has a lot of side effects, so hopefully, that approach will change as researchers discover new anti-inflammatory and immune-modulating treatments.

 Estrogen worsens endometriosis, but it does not cause endometriosis.

Both progesterone and progestins slow the growth of endometriosis lesions.

Diagnosis of Endometriosis

Currently, the only way to diagnose endometriosis is with laparoscopic (keyhole) surgery, which seems terribly outdated.

A pelvic ultrasound cannot usually detect endometriosis lesions, but it can sometimes detect endometriomas and a more severe form of endometriosis called *deep infiltrating endometriosis.*[304]

 Endometriosis cannot be ruled out by ultrasound.

The search is underway for a simple test that would use a *biomarker* found in blood, saliva, urine, menstrual blood, or the uterine lining.[305] A biomarker is a measurable indicator such as a protein or immune component. Once developed, it will mean that endometriosis can be diagnosed by a simple non-invasive test.[306] [307]

Before we move into the treatment section, it's important to make something clear. Endometriosis is a serious disease and there is currently no cure. Both conventional and natural treatments can relieve symptoms of endometriosis, but they cannot cure it.

Conventional Treatment of Endometriosis

Surgery

As well as being the standard diagnostic technique for endometriosis, surgery is currently the primary conventional treatment. Surgery does not cure endometriosis, but it does relieve pain and improve fertility. Furthermore, it reduces inflammatory cytokines in the pelvis, which makes endometriosis easier to treat with both conventional and natural treatments.

The procedure is laparoscopic or keyhole surgery to physically remove the endometriosis lesions. The success of the surgery depends on the skill and training of the surgeon and whether she manages to remove all of the lesions. A type of surgery called *excision surgery* is more successful in the long-term[308] and may come close to a cure for some women.

If you are contemplating surgery, please seek a surgeon who understands endometriosis and does excision surgery. I like how endometriosis expert Dr Iris Orbuch explains it: "Endometriosis shouldn't be the path of fifteen surgeries. It should be one surgery done right."[309]

There are downsides to surgery. The first, of course, is that it is surgery and requires general anesthetic and recovery. Another potential downside is that, like the disease itself, surgery can cause *adhesions* or scar tissue, which then cause pain. Finally, surgery does not cure endometriosis, although it can come close for some women. The rate of recurrence following surgery is 21 percent after two years and 40-50 percent after five years.[310] Recurrence can lead to more surgeries. The medical solution is to give hormone-suppressing drugs to try to prevent that.

I *do* recommend surgery for some of my patients. See Hannah's story later in this chapter.

Medical treatment

The drugs that suppress estrogen include the contraceptive pill, Depo-Provera®, Lupron®, and Danazol®. They have many side effects including depression and osteoporosis.

Another medical approach is to give a low dose progestin such as dienogest in the Visanne® pill or levonorgestrel in the Mirena® IUD. Low dose progestins drugs are gentler because they do not suppress ovulation or estrogen. Instead, they work by directly suppressing the growth of endometriosis lesions. I think these are *reasonable* solutions, but, in my experience, natural progesterone capsules work just as well—if not better—with fewer side effects. See Hannah's story.

Researchers are also actively looking for new *non-hormonal* treatments for endometriosis including the following:[311]

- angiogenesis inhibitors (drugs that inhibit *angiogenesis* or the growth of new blood vessels)
- anti-inflammatories (drugs that reduce inflammation)
- immunomodulators (drugs that alter the activity of the immune system).

A new non-hormonal treatment option would indeed be a welcome development!

In the meantime, there are many *natural* anti-inflammatory and immune-modulating treatments.

Diet and Lifestyle for Endometriosis

Diet is the most important part of natural treatment for endometriosis. It works by reducing inflammatory cytokines as explained in Chapter 6.

Avoid cow's dairy (A1 dairy)

Your first step is to avoid cow's dairy. My clinical observation is that stopping cow's dairy is effective for almost all patients. It's not a cure, but it can significantly reduce pain and inflammation. As I've described in other sections of the book, you can probably still have goat and sheep milk products.

Consider avoiding gluten

You may also want to try avoiding gluten. One study found that endometriosis improves after twelve months on a gluten-free diet.[312] As an endometriosis sufferer, you may be among the one in ten who have a major issue with gluten (see Chapter 6).

Consider avoiding eggs

Finally, you may want to try avoiding eggs, which are a common food sensitivity and therefore an inflammatory food for some of you. I estimate that egg sensitivity is a factor for about one in three of my endometriosis patients.

Until recently, few researchers had looked at dietary interventions for endometriosis. Then in 2017, a New Zealand clinical trial found that endometriosis symptoms improve on the low-FODMAP diet typically prescribed for irritable bowel syndrome.[313] (FODMAPs, as we saw in Chapter 6, are "fermentable carbohydrates" such as those found in wheat, legumes, and some types of dairy.) Such a study is a good first step and supports the idea that fixing digestion can help to reduce the inflammation of endometriosis.

And just a word about the low-FODMAP diet. It can be very helpful in the short term, but I do not recommend it in the long term because it can rob you of valuable dietary fiber. Instead, I recommend you identify and treat a condition called *small intestinal bacterial overgrowth* (SIBO), which I'll describe in the Digestive Health section in Chapter 11. You should then be able to tolerate FODMAPs, although you probably still want to avoid wheat and dairy.

Supplements and Herbal Medicines for Endometriosis

The best supplements for endometriosis are those that normalize immune function and reduce inflammation.

Turmeric reduces the size and activity of endometriosis lesions.[314] I prescribe turmeric capsules for almost all my endometriosis patients.

> **How it works:** Turmeric or curcumin works by several potential mechanisms.
>
> - It downregulates a proinflammatory transcription factor called NF-κappa B and accelerating healthy cell death or apoptosis in the lesions.[315]
> - It suppresses the local production of estrogen in endometriosis lesions.[316]
> - It inhibits angiogenesis or the growth of new blood vessels.[317]
>
> **What else you need to know:** If your endometriosis symptoms are severe, you will need a fairly high dose of turmeric. Take one or more high-dose capsules after every meal.

Zinc is a powerful immune-regulator and anti-inflammatory and researchers have proposed that zinc deficiency plays a role in the development of endometriosis.[318]

> **How it works:** It repairs intestinal permeability,[319] thereby improving immune function. Furthermore, it is anti-inflammatory[320] and reduces pain.[321] I recommend taking at least 30 mg per day directly after a large meal.

 You should not need a large number of supplements. Start with a dairy-free diet, turmeric, and zinc. And only then consider additional supplements.

Berberine is another anti-inflammatory herbal medicine that is currently being investigated as a treatment for immune dysfunction and inflammatory disease.[322] It has not yet been trialed for endometriosis, but I've included it here because I've seen good results with my patients.

How it works: It reduces inflammation by sheltering the immune system from the bacterial toxin LPS,[323] repairing intestinal permeability,[324] and downregulating pro-inflammatory genes.[325]

What else you need to know: There are a few precautions with berberine, including interactions with several medications. For safe use, refer to the Berberine section in Chapter 7. If in doubt, speak to your doctor.

Resveratrol is a phytonutrient found in grapes, berries, and other fruit. It's shown promise as treatment for endometriosis and was featured in a recent survey of new and upcoming pharmacological treatments for the disease.[326]

How it works: It reduces inflammatory cytokines and inhibits angiogenesis.[327] Resveratrol also downregulates aromatase, which is the enzyme that makes estrogen.[328]

What else you need to know: I normally recommend 100 to 400 mg per day with food. It is safe for long-term use.

N-acetyl cysteine (NAC) is an amino acid. It did well in a recent clinical trial for endometriosis. Of the 47 women in the NAC treatment group, 24 canceled their scheduled laparoscopy due to a disappearance of endometrioma cysts, a reduction in pain, or pregnancy.[329]

How it works: NAC is the precursor to glutathione which is the body's primary antioxidant and *immune regulator*. It reduces inflammation.

What else you need to know: NAC has the nice side benefit of reducing anxiety. Too much NAC can thin your stomach lining, so do not take if you have gastritis or stomach ulcers. I recommend 500 to 2000 mg per day.

Selenium is anti-inflammatory and having sufficient selenium has been correlated with a reduced risk of endometriosis.[330]

How it works: Selenium modulates and normalizes immune function. It is also essential for the production of progesterone.

What else you need to know: The therapeutic dose is 100 to 150 mcg per day. Higher amounts can be toxic, so do not exceed 200 mcg per day from all sources, including high-selenium foods such as brazil nuts.

Micronized progesterone or natural progesterone is another good treatment option for endometriosis.

How it works: Progesterone inhibits the growth of endometriosis lesions.[331]

What else you need to know: I have recently had the opportunity to see how much progesterone capsules have helped some of my endometriosis patients. It truly is a viable alternative to conventional progestin drugs such as Visanne® (dienogest). For more information, see the Natural Progesterone section in Chapter 10.

Your long-term outcome with endometriosis depends on many things including:

- location and severity of the endometriosis lesions
- effectiveness of the surgery
- presence of adhesions
- coexisting conditions such as adenomyosis, interstitial cystitis, and pelvic floor dysfunction.

---

 interstitial cystitis

Interstitial cystitis is also called painful bladder syndrome. It is the constant sensation of pressure or pain in the bladder and pelvis.

---

tip **Physical treatments** such as physiotherapy can be helpful for adhesions, pain, and pelvic floor dysfunction.

There's no easy fix for endometriosis, but natural treatment can give you a fighting chance.

Hannah: Second surgery for endometriosis

Hannah had always had painful periods, but she had her first real endometriosis attack when she was 23. The pain, nausea, and diarrhea were severe enough for her to go to the hospital where she was told she might have an ovarian cyst and was given antibiotics. Endometriosis was not mentioned by the doctors at that time.

Hannah then suffered two years of ongoing chronic abdominal pain and bloating and was diagnosed with irritable bowel syndrome (IBS). She tried various natural treatments including stopping dairy and wheat, which seemed to help.

When Hannah was 25, she had her second severe attack which turned out to be a burst endometrioma or chocolate cyst. She underwent emergency surgery during which extensive endometriosis was discovered and some of it was removed. She was prescribed the progestin drug Visanne® to try to prevent recurrence.

By the time I met Hannah at 27, she was not doing well. She had anxiety and yeast infections from the Visanne®. And she was still in pain almost every day. She had pain when waking in the morning and so much pain with sex that she could not have intercourse with her fiancé.

"I don't even recognize myself anymore," she said.

Hannah had spoken to her family doctor who advised her to "wait until she was ready to have a baby" and then have a second surgery. The doctor's reasoning was that surgery improves fertility for six to twelve months and so Hannah should not "waste" surgery by having it too soon.

"But this kind of pain is unacceptable," I said. "You can't go on like this. I think you should at least consider having the second surgery soon, but this time have it done properly by a doctor who can take the time to remove all the lesions. And then we'll use natural treatment to prevent recurrence."

I gave Hannah the name of a gynecologist who does excision surgery. I also asked Hannah to speak to him about using Prometrium® micronized progesterone capsules instead of Visanne® because natural progesterone has fewer side effects.

At the same time, I encouraged Hannah to continue to strictly avoid dairy and gluten, which she was already doing. I also prescribed 30 mg of zinc and a concentrated turmeric liquid that delivered 340 mg curcumin per dose. Even before she had the surgery five weeks later, Hannah's pain had already improved by 20 percent.

Hannah underwent "excision surgery" with the new surgeon, and it took two hours to remove a large number of lesions. Her doctor also agreed to prescribe Prometrium®.

Hannah experienced some pain for the few weeks after the surgery, but then she started to improve. By the time she was three months post-surgery, the pain was on average about 60 percent better.

I expect Hannah to continue to improve over the coming years. If not, I will recommend some of the additional treatments mentioned above.

Checklist for endometriosis

- Seek a referral to a gynecologist.
- Consider having excision surgery.
- Strictly avoid cow's dairy and maybe gluten and eggs.
- Consider taking zinc, turmeric, and NAC.

Period Pain

This section is about *normal* period pain—not the severe pain of adenomyosis or endometriosis discussed above. Normal period pain is mild pain for a day or two when your period starts. It responds to painkillers and does not prevent you from attending school or work.

Normal period pain also responds well to natural treatment. Essentially, it should *disappear* with natural treatment. If it doesn't, then it's not normal period pain.

By "normal" period pain, I mean *common* period pain that is not caused by an underlying condition. I don't mean that period pain is *normal*. In keeping with the message throughout this book, I will say that you have the right to *easy, pain-free periods*.

What Causes Period Pain?

As your uterine lining starts to break down at the end of your cycle, it releases prostaglandins. They stimulate your uterine muscle to contract to help to shed the lining. Prostaglandins are a normal part of the process, but *too many* prostaglandins can cause pain. The treatment is to reduce prostaglandins.

Conventional Treatment of Period Pain

Ibuprofen

Ibuprofen (Advil® or Nurofen®) blocks prostaglandins and relieves period pain. I don't have a problem with my patients taking the occasional ibuprofen if that's what they need to do. In fact, earlier in this chapter, I recommended ibuprofen as a treatment for heavy periods.

That said, once you get started on natural treatment, you will probably find that you don't need ibuprofen.

Diet and Lifestyle for Period Pain

Avoid cow's dairy

My clinical observation is that avoiding cow's dairy can eliminate period pain. I first discovered it 25 years ago during my training as a naturopathic doctor. When I stopped having dairy, I stopped having period pain. Since then, I've seen the same result with thousands of patients.

As explained in the Dairy section in Chapter 6, you can still have goat and sheep milk products.

Identify and treat histamine intolerance

Histamine intolerance is another cause of period pain. Recall from Chapters 6 and 8, that histamine intolerance is the condition of having too much of the inflammatory compound histamine. Histamine intolerance can cause or worsen headaches, anxiety, insomnia, brain fog, hives, and nasal congestion. It can also cause or worsen period problems because it increases both inflammation and estrogen. PMS and period pain are the two period problems most associated with histamine intolerance.

Supplements and Herbal Medicines for Period Pain

Magnesium is your number one supplement for period pain.

How it works: It reduces prostaglandins[332] and relaxes the uterus.

What else you need to know: Magnesium is both prevention and acute care for period pain. You can take magnesium throughout the month to prevent the formation of too many prostaglandins. You can also take more magnesium during your period to relieve acute pain. I recommend 300 mg magnesium glycinate per day.

Zinc prevents period pain. It's an immune-modulating treatment for endometriosis, but it also helps with normal period pain. Zinc has performed well in a couple of clinical trials.[333][334]

How it works: It inhibits prostaglandins and inflammation. See previous sections for dosing instructions.

Turmeric was listed as treatment for heavy periods, adenomyosis, and endometriosis. And here it is again for period pain. You can see that I prescribe turmeric quite frequently for period problems.

How it works: It reduces prostaglandins.

What else you need to know: The exact quantity of the herb depends on the concentration of the formula, so please use as directed on the bottle. For best effect, take the minimum recommended dose every day throughout your cycle. And then, when you have your period, take up to the maximum recommended dose.

Fish oil has been found to reduce period pain by 30 percent after two months.[335]

How it works: Omega-3 fatty acids reduce prostaglandins and inflammation.

What else you need to know: The standard dose is 2000 mg per day. You may also want to reduce your intake of inflammatory omega-6 fatty acids, as discussed in Chapter 6.

 You don't need *all* the supplements. I usually start with a simple prescription of dairy-free diet and zinc.

Checklist for period pain
- Avoid cow's dairy.
- Identify and treat histamine intolerance.
- Consider taking magnesium and zinc, and possibly one of the other supplements listed above.

Bleeding Between Periods

Bleeding or spotting between periods can occur for lots of different reasons.

Ovulation spotting
Ovulation spotting is typically bright red and happens because your estrogen dips a little just before your LH surge and egg release. Ovulation spotting is normal and does not require

treatment.

Premenstrual spotting

Premenstrual spotting is a darker color. It can mean you do not have enough progesterone to hold your uterine lining. In that case, the solution is to support progesterone with all the treatments discussed earlier in this book. And as we saw in the Roadmap to Progesterone section in chapter 4, your progesterone in any given cycle is the result of the health of your corpus luteum, which is the result of the health of your ovarian follicles during all their 100-day journey to ovulation.

Premenstrual spotting can also be a sign of an underlying thyroid problem. Please first read the Thyroid Disease section in Chapter 11, and then speak to your doctor about having a thyroid test. If you do have underactive thyroid or hypothyroidism, then your best treatment may be to supplement thyroid hormone.

Finally, spotting can mean you're having anovulatory cycles, such as occur with PCOS. Your best solution is to re-establish regular ovulation as described in Chapter 7.

Other causes of spotting

There are other reasons to bleed between periods. They include pregnancy, infection, endometriosis, an IUD, ovarian cysts (discussed below), and uterine polyps as we saw with Theresa's story in Chapter 5. If spotting is a new symptom for you, or if you notice other changes such as heavy bleeding, clotting, or pain, then check with your doctor.

Ovarian Cysts

Your ovaries always have "cysts" or fluid-filled sacs of some shape or size. Most of the time, they are your growing ovarian follicles and corpus luteum.

Every month, those normal cysts grow, burst, and are reabsorbed. Occasionally, there is a glitch, and one of your follicles becomes abnormally large and fluid-filled, forming an abnormal ovarian cyst. If your doctor suspects an ovarian cyst, she may order a blood test and a pelvic ultrasound to figure out what type of cyst it is.

Functional ovarian cyst

The most common type of abnormal ovarian cyst is a functional cyst. It forms when your ovarian follicle does not successfully rupture and release its egg. Instead, the follicle continues to grow and swell. Most functional cysts reach about 2 cm, but some can grow to 10 cm (4 inches) or more.

When they're small, functional cysts are harmless and symptomless. You can have them and never even know until they're picked up as an incidental finding on an ultrasound. Small functional cysts will usually reabsorb and go away on their own. They do not require treatment.

When they're large,functional cysts can cause symptoms such as pelvic fullness, pain, nausea, and spotting between periods. Rarely, they can rupture or twist and cause severe pain, which would require immediate medical attention.

Some functional cysts are the result of thyroid disease or hypothyroidism.[336] If you have recurrent ovarian cysts, please ask your doctor to rule out a thyroid problem. If you do have underactive thyroid or hypothyroidism, then thyroid hormone can prevent the formation of future ovarian cysts.

Chocolate cyst

Chocolate cysts are endometriosis lesions. See the Endometriosis section earlier in the chapter.

Dermoid cyst

Dermoid cysts are solid, benign (usually) ovarian tumors. They are strange in that they can contain hair or even teeth. Treatment is usually surgical removal, although some doctors may decide to watch and wait.[337] Once removed, dermoid cysts rarely grow back.

As strange as they are, dermoid cysts are reasonably common. I've had several patients with dermoid cysts over the years.

Polycystic ovaries

The multiple small "cysts" of PCOS are not true cysts in that they are *not* abnormally large follicles. Instead, they are abnormally *small* follicles that are in a state of partial development. They do not require the treatment discussed in this section. Instead, see the PCOS section in Chapter 7.

Conventional Treatment of Ovarian Cysts

Watch and wait

For cysts smaller than 5 cm, the medical approach is to watch and wait. They will usually disappear on their own.

Surgery

Cysts larger than 5 cm *may* require surgical removal, but please seek a second opinion before going under the knife. According to endocrinologist Dr Jerilynn Prior, ovarian cysts are rarely the cause of severe pain and rarely require removal.

Hormonal birth control

Hormonal birth control suppresses ovulation, thereby preventing the formation of any kind of cyst, normal or otherwise. It can prevent the formation of functional cysts, but it cannot treat them once they have formed.[338] One study found that the Mirena® IUD causes ovarian cysts in 5 percent of users.[339]

Diet and Lifestyle to Prevent Ovarian Cysts

Natural treatments work to *prevent* ovarian cysts. They cannot shrink a large cyst once it exists.

Avoid cow's dairy

My clinical observation is that dairy makes women more prone to ovarian cysts. It may be that inflammation hyper-sensitizes the follicles to estrogen or it may relate again to the histamine intolerance that some women experience from cow's dairy. Histamine plays a signaling role in the ovary.[340]

Identify and treat histamine intolerance

We discussed histamine intolerance in a few places in the book, including the PMS chapter and the period pain section earlier in this chapter. If histamine intolerance also plays a role in ovarian cysts, then your best strategy is to identify and treat histamine intolerance. Refer to the Histamine Intolerance sections in Chapters 6 and 8.

Supplements and Herbal Medicines to Prevent Ovarian Cysts

Iodine may help to prevent ovarian cysts. That is my clinical observation, but unfortunately, there are no studies at this stage.

> **How it works:** As we've seen in previous sections, iodine can downregulate and stabilize estrogen receptors. That can potentially prevent hyperstimulation of the ovarian follicles by estrogen.

> **What else you need to know:** Too much iodine can harm your thyroid, so do not exceed 500 mcg (0.5 mg) except under professional advice.

Selenium is another consideration for ovarian cysts.

> **How it works:** It promotes healthy ovulation and aids with the formation of a corpus luteum. Selenium also makes it safer to take iodine.

> **What else you need to know:** The therapeutic dose is 100 to 150 mcg per day. Higher amounts can be toxic, so do not exceed 200 mcg per day from all sources, including high-selenium foods such as brazil nuts.

Checklist for ovarian cysts

- Consider avoiding cow's dairy and taking a low dose of iodine and selenium.

- Polycystic ovaries are something different. See Chapter 7

A Final Word About Painful or Difficult Periods

You have the right to easy, pain-free, symptomless periods. With the right treatment, you should be able to get there—or at least much closer than you are now.

If you experience heavy periods or normal period pain, then you should expect complete resolution of your symptoms within a few months.

If you have endometriosis or adenomyosis, it might not be so easy. As discussed, endometriosis is a serious, whole-body inflammatory disease. It requires serious treatment, which sometimes includes surgery. That said, endometriosis can respond very well to natural treatments.

If you have the heavy, flooding periods of perimenopause, you're facing an even tougher battle. Read the next chapter.

Chapter 10

WHAT HAPPENS IN YOUR FORTIES

I N YOUR THIRTIES OR FORTIES? You may be experiencing symptoms you did not expect to see until your fifties: hot flashes, sleep problems, mood swings, and crazy heavy periods. Is this menopause already, and you're only 42? Not necessarily. Menopause may still be a decade away. This is *perimenopause*, which is the decade or more leading up to menopause.

Never heard of perimenopause? You're not alone. Researchers, journalists, and even doctors use the word "menopause" when, in reality, they're referring to perimenopause.

Menopause and perimenopause are *not* the same things. For example, menopause is a time of low estrogen. Perimenopause is a time of "estrogen on a roller coaster" when you can, at times, have *more* estrogen than ever before.

And yet your doctor may offer you estrogen replacement during perimenopause. Do you really want more estrogen when your own is already surging too high?

So, let's get our definitions straight.

Perimenopause is the two to twelve years before menopause and is when you're most likely to experience symptoms.

Menopause is the life phase that begins one year after your last period[341] and is when many symptoms will settle down.

You can expect to be healthy and symptom-free in menopause, which is good because you'll spend a third of your life there. You may encounter a few issues, which we'll look at in the Life After Periods section later in this chapter.

 Perimenopause is most likely to start in your 40s, but you may notice it as early as your late 30s.

What are the changes of perimenopause? According to Canadian endocrinologist Dr Jerilynn Prior, a midlife woman is likely to be in perimenopause if she has any three of the following nine changes, despite regular menstrual cycles:[342]

- new onset heavy and/or longer flow
- shorter menstrual cycles (less than 25 days)
- new sore, swollen, or lumpy breasts
- new mid-sleep waking
- increased menstrual cramps
- onset of night sweats, in particular premenstrually
- new or markedly increased migraine headaches
- new or increased premenstrual mood swings
- weight gain without changes in exercise or eating.

 Please see Dr Jerilynn Prior's book *Estrogen's Storm Season: stories of perimenopause* available from the CeMCOR website.[343]

Perimenopausal changes are not fun, and they can come on quite quickly. You may be going along in your busy life and then, suddenly, you find you just don't feel like yourself. If you seek help from your doctor, she may advise you just to ride it out, or offer the pill, estrogen, or an antidepressant. None are likely to be much help.

"There has to be a better way!" you say. And fortunately, yes, there is. It all starts with understanding what your hormones are up to.

Estrogen Goes on a Roller Coaster Ride

Contrary to what you've heard, your estrogen is not on a slow, gradual decline in your forties. It would be a lot nicer if it were, because then you could experience a slow, gradual transition to menopause. Instead, your estrogen is doing the worst possible thing: it's fluctuating wildly. It's soaring to twice what it was before[344] and then crashing down again to almost nothing. And it's doing that again and again—cycle after cycle.

I call it the *estrogen roller coaster* of perimenopause.

Symptoms of high estrogen include breast pain, heavy periods, fluid retention, and irritable mood. Symptoms of dropping estrogen include depression, night sweats, heart palpitations, and hot flashes.

 If you have ovaries, you will go through perimenopause—even if you've had a hysterectomy and do not have a uterus.

You might be okay

Not all of you will experience bad symptoms. Dr Prior estimates that only 20 percent of women go through such dramatic ups and downs of estrogen. Many of you will notice only a few mild changes that won't bother you much.

And some of you may be lucky enough to experience perimenopause as just a gradual lightening and fading away of your periods. In that case, yes, both your estrogen and progesterone are in decline, but you can definitely adapt to your new *normal* level of hormones.

Progesterone Becomes Seriously Deficient

At the same time that your estrogen is bouncing up and down, your progesterone is quietly exiting the scene. It's unfortunate because progesterone's soothing effects would have made estrogen's roller coaster a lot easier to bear. Remember, progesterone counteracts estrogen, thereby preventing estrogen excess symptoms such as heavy periods. Progesterone also shelters your nervous system from precipitous drops in estrogen.

Progesterone was hard enough to make in your twenties and thirties. It's even harder in your forties because your ovarian follicles are not as active or responsive.[345] The change to your follicles is genetically programmed and a natural, normal process. It's not because you've done something wrong, and it's probably not because you're running out of eggs.

Special Topic: Women May Not Run Out of Eggs

We used to think women are born with about 400,000 dormant eggs that get used up and eventually run out. New research suggests that this may be wrong.

You may, in fact, have ovarian stem cells that could continue to make new, viable eggs indefinitely,[346] which biologically, would make a lot more sense. According to researcher Jonathan Tilly: "There's no fathomable reason why a woman would have evolved to carry stale eggs around for decades before attempting to get pregnant while men evolved to have fresh sperm always available."[347]

If you have ovarian stem cells, then you do not simply run out of fertility because you're old. You *could* keep reproducing, but you won't, and scientists think they know why. It's because you're genetically programmed to stop reproducing while still relatively young so you can dedicate time and resources to your descendants. It's called the "grandmother theory"[348] and has been proved in orca whales, one of the only other species to undergo menopause.[349]

Yes, it's sad to lose progesterone, but at the same time, it was great to have it for even those few short decades.

Here's how I see it: The fact that we have to lose progesterone eventually should make us more grateful to have ever had it at all. And more determined to *not* switch it off with hormonal birth control.

What can you do to ease your way through perimenopause? As it turns out, your best strategy is the one we've used again and again throughout the book:

- Support progesterone
- Metabolize estrogen
- Reduce inflammation

The main difference with perimenopause is that you may need to work a little harder at it. You may also need to supplement progesterone.

Let's have a look.

Perimenopausal Mood, Sleep, and Hot Flashes

The most troubling symptoms of perimenopause are mood swings, sleep disturbance, and hot flashes. All three symptoms stem from the same underlying destabilization of your HPA axis. And, fortunately, all three symptoms respond to the same treatments.

Let's start with mood and sleep. You are at greater risk of depression and insomnia during perimenopause and it happens for a couple of different reasons. First, you're probably pretty busy. You have more career and family obligations than at any other time in your life, and that means you're dealing with more stress than at any other time in your life. As if that wasn't enough, your changing hormones make you less able to cope with stress. It all comes back to the loss of progesterone, which is a loss of stability for your stress response system or HPA axis.[350] Recall from Chapter 6 that progesterone every month helped to regulate your HPA axis and progesterone every month is what your nervous system was *used to*.

Now, in your forties, you're losing progesterone so you are more vulnerable to anxiety, depression, and insomnia.[351]

The good news is that it won't last forever. Eventually, you will reach menopause, and then your mood should be at least as good as it was when you were younger, and maybe even better.[352] As Dr Jerilynn Prior puts it: "Women need to know that perimenopause ends in a kinder and calmer phase of life appropriately called menopause."[353]

For example, one Australian study tracked 400 menopausal women over twenty years and discovered that mood scores steadily improve with age.[354] The researchers concluded that "women report feeling pretty fantastic after menopause."[355]

Hot flashes and heart palpitations are other symptoms of the same temporary dysregulation of your HPA axis. They respond to the same treatment that I'm going to describe below.

Special Topic: Perimenopause and Histamine Intolerance

During perimenopause, you may notice other strange allergy-like symptoms such as brain fog, hives, and nasal congestion. Or you may experience a worsening of existing allergies such as hay fever. You're not imagining things. The combination of high estrogen and low progesterone can worsen the *histamine intolerance*[356] we discussed in Chapters 6 and 8.

Conventional Treatment of Perimenopausal Mood, Sleep, and Hot Flashes

Conventional treatments are antidepressants, the pill, or estrogen treatment—none of which are all that effective.[357] I advise against taking the pill and/or estrogen during perimenopause because it's already a time of high estrogen. And there's no evidence that taking estrogen can prevent the estrogen surges that characterize perimenopause. Progesterone is a better option, as we'll see.

Low-dose estrogen may be appropriate after your periods finally stop. See the Life After Periods section later in this chapter.

Diet and Lifestyle for Perimenopausal Mood, Sleep, and Hot Flashes

Rest and self-care

You are at a vulnerable time. You have permission to slow down and look after yourself, at least until you arrive safely in menopause. For example, you might want to look at temporarily cutting back your work hours, or seeking more help at home. Sign up for a yoga class. Book a massage. Being in my late forties finally convinced me to meditate regularly.

Reduce alcohol

Alcohol impairs the healthy metabolism of estrogen, and that can be a problem when your estrogen is already soaring to twice what you had before. Alcohol also lowers progesterone[358] and interferes with progesterone's calming action in the brain.[359] You might be able to get away with four or five standard drinks per week, but my experience with perimenopause is that I feel better with no alcohol.

Supplements and Herbal Medicines for Perimenopausal Mood, Sleep, and Hot Flashes

Magnesium is a powerful stress-reliever. If you take one supplement during perimenopause, let it be magnesium.

How it works: It calms the brain, regulates the HPA axis, and promotes sleep.

What else you need to know: I recommend 300 mg magnesium glycinate with food. I prescribe magnesium for almost every perimenopausal patient, and I usually prescribe it together with the amino acid taurine.

Taurine is an amino acid that calms the brain and stabilizes the HPA axis.

How it works: It has a tranquilizing effect similar to the neurotransmitter GABA.

What else you need to know: Taurine can only be obtained from animal products, so you are at risk of deficiency if you are vegetarian. Also, it's depleted by estrogen so, as a woman, you need more taurine than men.[360] You may need to supplement. I recommend 3000 mg per day together with magnesium.

Vitamin B6 is the amazing PMS treatment we discussed in Chapter 8. It has similar benefits for perimenopausal mood symptoms.

How it works: It promotes healthy estrogen metabolism and boosts GABA.

What else you need to know: I recommend 20 to 150 mg daily.

Ashwagandha (*Withania somnifera*) is a herbal medicine that dials down the stress response.

How it works: It stabilizes the HPA axis, and also has direct anti-anxiety and sleep-promoting effects (hence the Latin name *somnifera* or "sleep-inducing").

What else you need to know: The exact quantity of the medicine depends on the concentration of the formula, so please take as directed on the bottle. Doses range from 300 to 3000 mg and may be taken in a formula that contains other adaptogens such as Rhodiola.

Ziziphus is a herbal sedative traditionally prescribed for perimenopause.

How it works: It's a non-addictive sedative.[361]

What else you need to know: It's often combined with magnolia (*Magnolia officinalis*) for a stronger effect.[362] Dose as directed on the bottle.

Micronized or natural progesterone is helpful for both perimenopausal insomnia and hot flashes.[363]

How it works: It dramatically improves sleep by reducing anxiety[364] and by acting directly on the sleep centers of the brain.[365] Progesterone can also relieve hot flashes by modulating the activity of the hypothalamus.

What else you need to know: You can use cream or capsule, but a capsule works better for sleep. Ingesting progesterone means that more of it converts to the sedating metabolite allopregnanolone (ALLO). Progesterone capsules are called micronized progesterone and can be prescribed as a compounded capsule or the brand Prometrium®.

Take it for the last two weeks of your expected cycle and take it at bedtime because it will make you sleepy. For more information, see Dr Prior's paper, "Progesterone for Symptomatic Perimenopause Treatment."[366]

Checklist for perimenopausal mood, sleep, and hot flashes

* Make more time for yourself.
* Reduce or eliminate alcohol.
* Consider taking magnesium, taurine, and micronized progesterone.

 My "*rescue prescription*" for perimenopausal mood and sleep problems is magnesium plus taurine plus micronized progesterone.

 Lori: Rescue prescription for perimenopause

Lori was 47 when she hit what she called "the wall."

"I've started feeling anxious," she told me. "Out of nowhere. And suddenly, I can't sleep. I fall asleep but then jolt awake a few hours later."

Lori had a busy life, so it didn't take long for her to start feeling pretty desperate. She saw her doctor who offered an antidepressant.

"I don't think I'm depressed," she said. "I've never had a problem before. I feel like something's really changed in my body."

I asked Lori about her periods, and she said they were coming closer together and were heavier than they used to be. I had a pretty good idea what was going on.

I ordered a couple of blood tests. The first was thyroid, which was normal, and the second was a Day 3 FSH or follicle-stimulating hormone. It's the test for menopause, and it was normal at 18 mIU/mL.

We talked a bit more about her symptoms. Lori had the new symptom of breast pain before her periods, and she'd noticed a bit of weight gain.

"You're in perimenopause," I said. "Your hormones are fluctuating pretty dramatically, but menopause itself could still be five years away."

Lori: "I can't go through five more years of this."

Lori ate well; she exercised, and even meditated fifteen minutes per day. I felt Lori was already doing everything right, but she needed something more. I offered her my "rescue prescription," which is a powder with magnesium and taurine, and asked her to talk to her doctor about obtaining Prometrium® in accordance with Professor Prior's guidelines for perimenopause. The first night that Lori took Prometrium® she slept eight solid hours and then continued to feel a steady return to her normal self.

Did you notice that Lori's FSH blood test for menopause was "normal?" She wasn't in menopause, but she was in perimenopause, which can't be detected with a blood test. If Lori's FSH had been high at 80 mIU/mL, then I would have predicted that her periods would soon stop. As it was, her FSH test was normal so I knew she was probably going to keep menstruating for a few more years. But that didn't mean everything was okay. She had symptoms of perimenopause, and she was 47. She needed help.

The main reason I ordered blood tests for Lori was to check her thyroid.

Is It Perimenopause or Thyroid or Both?

Thyroid disease can look and feel a lot like perimenopause. For example, both conditions can cause depression, insomnia, weight gain, irregular periods, heavy periods, hot flashes, and especially brain fog or difficulty concentrating.

You could have perimenopause, or you could have thyroid disease, or quite possibly you could have both. About 26 percent of perimenopausal women also have autoimmune thyroid disease.[367]

If you think you're suffering symptoms of perimenopause, you also need to rule out thyroid.

Rae: Am I in early menopause?

I could see that Rae was worried. She'd brought her partner Sam to our appointment, and he looked pretty worried too.

"My periods have gone all haywire," she told me (meaning her periods had become irregular.) "I'm losing hair, and I'm having night sweats—" Rae paused, then finally asked me: "Am I in early menopause?"

Rae was only 34.

"Probably not," I said, because premature menopause is not common. "But let's do a blood test to find out."

As I suspected, Rae's FSH was fine at 8 mIU/mL. Her TSH, on the other hand, was 45 mIU/L which meant she had hypothyroidism or underactive thyroid.

I explained to Rae that hypothyroidism or low thyroid was the cause of her irregular periods and night sweats, and I recommended she see her doctor, who prescribed thyroxine, or thyroid hormone. After two weeks on thyroid medication, Rae's night sweats disappeared. After three months, she regained a regular period.

 TSH

TSH (thyroid stimulating hormone) is the pituitary hormone that stimulates the thyroid gland. It's the standard test for thyroid dysfunction and should be between 0.5 and 4 mIU/L.

Rae did well with basic thyroid testing and the basic thyroid medication thyroxine. Depending on your situation, you may require additional thyroid testing and a different kind of thyroid medication. Refer to the Thyroid Disease section in Chapter 11.

(tip) **Progesterone supports thyroid.** If you're perimenopausal and your thyroid is just a little bit low, you may benefit from natural progesterone, which increases thyroid hormone.[368]

The Heavy Menstrual Bleeding of Perimenopause

Heavy menstrual bleeding is defined as blood loss of greater than 80 mL (sixteen regular tampons) or lasting longer than seven days. It can happen at any age, but it can be particularly bad during perimenopause when it can turn into *menstrual flooding,* which is flow so heavy you bleed through your tampon or pad.

Do you have a medical condition?

Heavy menstrual bleeding can be secondary to a medical condition such as thyroid disease, coagulation disorders, fibroids, or adenomyosis. We discussed those common conditions in Chapter 9, and it's not unusual for them to go undiagnosed.

It's worth asking your doctor outright: "Have I been tested for thyroid disease? Have I been screened for a coagulation disorder?" And finally, "Do I have adenomyosis? May I please see a copy of my ultrasound report?"

See the How to Talk to Your Doctor section in the next chapter.

The stakes are high

The heavy menstrual bleeding of perimenopause can become quite serious and, if untreated, can escalate to the point of requiring surgery. When I started practicing twenty years ago, way too many of my forty-something patients had lost their uteruses to hysterectomy as a treatment for heavy bleeding.

Fortunately, there are better options today—both conventional and natural.

Conventional Treatment of the Heavy Menstrual Bleeding of Perimenopause

Ibuprofen

As we saw in the Heavy Periods section of the last chapter, ibuprofen can reduce your menstrual flow by half. It's a simple and practical solution and a good first step while you work on the other treatments. Take it on your heavy days, and take it with food to decrease the risk of stomach irritation.

Hormonal birth control

Conventional treatment includes the pill and the Mirena® IUD. They work because progestins thin the uterine lining. It's worth noting that micronized or natural progesterone does the same thing, but without the many side effects of synthetic progestins.

> (tip) **The combination of ibuprofen plus micronized progesterone** is highly effective for the heavy periods of perimenopause and will work for most of you. See *Managing Menorrhagia without Surgery* on Dr Prior's CeMCOR site.[369]

You should see results with micronized progesterone and the natural treatment discussed later in the chapter. If not, and if you feel you need some kind of hormonal birth control, then consider the Mirena® IUD. It's better than the pill for the reasons I discussed in Chapter 2. Dr Jerilynn Prior says the oral contraceptive pill should be avoided during perimenopause.

D and C (dilation and curettage)

D and C is the surgical removal of part of your uterine lining. It is done under general anesthetic.

The idea is that removing the thickened uterine lining will reduce flow, but it gives no lasting benefit. As soon as the uterine lining grows back, your flow will increase again. I do not recommend it.

Tranexamic acid (Lysteda®)

Tranexamic acid is a medication that increases blood clotting. Your doctor may give it to you as emergency medicine during very heavy flow, or she may ask you to take it every period. It carries a small risk of pulmonary embolism and deep vein thrombosis (blood clots).

Endometrial ablation

Endometrial ablation is the surgical destruction of your uterine lining. It's done under general anesthetic and destroys fertility, so will only be offered if you do not want more children.

Your hormones still cycle normally after ablation, but you don't build up a uterine lining, so you will bleed lightly or not at all. It doesn't work for everyone, and the effect lasts only about five years, after which time your lining may grow back. About 22 percent of women require a repeat procedure, and many go on to require a hysterectomy anyway.[370]

Ablation can trap blood behind scar tissue, which can cause long-term pelvic pain. That complication is more likely to occur after tubal ligation and is estimated to affect up to 10 percent of women who have undergone ablation.[371]

Endometrial ablation is not ideal, but in my view, it's preferable to hysterectomy.

Hysterectomy

Hysterectomy (surgical removal of your uterus) has been the standard medical treatment for heavy bleeding for generations. It is still sometimes necessary, but I encourage my patients to keep their uterus, if at all possible.

One study indicated that hysterectomy doubles your long-term risk of vaginal prolapse and urinary incontinence.[372] It can also adversely affect your sexual response and ability to orgasm, especially if your ovaries were also removed.

On the other hand, if a hysterectomy relieves severe pain and bleeding, then it may improve your sexual enjoyment.

Remember, there are two types of hysterectomy: *total hysterectomy*, when the surgeon removes your uterus and cervix and possibly your ovaries; and *partial hysterectomy* when the surgeon removes your uterus but leaves your cervix.

Removal of your ovaries causes surgical menopause, which we'll discuss later in the chapter. It's different from normal menopause and can put you at risk of depression, heart disease, and many other long-term complications. The Mayo Clinic recommends that ovaries should *not* be removed except in very high-risk cases.

Removal of your uterus, but not your ovaries, does *not* alter your hormones or cause menopause. You will still benefit from natural period repair.

Special Topic: Tracking Your "Virtual Periods" After a Hysterectomy

If you still have ovaries, then you still cycle, and have a "virtual period."

For example, you could still ovulate and go through a premenstrual phase when you feel a bit irritable and headachy. You will then reach a *relief day,* which is when your hormones drop, and you would bleed if you had a uterus.

That relief day is your "day 1", and you can try tracking it with your period app.

At some stage after a hysterectomy, you will reach menopause. It will probably happen at the age you would have gone through menopause anyway.

Since you don't bleed, you may not recognize that you've reached menopause. Watch for symptoms such as hot flashes and vaginal dryness, and ask your doctor to test FSH. An FSH greater than 40 IU/L marks the onset of menopause.

It's okay to resort to conventional treatment

Despite all your best efforts, you may require surgery or medical treatment for heavy menstrual bleeding. It's not a failure on your part. You cannot be expected to endure very heavy periods for long. It's still worth trying natural treatment because there's a good chance it will work and, even if it does not, you will still benefit from its hormone-balancing effects.

Now let's look at the natural treatment options. Many are the same as the ones we discussed in the Heavy Periods section in the last chapter.

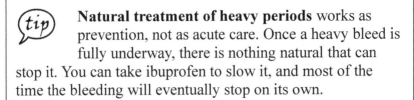

Natural treatment of heavy periods works as prevention, not as acute care. Once a heavy bleed is fully underway, there is nothing natural that can stop it. You can take ibuprofen to slow it, and most of the time the bleeding will eventually stop on its own.

If you feel dizzy or unwell, please see your doctor. You may need the clotting drug tranexamic acid (Lysteda®).

Diet and Lifestyle for the Heavy Menstrual Bleeding of Perimenopause

Avoid cow's dairy

As we discussed in Chapter 9, dairy can make periods heavier.

Reduce alcohol

Alcohol increases your exposure to estrogen by impairing your liver's ability to metabolize it. More estrogen means a heavier period.

Maintain healthy gut bacteria

Healthy gut bacteria escort estrogen safely out of your body. You want healthy estrogen metabolism, not just to reduce menstrual flow, but also to relieve other symptoms of estrogen excess, such as irritability and breast pain.

For a full discussion of breast pain and fibrocystic breasts, refer to Chapter 8.

Eat phytoestrogens

Phytoestrogens shelter you from estrogen by blocking estrogen receptors and promoting the healthy metabolism of estrogen.

Correct insulin resistance

Insulin resistance increases your risk of heavy periods in two ways:

- Elevated insulin directly thickens the uterine lining.
- Elevated insulin can impair ovulation and therefore cause low progesterone.

For treatment, refer to the section about insulin resistance in Chapter 7.

 If you had insulin resistance and PCOS when you were younger, you are likely to still have it now. PCOS does not end with menopause.

Exercise

Exercise improves insulin sensitivity and promotes the healthy elimination of estrogen through perspiration.

Supplements and Herbal Medicines for the Heavy Menstrual Bleeding of Perimenopause

Turmeric lightens periods, as explained in Chapter 9.

Iron corrects the iron deficiency caused by your heavy periods and also *lightens* your period.

Calcium d-glucarate promotes healthy estrogen metabolism. We first met it in Chapter 8 as a treatment for PMS.

How it works: Glucarate assists with estrogen detoxification in two ways. First, it binds to estrogen in the liver and deactivates it. Second, it inhibits *beta-glucuronidase*, which is the enzyme made by gut bacteria that causes estrogen to be reabsorbed.

What else you need to know: I recommend 1000 to 1500 mg per day. It may also help to prevent breast cancer.[373]

Micronized or natural progesterone makes periods lighter.

How it works: It thins your uterine lining, as do synthetic progestins such as noresthisterone (Primolut®) and medroxyprogesterone (Provera®). But progesterone is a far nicer treatment because it is also soothing for mood and sleep.

What else you need to know: A progesterone capsule such as Prometrium® works better than a topical cream. The standard dosing according to Dr Jerilynn Prior is to take a progesterone capsule at bedtime during the last two weeks of your cycle. For more information, see Dr Prior's paper, "Progesterone for Symptomatic Perimenopause Treatment."[374]

Checklist for perimenopausal heavy periods or flooding

- Rule out a medical cause such as thyroid disease or adenomyosis.
- Consider taking ibuprofen on your heavy days.
- Reduce or eliminate alcohol.
- Avoid cow's dairy.
- Consider taking iron, turmeric, and calcium d-glucarate.
- Consider taking micronized or natural progesterone.
- See the Heavy Periods section in Chapter 9.

Life After Periods

If you have the impression that menopause is difficult, it's because the *transition* to menopause can be difficult. Menopause itself can be easy and fine and may not require any treatment at all.

During menopause, you will have far less estrogen and progesterone than you had before—but you'll still have *some*. For example, you'll still make a small amount of both estrogen and progesterone from both your ovaries and adrenal glands. You'll also make estradiol *inside your cells* from the adrenal hormone DHEA.[375]

Altogether, that should be enough hormone to keep you well, especially once you've had a chance to adapt.

The same cannot be said for premature menopause or surgical menopause. They are unique circumstances which almost always require hormone treatment.

Premature Menopause

Premature menopause, also called *premature ovarian failure* or *primary ovarian insufficiency,* is defined as the loss of ovarian function before age 40. It's diagnosed by the blood test FSH and affects about one in 100 women.[376]

Factors contributing to primary ovarian insufficiency are genetics, autoimmune disease, and endometriosis.[377] In most cases, the cause is not known.

If you've entered premature menopause, then you probably need menopausal hormone therapy.

Surgical Menopause

Losing your ovaries to surgery is not normal menopause. For one thing, you'll experience a rapid decline in hormones that is very different from menopause and can cause strong symptoms, such as hot flashes.

Also, with surgical menopause, you'll go on to have lower levels of hormones compared to women in natural menopause. That will put you at greater long-term risk of heart disease,[378] dementia,[379] osteoporosis,[380] and some cancers.[381] You'll also likely suffer a greater reduction in libido and sexual function compared to menopausal women with ovaries.[382] Hormone therapy can help, but it can't entirely compensate.[383]

Hold on to your ovaries, if you can. I know it's not always possible. Speak to your doctor.

Problems That Can Arise in Menopause

Hot flashes

Hot flashes can start during perimenopause or after your last period. If your flashes start during perimenopause, then they could last as long as ten years.[384] If they start after your last period, they will probably last only a couple of years. Either way, you may need treatment.

The magnesium plus taurine plus progesterone combination works well for menopausal hot flashes,[385] as do the herbal medicines black cohosh and sage. If your flashes are bad enough, you may need a low-dose estrogen supplement such as a natural estradiol patch (see below).

Vaginal dryness, reduced libido, and bladder infections

After menopause, you may experience something called *vaginal atrophy*, which means the tissue of your vaginal wall becomes thinner and drier. It can cause a range of symptoms including:

- reduced desire, arousal, and orgasm
- painful intercourse
- increased frequency of bladder infections
- leaking urine
- pelvic prolapse.

The conventional treatment is a vaginal pessary of low dose estradiol (Vagifem®) which I do recommend. There's also the option of a vaginal cream with the hormone DHEA.[386] See the Resources section for a link to a DHEA pessary called Julva®.

A non-hormonal treatment for vaginal atrophy is the nutritional supplement sea buckthorn oil, to be taken orally.[387]

Weight gain

In menopause, you may gain weight around your middle. It's because you've lost the insulin-sensitizing effect of estradiol and are therefore at greater risk of insulin resistance.[388] To combat this, please implement the treatment strategies discussed in the Insulin Resistance section of Chapter 7. You can also try a low-dose estradiol patch (see below) to improve insulin sensitivity.

Insulin resistance after menopause can also cause symptoms of androgen excess similar to PCOS. For treatment ideas, see the Anti-Androgen Treatment section in Chapter 7.

Osteoporosis

Your risk of osteoporosis will increase during the final year of perimenopause and the first five years of menopause. During that time, you could lose up to 10 percent of your bone density and be at greater risk of osteoporotic fracture.[389]

Please keep in mind, however, that your *absolute risk* of osteoporosis depends on many things including a history of any of the following:

- celiac disease (gluten sensitivity)
- smoking
- high alcohol intake
- corticosteroid medication
- SSRI antidepressant medication
- PPI stomach acid medication
- eating disorder
- amenorrhea
- total hysterectomy including removal of the ovaries
- deficiency of vitamin D, zinc, vitamin K2, magnesium, or protein.

Many of these factors increase your osteoporosis risk by at least as much as menopause, if not more. For example, an SSRI antidepressant can double your risk of osteoporotic fracture.[390]

Osteoporosis is a frightening diagnosis, but please think it through before submitting a medication such as Fosamax® or the injection Prolia®. They have significant side effects and risks.

The first thing to consider is whether you have osteoporosis or only *osteopenia* which is not a disease but can be interpreted as the healthy, normal aging of bone.[391]

The next thing to understand is that your risk of osteoporotic fracture *may not* be accurately predicted by a bone density scan, [392] so please don't put too much faith in such a test.

The best way to maintain healthy bones is to address any underlying risk factor such as smoking or antidepressant use. Beyond that, you can get results with eating well and exercising and taking the nutritional supplements vitamin D, vitamin K2, calcium, and magnesium.

You can also look at supplementing the bone-building hormones estrogen and progesterone.

A full discussion of osteoporosis is beyond the scope of this book. Speak to your doctor for advice.

Bioidentical Hormone Therapy

You may not require supplementary hormones in menopause. If you do, please make sure they are bioidentical.

Bioidentical hormones are derived from plant sterols such as wild yam, but so are most types of hormone drugs. That's *not* why bioidentical hormones are better.

Bioidentical hormones are better because they're structurally identical to your own human hormones. In that way, they are different from the pseudo-hormones or "horse hormones" of hormonal birth control or old styles of hormone therapy. Until recently, bioidentical hormones were available only from a compounding chemist. Now, they are available as a conventional prescription. Bioidentical prescriptions include the products Estradot®, Climara®, Estraderm®, and Prometrium®.

 Bioidentical means "body identical" or "nature identical."

Micronized or Natural Progesterone

Natural progesterone is also called bioidentical progesterone or micronized progesterone. Your doctor prefers the last term. I recommend you *not* use the words natural or bioidentical when speaking with your doctor. In the case of progesterone, say instead *oral micronized progesterone* or the brand name Prometrium®.

Micronized progesterone is the same progesterone you would normally make after ovulation. If you cannot make enough progesterone, then you can supplement it. Taking progesterone is a way to compensate for progesterone deficiency and relieve symptoms. It cannot increase production of your *own* progesterone. To do that, you need to follow the many guidelines discussed in this book.

Micronized progesterone is different from the progestins norethisterone in Primolut® and levonorgestrel in the Mirena® IUD and many other types of hormonal birth control.

I've mentioned micronized progesterone a few times in the book. It's helpful for PCOS, PMS, migraines, heavy periods, adenomyosis, endometriosis, perimenopause, menopause, and osteoporosis.[393]

Cream versus capsule

You can take progesterone as a cream or capsule. A cream works well for mild problems, such as PMS. A capsule is better for heavy periods, adenomyosis, endometriosis, and perimenopausal mood and sleep symptoms. Progesterone is also available as a vaginal pessary, which is typically given as part of fertility treatment.

Dose and timing

An over-the-counter progesterone cream is 2 percent progesterone, so one gram (a quarter teaspoon) delivers 20 mg of progesterone. That's a good starting dose for conditions like PMS. Apply at bedtime to your face, inner arms, or behind your knees—all places where your blood vessels are close to the surface. That way, the hormone goes directly into your blood and is not stored in fat.

A progesterone capsule is typically 100 mg which is suitable for heavy periods and perimenopause. Take only at bedtime as it can be very sedating.

If you ovulate regularly, take progesterone after ovulation during your luteal phase. If you do not ovulate, then speak to your doctor about the best time to take progesterone. (And also find a way to ovulate, if possible.)

Safety and precautions

At an appropriate dose, micronized progesterone should have no side effects. At a high dose, it can cause drowsiness, abdominal bloating, and breast tenderness. If you experience such side effects, then reduce your dose or stop it.

Unlike progestin drugs, micronized progesterone does *not* increase the risk of breast cancer or heart disease. Instead, it may reduce the risk of both conditions.[394][395]

Progesterone on its own is helpful for most symptoms, even once you are in menopause. However, you may find that you need the addition of estrogen.

Estrogen

Taking estrogen can be a lifesaver for menopausal mood, sleep, hot flashes, and vaginal dryness.

Yes, estrogen therapy does carry some risk, but not as much as you might think. The highest risk from hormone therapy was from the drugs Premarin® and Provera® back in the 1980s and 1990s. Those drugs were *not* bioidentical hormones. Instead, they were a mix of the horse estrogens estrone sulfate, equilin sulfate, equilenin sulfate, and a progestin called medroxyprogesterone. Those drugs caused numerous side effects and problems.

It's all changed now.

Today, most (not all) estrogen prescriptions are low-dose bioidentical estradiol, which is a lot safer than Premarin®.

What type of estrogen?

For vaginal atrophy symptoms, I recommend the estradiol vaginal pessary Vagifem®. It relieves dryness, and I observe that it can relieve other menopausal symptoms such as insomnia. Because it's such a low dose, you can use Vagifem® on its own, without progesterone.

For severe hot flashes and menopausal insomnia, I recommend an estradiol patch such as Estradot® or Climara®. If you take an estradiol patch, you'll also need progesterone. That's true even if you don't have a uterus.

Special Topic: Why Your Doctor Says You Don't Need Progesterone If You Don't Have a Uterus

Conventional medicine does not necessarily recognize the many benefits of natural progesterone. In conventional thinking, the only purpose of a progestin is to prevent the unwanted buildup of the uterine lining. That's true for synthetic progestins, because they have no additional benefits. Progesterone is different. It protects the uterine lining *and* it helps mood, bones, brain, and thyroid. It may even help to prevent breast cancer.

Watch for signs of another period

In the early stages of the menopause transition, you may experience several months of estrogen deficiency when you benefit from taking estrogen. But then, suddenly, things can change. Your body starts moving towards another period and making its own estrogen.

If that happens, you'll experience breast swelling and what feels like new premenstrual irritability. That means you now have too much estrogen and should stop the estrogen patch until things settle down again. You can still take progesterone.

 It's normal for your period to stop and start during the menopause transition.

In summary, natural progesterone and other bioidentical hormones are possible treatment options for perimenopause and beyond. Some bioidentical products are available without a prescription in the USA, but they require a prescription in other countries.

Bioidentical hormones cannot be used to prevent pregnancy.

A Final Word About Life After Periods

Because our society values young women of reproductive age, some of us entering menopause can feel a loss of power and worth.

It doesn't have to be that way. As I approach menopause myself, I am waking up to a new kind of power—one of wisdom and a strong desire to help others. I also feel a camaraderie with other older women. By the year 2030, there will be 1.2 billion menopausal women in the world[396]—more than ever before.

Surely, we can be a force for good.

Chapter 11

ADVANCED TROUBLESHOOTING

Putting It All Together

TIME FOR A REVIEW.

What should your period be like? Your period should be regular. It should arrive without premenstrual symptoms and without pain. It should not be heavier than 80 mL (sixteen filled tampons) over all the days of your bleed.

You have the right to this kind of ease with your periods. No pain. No flooding. No PMS. It *is* possible.

Your period is your monthly report card. Your symptoms are your clues.

What are *your* clues? What are they trying to tell you about your underlying health?

When interpreting your period clues, please always come back to these three questions:

- Do you ovulate regularly? If you *do not* ovulate, then why not?
- Do you metabolize or detoxify estrogen well? If not, why not? And what can you do to improve that?
- Do you suffer chronic inflammation that is interfering with your hormonal communication? What can you do to reduce inflammation?

These are the questions to ask yourself. They're not the questions to ask your doctor, because she may not be as familiar with concepts such as estrogen metabolism and chronic inflammation. I'll provide a list of doctor-speak questions later in this chapter.

Do You Ovulate?

We have asked this question again and again throughout the book. Ovulation is essential for period health because it's how you make progesterone.

Failure to ovulate and make progesterone is the main reason for many period problems, including irregular periods, PCOS, and heavy periods.

How do you know if you ovulate and make progesterone?

Signs of *possible* ovulation include fertile mucus and a regular cycle. Evidence of *definite* ovulation includes a rise in basal body temperature and an increase in progesterone as measured by a mid-luteal phase blood test. A period itself is not a definite sign of ovulation because it is possible to have an anovulatory cycle. For more information, see the Physical Signs of Ovulation section in Chapter 3 and Progesterone Testing in Chapter 5.

Why do you not ovulate?

Here are some possibilities:

- PCOS
- insulin resistance
- deficiency of zinc, selenium, iodine, or vitamin D
- undereating

- low-carb diet
- too many phytoestrogens, such as soy
- stress
- elevated prolactin
- perimenopause
- celiac disease
- thyroid disease (see below).

This is not an exhaustive list, but it's a good starting place. It should help you to ask your doctor more targeted questions.

Once you have identified *why* you do not ovulate, your best treatment is to correct *that* issue. We explored a variety of treatments in Chapter 7.

Do You Metabolize Estrogen Well?

Estrogen excess is a key factor in PMS, fibroids, and heavy periods.

How do you know if you have estrogen excess?

Look for symptoms such as premenstrual irritability, breast tenderness, heavy periods, and fibroids. Ask your doctor to test estrogen with a blood test in your luteal phase when both estrogen and progesterone are high.

Why do you not metabolize estrogen well?

Common reasons for impaired estrogen metabolism or detoxification include:

- alcohol
- digestive problems
- environmental toxins
- nutrient deficiency
- chronic inflammation.

For a full discussion, review the Estrogen Excess section in Chapter 5.

Do You Suffer Chronic Inflammation?

In many sections of this book, we saw how inflammation distorts hormonal communication. For example, chronic inflammation blocks hormone receptors. It also impairs estrogen metabolism and prevents ovulation and the production of progesterone.

> **Chronic inflammation** could be the main reason for your period problems.

How do you know if you have chronic inflammation?

Look for signs such as headaches, joint pain, or chronic skin conditions such as eczema and psoriasis. Those are your clues.

Fatigue is another symptom of inflammation, but one you should be careful interpreting because fatigue can be caused by many different things. Your first step is to see your doctor to rule out common causes such as iron deficiency and thyroid disease. Then, please consider whether you get enough sleep. Once you have ruled out those common issues, you are left with the possibility that chronic inflammation is the cause of your fatigue.

There's no simple blood test for inflammation. Your doctor can test for inflammatory markers such as CRP, ESR, thyroid antibodies, and gluten antibodies. But you could have chronic inflammation *even if those tests are normal.*

Chronic inflammation can be the result of stress, insulin resistance, infection, environmental toxins, and digestive problems. Your strategy is to address those underlying problems.

Environmental Toxins

I wish I didn't have to include this section. It makes me sad just to think about it. Still, it must be faced: environmental toxins can play a significant role in period problems.

Environmental Working Group (EWG)

The best resource for information about environmental toxins is the nonprofit organization Environmental Working Group (www.ewg.org). The people behind it have been working in this field for over two decades and provide regular updates about the environmental toxins in our food, cosmetics, and household products. They also publish new research.

Toxic at low dose

We used to think that environmental toxins are only a problem when they are present at a dose high enough to kill a mouse in a lab study. We now know that environmental toxins can be a problem at a frighteningly low dose. Why? Because many environmental toxins are *endocrine disruptors* or *endocrine-disrupting chemicals* (EDCs).

📖 endocrine disrupting chemicals

Endocrine disrupting chemicals (EDCs) are substances that cause adverse health effects by altering the function of the endocrine or hormonal system. They include pesticides, metals, industrial pollutants, solvents, food additives, and personal care products.

Your body is *accustomed* to responding to hormones at a low dose. Therefore, it makes sense that your body will respond to endocrine disruptors at a low dose. Even at a few parts per million, environmental toxins can disrupt your hormonal system. For example, they can stimulate more of certain hormones and fewer of others. They can directly damage glandular tissue such as thyroid and ovaries. Finally, they can impair estrogen metabolism and block and disrupt hormone receptors.

Not all environmental toxins are hormone disruptors, but many are.

Dirty Dozen Endocrine Disruptors

According to a 2013 EWG report, the most concerning endocrine disrupting chemicals (EDCs) are the following:[397]

1. **Bisphenol A (BPA)** is used to make some types of plastic. It mimics estrogens and disrupts estrogen metabolism. Other bisphenols (such as bisphenol S) may be just as harmful.

2. **Dioxins** are an industrial byproduct and accumulate in animal foods like meat, fish, milk, eggs, and butter. They interfere with hormonal signaling and are implicated in the causation of endometriosis.[398] They can also have a devastating effect on sperm.

3. **Atrazine** is a widely used herbicide. It's been linked to reproductive cancers.

4. **Phthalates** are used in the manufacture of plastic, food containers, shampoos, and other household products. They disrupt many hormones including thyroid. A recent study linked phthalate exposure to underactive thyroid in girls.[399]

5. **Perchlorate** is a component of rocket fuel that can end up in food and drinking water. It disrupts thyroid function.

6. **Fire retardants** are applied to furniture, mattresses, and carpets. They disrupt thyroid function.

7. **Lead** is a powerful nerve toxin, and it also lowers sex hormones and disrupts the HPA axis.

8. **Arsenic** is a breakdown product of some pesticides and also occurs naturally in some soils. It can end up in drinking water and rice and can cause acne and insulin resistance.

9. **Mercury** is a powerful nerve toxin. It also directly alters levels of FSH, LH, estrogen, progesterone, androgens, and thyroid hormone.[400] It's the ultimate endocrine disruptor.

10. **Perfluorinated chemicals (PFCs)** are used to make non-stick cookware and water-resistant clothing. They appear to be "completely resistant to biodegradation," which means they may never break down or leave the body.

They may alter levels of thyroid and ovarian hormones.

11.**Organophosphate pesticides** are the most common type of pesticide. They affect thyroid and ovarian hormones.

12.**Glycol ethers** are common solvents in paints, cleaning products, and cosmetics. They may damage fertility.

Period Problems

Can all of those hormone-disrupting effects actually contribute to period problems? Recent research indicates they can.

Research has linked BPA, phthalates, and mercury to PCOS,[401] [402] and dioxins, phthalates, and polychlorinated biphenyls (PCBs) to endometriosis. Phthalates, pesticides, and dioxins have also been demonstrated to advance the onset of menopause by up to four years.[403]

Experts are concerned. In 2013, two major medical organizations raised a cautious alarm. Together, the American College of Obstetricians and Gynecologists (ACOG) and the American Society for Reproductive Medicine (ASRM) stated:

> "Scientific evidence over the last 15 years shows that exposure to toxic environmental agents...can have significant and long-lasting effects on reproductive health."[404]

Then just over a year later, based on a review of more than 1300 studies, the Endocrine Society stated that "it's time for doctors to start talking to their patients about endocrine disrupting chemicals."[405]

The Endocrine Society stopped short of advising individuals to take specific measures to protect themselves. They say the onus is on government and industry to reduce pollutants and protect the public. I wholeheartedly agree that industry should make changes to protect us. Hopefully, that will improve the health of future generations. In the meantime, what can you do to help yourself now?

Are you affected by environmental toxins?

If you live in the modern world, you have environmental toxins in your body. All of us do. But that doesn't necessarily mean they are the biggest cause of your period problems. For example, if you have insulin-resistant PCOS, then sugar is more likely to be the thing you need to change.

But if you suspect that environmental toxins are affecting you, then here are some things to consider.

Consider your exposure

Do you work in a setting such as a hair salon, craft studio, or dentist's office where you regularly breathe chemical fumes? Do you live near a golf course, or in an agricultural area where you're exposed to pesticides? Finally, do you eat a lot of tuna, which contains mercury?

These are just a few examples where you might have higher than average exposure.

Consider your symptoms

Do you have unexplained fatigue, headaches, anxiety, or joint pain? Those could be signs of exposure to environmental toxins.

Look at your standard blood test

Your doctor may have ordered something called a complete blood cell count and liver function test. Take a closer look. Do you have a high number of white blood cells that cannot be explained by an infection or other condition? That could be a sign of exposure to pesticides. Do you have low platelets? That could be a sign of exposure to mercury.

 platelets

Platelets are blood cells whose function is to stop bleeding.

Also, look at your liver function panel, and in particular, at something called GGT (*gamma-glutamyl transpeptidase*). Your GGT should be less than 30 IU/L. If it is higher than 30, then it means you are burning through your glutathione, which is your body's primary detoxifying molecule. High GGT can mean you've been exposed to a toxin, such as alcohol or an environmental toxin.

Testing for Environmental Toxins

Toxic metals

If you've been exposed to toxic metals, then talk to your doctor about a blood test for mercury, lead, or cadmium. When interpreting your result, ignore the reference range. Its purpose is to assess *industrial* exposure, but you are an individual in a non-industrial setting, so you should come back with essentially no mercury, cadmium, or lead. If you show a reading, then you could have a problem with toxic metals.

Unfortunately, a negative blood test is not a guarantee that metals are not a problem. A blood test can only detect toxic metals that are floating freely in your blood that day. It cannot detect metals sequestered in your organs, brain, and bones, as they commonly are.

There is also a "challenge test" for mercury, which is done by first injecting a substance to liberate it from storage and then testing your urine. I do not recommend challenge testing because it can expose you to a lot of mercury all at once. I hope the future will bring better, more reliable, and safer methods of metal testing.

Plastics, pesticides, and other toxins

Some doctors test for plastics, pesticides, PCBs, and flame retardants. Such a test might be helpful if it alerts you to a source of exposure of which you were not aware. But if you already *know* you have toxic exposure, then you won't gain much from knowing your exact level.

For all kinds of toxins, it's simpler to just proceed with a gentle detoxification lifestyle such as the one described below. That's what I recommend for my own patients.

Minimize Your Exposure

We are all exposed to toxins, so we all have to make the best of a bad situation. Until our governments legislate tougher restrictions, we can only minimize our individual exposure. We cannot completely avoid toxins.

With that in mind, please make sensible, obvious choices *when you can*. For example, choose organic if you can afford it. If you cannot afford it, then it's okay. You do not need to fear non-organic food. It's better to eat non-organic vegetables than to eat no vegetables at all.

Plastics, solvents, pesticides

Avoid as much as possible the toxic chemicals used in farming, gardening, and building materials. For example, reject unnecessary domestic products such as air fresheners, dryer sheets, and chemical carpet cleaners. And if you can, use an activated carbon water filter to remove pesticides from your drinking water—especially if you live in a rural, agricultural area.

Choose cosmetics and body products that do not include phthalates, arsenic, or other toxins (see the EWG website for more information). And always wash your hands after handling cash register receipts, because they're high in BPA.

Mercury

Mercury comes from fish and dental amalgams.

Reduce your intake of large fish. The mercury in fish ultimately comes from the pollution from coal-fired power plants throughout the world. Mercury enters the air and then falls into the water. There, bacteria convert mercury to methylmercury, which enters the fish's food supply. Little fish eat mercury, then bigger fish eat the little fish. That's how mercury becomes more and more concentrated as it goes up the food chain. And that's why big fish such as tuna, swordfish, and marlin have the most mercury. Small fish such as salmon, oysters, sardines, flounder, squid, anchovies, and herring have the *least* mercury. Small fish are a healthy food.

Consider having your amalgam fillings removed. You do not necessarily have to remove every amalgam. It's only something to think about if you have more than two amalgams and if your health problems are not improving with other treatments. The removal of amalgams is best done by a dentist who understands the correct protocol. Done incorrectly, amalgam removal can expose you to more mercury than if you just left them in your teeth.

Pesticides on food

Foods with the highest pesticide residues include animal fat, grains, and certain types of fresh produce.

Every year, the EWG publishes a list of the produce with the highest level of contamination.

Diet and Lifestyle to Support Detoxification

Your body is made to detoxify. Detoxification is the biggest and most energy-consuming activity your cells undertake, and they do it *every minute of every day.*

How can you support healthy detoxification on an ongoing basis?

- **Maintain healthy gut bacteria,** because they play a key role in escorting toxins out of your body. See the Digestive Health section below.
- **Avoid food sensitivities** like gluten and cow's dairy. They create inflammation in the gut, which can impair healthy detoxification.
- **Reduce or eliminate alcohol** to maintain a healthy liver. Remember, your liver is your primary detoxification center.
- **Get enough sleep**, because deep sleep is when you

recycle glutathione to its active form.
- **Sweat** in the sauna or during exercise to mobilize and eliminate stored toxins. Be sure to drink plenty of water.

Supplements and Herbal Medicines to Aid Detoxification

The best supplements for detoxification are those that support the production of glutathione. We met glutathione in Chapter 6. It's your body's master antioxidant and detoxifying molecule. It also regulates your immune system and reduces inflammation. The more glutathione you have, the healthier you will be and the better equipped to detoxify mercury, pesticides, and other toxins.

The best supplements to boost glutathione are:

Liposomal glutathione, which is an absorbable preparation of glutathione itself.

> **What else you need to know:** Taking glutathione in this way has been shown to raise the blood level of glutathione and reduce oxidative stress.[406] The standard dose is 100 to 400 mg per day taken on an empty stomach.

Milk thistle (silymarin) is a herbal medicine traditionally used for liver health.

> **How it works:** It boosts glutathione and protects liver cells from toxic damage.

> **What else you need to know:** The exact quantity of the herb depends on the concentration in the formula, so please use as directed on the bottle.

Turmeric or **curcumin**. I've already recommended turmeric for its anti-inflammatory properties, and its effectiveness for heavy periods and endometriosis (Chapter 9). We now come to its hidden power: it also boosts glutathione.[407]

> **How it works:** It reduces inflammation, boosts glutathione, and protects liver cells from toxic damage.

> **What else you need to know:** Turmeric is better absorbed when taken directly after a meal.

N-acetyl cysteine (NAC) is one of my favorite supplements for supporting healthy detoxification. We've already looked at it as a treatment for inflammatory PCOS and endometriosis.

> **How it works:** It boosts glutathione and also binds to mercury to draw it out of your body.

> **What else you need to know:** NAC has the nice side benefit of reducing anxiety. Too much NAC can thin your stomach lining so do not take it if you have gastritis or stomach ulcers. I recommend 500 to 2000 mg per day.

Alpha-lipoic acid is helpful for detoxification. We also saw it as a treatment for insulin-resistant PCOS in Chapter 7.

> **How it works:** It improves insulin sensitivity and boosts glutathione.

> **What else you need to know:** Alpha-lipoic acid is safe, but doses greater than 1000 mg can decrease thyroid hormone. I recommend 300 to 600 mg per day with food.

Selenium is an important anti-inflammatory and detoxifying mineral. We've already seen it a few times for PMS, ovarian cysts, and endometriosis.

> **How it works:** It boosts glutathione.

> **What else you need to know:** The therapeutic dose is 100 to 150 mcg per day. Higher amounts can be toxic, so please do not exceed 200 mcg per day from all sources, including high-selenium foods such as brazil nuts.

Magnesium aids with detoxification.

> **How it works:** It supports detoxification pathways through your liver and kidneys. It also actively pushes out toxic metals such as lead and cadmium. See previous magnesium sections for dosing instructions.

Digestive Health

You cannot have truly healthy periods until you have a healthy digestive system. It is really that simple. One way that digestive problems affect periods is by forcing you to undereat which, as we saw in Chapter 7, can then cause you to lose your period. The other way that digestive problems affect periods is by impairing your gut microbiome.

Gut Microbiome

Recall that your gut microbiome is the genetic material of the bacteria that live in your gut. When you have a friendly gut microbiome, it does many good things for your hormonal health. For example, it regulates your HPA axis, activates thyroid hormone, reduces inflammation, and metabolizes estrogen.

When you have an unfriendly microbiome, then you have a condition called *dysbiosis*, which means an unhealthy change to your normal bacterial ecology. Dysbiosis can disrupt your HPA axis, interfere with thyroid hormone, and impair estrogen metabolism.

Dysbiosis is a common reason for many period problems. It can also affect your vaginal microbiome, which we'll discuss later in the chapter.

Fortunately, there are many things you can do to improve your gut health.

How to maintain a healthy gut microbiome

- **Avoid, as much as possible, drugs that damage gut bacteria.** That includes hormonal birth control, stomach acid medication, and *antibiotics*. I cannot emphasize this enough. See Kate's story below.
- **Avoid concentrated sugar**, because it feeds unfriendly bacteria.
- **Avoid food sensitivities such as wheat and dairy**, because they create inflammation.
- **Eat vegetables and healthy starches**, because they feed friendly bacteria.
- **Reduce alcohol**, because alcohol causes dysbiosis.
- **Get enough sleep**, because sleep deprivation causes

dysbiosis.
- **Reduce stress**, because stress causes dysbiosis.
- **Eat fermented foods** such as natural yogurt and sauerkraut, because they support friendly bacteria.
- **Ensure adequate stomach acid** because you need stomach acid to kill unfriendly bacteria and digest protein. If you experience digestive bloating and heartburn, then you may have *low stomach acid*. Consider taking a digestive enzyme that supports stomach acid.
- **Consider taking a probiotic** which is a capsule containing beneficial bacteria.

 ## Kate: Recurrent chest infections and antibiotics

Kate came to me for help with fatigue, PMS, and chronic yeast infections.

"The yeast infections are from antibiotics," she told me. "I have to take them every few months for bronchitis."

Me: "Every few months!"

Kate: "Yes, my doctor says I need them because one time my chest got so bad, it turned into pneumonia. I don't want that to happen again, so I take the antibiotics. But I always take a probiotic after."

"A probiotic can help," I said. "But it isn't enough. It cannot replace the species of good bacteria you lose every time you take antibiotics."

I then went on to explain how *dysbiosis* (a problem with her gut bacteria) could be contributing to her fatigue and PMS.

"Dysbiosis impairs your ability to metabolize and detoxify estrogen," I said. "That means you end up having *too much estrogen*. Dysbiosis also generates a lot of inflammation, which can interfere with progesterone and other hormones."

"Is there a better probiotic I could take?" Kate asked.

"I have a different plan," I said. "Let's find a way for you to *not* need the antibiotics."

Kate had never considered that as a possibility.

I suggested we work on her immune system to prevent the future use of antibiotics and therefore give her gut microbiome a chance to recover.

"I consider immune treatment to be the key part of your hormonal treatment," I said.

I asked Kate to stop having normal cow's milk because I felt it was disrupting her immune function and putting her at risk of chest infections. I prescribed zinc, vitamin D, and a medicinal mushroom extract to improve her immunity. I also prescribed a probiotic with the strains *Lactobacillus rhamnosus* (LGG®) and *Lactobacillus plantarum* (HEAL 9), which have been clinically demonstrated to support immunity and reduce the severity of acute viral infections.[408]

Kate did get one more mild chest infection but managed to avoid antibiotics. By the time we met six months later, she'd had no more chest infections. Her energy and her PMS were also improved.

Kate stopped the mushroom extract and the probiotic but continued the zinc, vitamin D, and dairy-free diet as ongoing immune support.

 Antibiotics are amazing life-saving drugs. But if you're healthy, you should not expect to need them more than three or four times in your *lifetime*.

As you can see, I prescribed a probiotic for Kate, but I chose one with the particular purpose of supporting her immune function so she could avoid future antibiotics. Later in the chapter, I'll refer to other specific strains of probiotic bacteria that are helpful for intestinal permeability and the vaginal microbiome.

At this stage in my clinical practice, I lean more and more toward choosing a probiotic that contains a strain, or strains, of microorganisms that have been clinically trialed for a particular purpose. Gone are the days of the shotgun twelve-strain probiotic.

How to choose a probiotic

Our understanding of the gut microbiome is still in its infancy.

At this stage, we know that *certain strains* of probiotics work for *certain conditions*, but we *cannot* say there is one best probiotic that works for everyone. And research is moving so quickly that we're likely to see countless new strains of probiotics in the coming years. My selection of the best probiotic changes as new research comes to light.

Here are some things to understand:

- Probiotic species *do not* colonize your gut. In other words, they do not become established as permanent residents in your intestine. Instead, they exert beneficial effects on your microbiome, intestinal wall, and immune system as they *pass through*.
- Clinical benefits have been demonstrated for specific *strains* (or subtypes) of bacteria. You may not get the same benefit from another strain of the same species.
- Different probiotic strains work for different conditions. For example, the probiotic strain *Lactobacillus plantarum 299v* is clinically proven to treat irritable bowel syndrome (see below). The strains *Lactobacillus rhamnosus*, GR-1 and *Lactobacillus reuteri*, RC-14 can normalize vaginal microbiome and relieve yeast infections (see below).
- It's better to choose a product with many individual bacteria but *fewer* strains or types of bacteria. That way, each strain can have a more targeted effect.
- Probiotics work better in combination with a prebiotic or fiber supplement. Such products are called *synbiotics*.

- Diet has a more powerful effect on the microbiome than any probiotic.
- If you experience digestive bloating from a probiotic, then it could be a sign you have SIBO. With SIBO, you may benefit more from a course of a herbal antimicrobial than you do from a probiotic.

Intestinal Permeability

I referred to intestinal permeability when we discussed food sensitivities in Chapter 6 and endometriosis in Chapter 9. It's an important topic because it's a potential cause of inflammation.

Intestinal permeability is a condition in which tiny microscopic gaps or leaks form between the cells of your intestinal wall. Normally, your intestinal cells should be tightly joined to create a barrier to prevent bacteria and food proteins from entering your body. Intestinal permeability occurs when that barrier is breached by infection, antibiotics, hormonal birth control, SIBO, or inflammatory foods such as gluten.

When you develop intestinal permeability, food proteins and bacterial toxins enter your body and can stimulate your immune system to make inflammatory cytokines.

How to treat intestinal permeability

- Consider avoiding gluten, because it can cause or worsen intestinal permeability.
- Improve the health of your gut microbiome (see above) and treat SIBO (see below).
- Consider a short course of treatment with the herbal medicine berberine (see the IBS and SIBO section below).
- Supplement zinc, because it repairs the integrity of the intestinal barrier.[409]
- Supplement with a strain of probiotic such as *Lactobacillus rhamnosus* (LGG®), because it can help to repair the integrity of the intestinal barrier.[410]

Inflammatory Bowel Disease (IBD)

The most serious digestive problem is *inflammatory bowel disease* which includes Crohn's disease, ulcerative colitis, and celiac disease. Treatment of IBD is beyond the scope of this book. Please seek professional advice.

Irritable Bowel Syndrome (IBS) and Small Intestinal Bacterial Overgrowth (SIBO)

A less serious digestive problem is *irritable bowel syndrome* (IBS), which causes pain, bloating, diarrhea, and constipation. IBS can be the result of SIBO, which is the overgrowth of normal bacteria in the small intestine.

Your gut bacteria are supposed to live down in your *large* intestine. Various perturbations can cause them to move up into your small intestine, resulting in SIBO. Common perturbations include infection, antibiotics, stomach acid drugs, thyroid disease,[411] and the oral contraceptive pill.

Once bacteria move up into your small intestine, they can cause IBS, intestinal permeability, and inflammation. That inflammation can then cause or worsen your period problems.

Natural treatment of IBS and SIBO

Consider a short-term low FODMAP diet. As we saw in Chapter 6, FODMAPs are fermentable carbohydrates. Bacteria ferment FODMAPs, which is fine as long as the bacteria are in the large intestine where they're supposed to be. If bacteria are in your small intestine (SIBO), the fermentation of FODMAPs can cause bloating and inflammation.

A low-FODMAP diet can give short-term relief, but I don't see it as a solution in the long-term. For one thing, a low-FODMAP diet is restrictive and may cause you to undereat. Also, a low-FODMAP diet can starve the bacteria in your large intestine of the fiber they need to keep you healthy.

A better plan is to do a short-term low-FODMAP diet, but to also treat the underlying SIBO with a herbal antimicrobial.

Berberine is one of several antimicrobial herbal medicines that were used in a John Hopkins University study to treat SIBO.[412] The researchers concluded that the berberine combination is as effective as antibiotics for treating SIBO.

How it works: Berberine is antimicrobial and reduces the overgrowth of bacteria in the small intestine. It also repairs intestinal permeability.[413]

What else you need to know: I usually prescribe an eight-week course of berberine in combination with other herbal antimicrobials, such as oregano oil. Metagenics® Candibactin-BR is an example of a product with berberine and oregano. Please do not take berberine for more than eight weeks continuously except under professional advice. Refer to the berberine section in Chapter 7 for further precautions and dosing instructions. Sometimes one course of treatment with an antimicrobial is enough to resolve SIBO. But sometimes a second course is required.

Even once you've addressed SIBO and resolved your IBS symptoms, you are at risk for recurrence. Here are some ways to prevent that:

- Avoid food sensitivities such as wheat and dairy, because they can create inflammation that impairs bowel motility.
- Identify and treat an underlying thyroid problem, because underactive thyroid can cause SIBO.
- Avoid as much as possible drugs that cause SIBO. They include antibiotics, stomach acid medication, and the oral contraceptive pill.
- Consider taking a digestive enzyme to support stomach acid, because stomach acid promotes healthy bowel motility.
- Consider taking the probiotic strain *Lactobacillus plantarum 299v*, which treats IBS.
- Consider taking milk thistle, because it promotes bowel motility.

Some probiotics can *worsen* the digestive bloating associated with SIBO.

Digestive health is a complex topic. A full discussion is beyond the scope of this book. If your symptoms do not improve, then seek professional advice.

Yeast Infections and Bacterial Vaginosis

As we saw in Chapter 5, both yeast infections and bacterial vaginosis (BV) are caused by a disrupted vaginal microbiome. That means, ultimately, that they're caused by a disrupted gut microbiome. The two populations of bacteria are connected. Think of it as your *whole-body ecosystem.*

The best way to treat yeast infections and vaginosis is to do all the things described above to maintain a healthy gut microbiome *plus* these additional recommendations for vaginal microbiome:

- Supplement with the probiotic strains *Lactobacillus rhamnosus*, GR-1 and *Lactobacillus reuteri*, RC-14 which have been clinically proven to improve yeast and bacterial vaginosis.[414] The probiotic combination works when taken orally, but you can also insert it vaginally for additional benefit.
- Do not use a feminine wash or douche, because it depletes your friendly vaginal bacteria.
- Do not use spermicide, because it depletes your friendly vaginal bacteria.
- Consider whether your IUD is contributing to the problem. The copper IUD doubles the risk of bacterial vaginosis (BV).[415] The main symptom of BV is vaginal discharge with a fishy odor.

Thyroid Disease

Looking back, you'll see that I've mentioned thyroid disease in almost every chapter in the book. You will not be surprised when I say that thyroid health is a major factor in period health.

Your thyroid is a butterfly-shaped gland in the front of your throat. It manufactures thyroid hormone, which is a small protein hormone made from tyrosine and iodine. Thyroid hormone is the ignition switch for each and every cell. It stimulates the burning of calories and the manufacture of proteins.

Thyroid hormone is essential for all metabolic activity, including healthy digestion, detoxification, and ovulation.

How Thyroid Disease Causes Period Problems

The most common type of thyroid disorder is hypothyroidism (underactive thyroid), which occurs when the thyroid does not make enough hormone. Hyperthyroidism (overactive thyroid) can also affect periods, but it is less common.

Hypothyroidism interferes with period health in the following ways:

- It stimulates prolactin which suppresses ovulation (Chapter 7).
- It worsens insulin resistance and increases your risk of PCOS (Chapter 7).
- It impairs the healthy metabolism of estrogen, and so causes estrogen excess.
- It robs your ovaries of the cellular energy they need to ovulate, and so causes anovulation and low progesterone.
- It decreases coagulation factors, and so causes heavy bleeding (Chapter 9).

Hypothyroidism affects at least one in ten women. It is often overlooked because it's difficult to detect with a standard blood test.

Diagnosis

The standard test for thyroid disease is a blood test for thyroid-stimulating hormone (TSH).

When your thyroid gland is making enough thyroid hormone, it signals your pituitary to make *less* TSH.

When your thyroid gland is *not* making enough thyroid hormone, it signals your pituitary to make *more* TSH.

Therefore, insufficient thyroid hormone causes a high TSH reading on a blood test. High TSH means you have underactive thyroid or hypothyroidism.

TSH controversy

There is some debate about what should be considered "high" TSH. Under current guidelines, your doctor cannot diagnose underactive thyroid until your TSH is greater than 5 or 6 mIU/L. In other words, until your TSH is greater than 5 mIU/L, you are considered to have *normal* thyroid function.

Fifteen years ago, the American National Academy of Clinical Biochemistry dropped the upper limit of TSH to 2.5 mIU/L, and the American Association of Clinical Endocrinologists (AACE) quickly followed suit.[416] Under those proposed guidelines, your doctor could diagnose underactive thyroid when your TSH was only 2.5 mIU/L. It was a game-changer because, suddenly, thousands of people with a borderline thyroid problem could be treated with thyroid hormone.

That would have been particularly important for women because women have better outcomes with fertility and pregnancy when their TSH is *less* than 2.5 mIU/L.[417]

Unfortunately, the new 2.5 TSH guideline was not widely adopted by labs or doctors, and so most doctors today still adhere to the old 5 mIU/L cutoff. It means that doctors today are missing opportunities to treat thyroid disease and help women with period and fertility problems.

With my own patients, I suspect thyroid to be a possible issue if the TSH reading is consistently greater than 3 mIU/L.

There's another problem

If your TSH is less than 3 mIU/L, then it should mean you have normal function. However, TSH can be artificially suppressed by many things including stress and chronic inflammation. In other words, you could have a normal TSH but still be suffering underactive thyroid.

You need to consider symptoms.

Thyroid symptoms

The most common symptoms of underactive thyroid include:

- fatigue
- irregular periods
- heavy periods
- infertility
- hair loss
- dry skin
- cracked heels
- fluid retention
- high cholesterol on blood test
- feeling cold all the time
- digestive problems including SIBO
- brain fog
- depression.

 Up to 20 percent of depression may be due to an undiagnosed problem with thyroid.

Of course, many of those same symptoms can be due other causes. For example, fatigue could be the result of iron deficiency or sleep problems. But if you suffer from the majority of these symptoms, and especially if you have thyroid disease in your family, then speak to your doctor about another test for thyroid disease called *thyroid antibodies*.

Thyroid antibodies

Thyroid antibodies are an autoimmune response against your thyroid gland. It's a type of inflammation and is one of the best tests for identifying a thyroid problem.

If you test positive for thyroid antibodies, you may have an autoimmune disease called Hashimoto's thyroid disease, which accounts for 90 percent of hypothyroidism in Western countries.

Hashimoto's thyroid disease runs in families, so you are more likely to suffer it if your mother or sister had it.

Conventional Treatment of Thyroid Disease

Thyroid hormone

The conventional treatment of thyroid disease is to give thyroid hormone usually in the form of levothyroxine, which is natural T4 hormone. Levothyroxine will return your TSH to the normal range, and for most of you, it will improve symptoms. For some of you, it will not improve symptoms. Up to 10 percent of thyroid patients continue to have symptoms on thyroxine, even when their TSH is normal.[418] If that's happening to you, ask your doctor for a combination of T4 and T3 hormone. T3 is the active form of thyroid hormone, and there's growing evidence it's better for symptoms.[419] More and more doctors are willing to prescribe it.

Desiccated thyroid gland (from a pig) is another popular type of thyroid hormone supplement, and was the type historically used before the popularity of levothyroxine. It naturally contains both T4 and T3. A 2013 clinical study concluded that desiccated thyroid is safe and preferred by the majority of patients.[420]

I consider thyroid hormone (even levothyroxine) to be a natural and highly beneficial treatment. If your blood test says that you require it, I encourage you to take it. You can also implement some of the natural thyroid treatments described below.

All types of thyroid hormone (including desiccated thyroid) must be prescribed by your doctor.

Diet and Lifestyle for Thyroid Disease

Avoid gluten

The best natural treatment for thyroid disease is to reduce

autoimmunity by avoiding inflammatory foods, especially gluten. A gluten-free diet has been shown to reduce thyroid antibodies and improve thyroid function in patients with celiac disease.[421]

Correct intestinal permeability

By correcting intestinal permeability, you can protect your immune system from the bacterial toxins and other proteins that can worsen autoimmune thyroid disease. Refer to the Intestinal Permeability section earlier in the chapter.

Identify and treat the Epstein-Barr virus

Infection may play a role in autoimmune thyroid disease. For example, the Epstein-Barr virus has been identified as a possible cause of Hashimoto's disease.[422] Epstein-Barr virus is common, and is dormant in most of us from a prior infection. If the virus reactivates, it can trigger or worsen thyroid disease. The best treatment for Epstein-Barr is to support the immune system with natural anti-viral treatments such as zinc, selenium, and vitamin D.

Supplements and Herbal Medicine for Thyroid Disease

Ashwagandha (*Withania somnifera*)is the herbal medicine we considered as a treatment for hypothalamic amenorrhea in Chapter 7 and perimenopause in Chapter 10. It also helps thyroid.

> **How it works:** Ashwagandha stimulates the healthy production of thyroid hormone.[423] It also reduces inflammation and stabilizes the HPA axis or stress response system.

> **What else you need to know:** The exact quantity of the medicine depends on the concentration of the formula, so please take as directed on the bottle. Doses range from 300 to 3000 mg and may be taken in a formula that contains other adaptogens such as Rhodiola. Ashwagandha works best when taken for at least three months.

Selenium is a key nutrient for thyroid.

How it works: It reduces inflammation and thyroid antibodies.[424][425] It also aids with the activation of T4 to T3 and can protect your thyroid from iodine.

What else you need to know: The therapeutic dose is 100 to 150 mcg per day. Higher amounts can be toxic, so please do not exceed 200 mcg per day from all sources, including high-selenium foods such as brazil nuts.

Iodine is controversial for thyroid disease. Your thyroid needs iodine, and iodine deficiency is the primary cause of thyroid disease in some parts of the world. Iodine deficiency is not the primary cause of thyroid disease in Western countries— autoimmunity is. And unfortunately, too much iodine can cause or worsen thyroid autoimmunity.

If you do *not* have thyroid antibodies, then you can take a small amount of iodine and it may promote healthy thyroid function. Refer to the Iodine section in Chapter 6 for safe dosing instructions.

If you *do* have thyroid antibodies, then you should not take iodine for your thyroid.

How it works: Iodine is an essential part of thyroid hormone.

What else you need to know: Do not exceed 500 mcg (0.5 mg) except under professional advice.

Thyroid disease is a complex topic. A full discussion is beyond the scope of this book. Please seek professional advice.

Hair Loss

Hair loss is a common symptom that can sometimes result from a problem with female hormones, but can also be due to a large number of causes including:

- post-partum
- illness

- undereating
- low-carb diet
- celiac disease or gluten sensitivity
- stress
- thyroid disease
- iron deficiency
- zinc deficiency
- protein deficiency
- hormonal birth control
- stopping hormonal birth control
- antidepressant medication
- alopecia areata (autoimmune disease that causes patchy hair loss)
- PCOS or androgen excess.

Yes, it's a long list, but your only hope to recover your hair is to identify the cause (or causes) and correct *that*. For example, if you have iron deficiency, then take iron. If you have PCOS, then treat PCOS.

When considering the cause of your hair loss, keep in mind that the cause comes first and then the hair loss about three months later. With my own patients, I often draw out a timeline to figure out what is going on. See the Time Lag section below.

Depending on the cause and type of hair loss, your doctor will diagnose you with either *telogen effluvium* or *androgenetic alopecia*, or a combination of the two. According to the American Hair Loss Association, the early stages of androgenetic alopecia are effectively telogen effluvium.[426]

Telogen effluvium means "hair falling out" due to *something*. That *something* is one of the things listed above such as after childbirth (post-partum), stress, illness, dieting, or stopping birth control. That something could also be exposure to androgens or male hormones, in which case telogen effluvium will develop into androgenetic alopecia.

Androgenetic alopecia (female pattern hair loss) is progressive hair loss caused by male hormones or a *sensitivity* to male hormones. It causes a widening of the part and a diffuse thinning and miniaturization of the hair follicles. It can go on for years and is not easy to reverse.

We discussed androgenetic alopecia in two places in the book. First, in Chapter 2 where we saw that hormonal birth control with a high androgen index can cause androgenetic alopecia, and then again in the Female Pattern Hair Loss treatment section in Chapter 7.

I know from my conversations with many patients that hair loss is distressing. It's distressing because it takes a long time to improve, and also because it's difficult to resolve with any treatment, including conventional treatments.

Conventional Treatment of Hair Loss

Hormonal birth control

Progestins with a low androgen index (see Chapter 2) can, in theory, be helpful for androgenetic alopecia because they block androgens. Unfortunately, my experience with patients is that they don't work all that well, probably because they also suppress progesterone. Remember, progesterone is great for hair!

Spironolactone (Aldactone®)

We met this androgen-suppressing drug as a treatment for PCOS in Chapter 7. It's almost the same drug as the progestin drospirenone used in the birth control pill Yasmin®. My observation is that stopping the drug can result in even worse hair loss.

Minoxidil (Rogaine®)

It's a blood pressure drug that has been "repurposed" to be applied topically and improve blood supply to the hair follicles. Paradoxically, one of its side effects is hair loss.

Natural Treatment of Hair Loss

The only way to treat hair loss is to identify the underlying cause (or causes) and treat that.

I know it can be overwhelming, so I've broken it down into eight simple questions:

Is it your medication?

Many medications cause hair loss including antibiotics, antifungals, acne medication, antidepressants, and hormonal birth control. And remember, your hair loss would have started at least three months *after* starting the medication. Speak to your doctor about an alternative.

Are you eating enough?

Your hair needs you to be fully nourished in every respect, including all the macro- and micronutrients we discussed in Chapter 6. You're at risk for hair loss if you follow a vegan or low-carb diet.

Is it your thyroid?

Both underactive and overactive thyroid can cause hair loss. Keep in mind that your doctor may have missed a thyroid diagnosis. Refer to the Thyroid Disease section earlier in this chapter.

Do you ovulate?

Your hair *loves* estrogen and progesterone, and the only way to make those hormones is to ovulate each month and have a natural, healthy menstrual cycle.

 Your period is the report card of your health. Your hair is *also* a report card—to an even greater degree if that's possible.

Do you need zinc?

Zinc is great for hair because it promotes ovulation, reduces inflammation, and blocks androgens. It also directly stimulates hair growth. Common causes of zinc deficiency include a vegetarian diet and hormonal birth control.

Do you need iron?

Hair needs iron. So, no matter the cause of your hair loss, you will need sufficient iron to recover it. Ask your doctor to test serum ferritin, which should be at least 50 ng/mL. If it's lower than 50, then consider supplementing with 25 mg of a gentle iron such as iron bisglycinate.

Do you have PCOS?

Do you have the androgen excess condition PCOS? Are you sure? Remember, PCOS cannot be diagnosed or *ruled out* by ultrasound. If you *do* have PCOS, then you need to treat the driver of your type of PCOS, as well as consider taking an anti-androgen supplement such as DIM. You can also use a topical treatment such as rosemary, which has a local anti-androgen effect,[427] or melatonin, which reduces inflammation.[428] For a full discussion of PCOS and anti-androgen treatments, refer to Chapter 7.

Do you have chronic inflammation?

Chronic inflammation *hyper-sensitizes* hair follicles to androgens, which is why it can worsen androgen hypersensitivity and androgenetic alopecia. You'll have a clue that inflammation is an issue if you suffer chronic dermatitis or irritation of your scalp. Treatment is to remove inflammatory foods from your diet, and also to correct any underlying digestive problems. You can also consider the topical rosemary treatment described in the Female Pattern Hair Loss section in Chapter 7.

Time Lag

Even with the best treatment, you cannot expect to see any improvement for at least three to six months. Why? Because your hair has a telogen (resting) phase, which is like a "hair waiting room." Once your hairs have entered the telogen phase, they are destined to fall out one to four months later—*no matter what you do.*

> *telogen phase*
>
> Hairs in the telogen phase are dormant or resting before they fall out. The telogen phase has a fixed duration of one to four months. In contrast, hairs in the anagen phase are actively growing. The anagen phase has a variable duration of years.

For example, you may currently have a lot of hair in the telogen phase because of something that happened months ago. Those hairs are going to fall out, and there's nothing you can do to stop them. You can only work to prevent further hair loss three to six months from now.

Stay calm, be patient, and stick with your treatment.

How to Come Off Hormonal Birth Control

As we saw in the Coming Off the Pill section in Chapter 2, you will probably feel better when you stop hormonal birth control. Better mood, more energy, fewer headaches, and regular cycles. That is the most common experience.

You may, however, develop problems such as post-pill acne, PMS, PCOS, amenorrhea, anxiety, heavy periods, painful periods, and facial hair.

What causes post-pill symptoms? It's not the drugs themselves because they leave your body pretty quickly. Instead, post-pill syndrome is the result of:

- withdrawal from the strong synthetic estrogen
- surge in androgens (especially if you have a tendency to PCOS)
- real periods for the first time in years
- delay in establishing regular ovulation.

Estrogen withdrawal

The estrogen in the pill (ethinylestradiol) is four times stronger than your own lovely estradiol.[429] That much estrogen has a strongly stimulating effect on brain chemistry, which you will miss when you stop taking it. It's like coming off a drug.

What to do: Find a way to ovulate so you can make your own estrogen and progesterone. Refer to Chapter 7 for treatment strategies. You can also try a small amount of natural progesterone cream for its soothing effects on the brain. See the Natural Progesterone section in Chapter 10.

Surge in androgens

Your androgens (male hormones) will increase when you stop the pill. A small increase is beneficial for mood and libido, but a large increase can cause the unwanted androgen symptoms of acne, hair loss, and hirsutism. There are several reasons why you can end up with a large post-pill surge in androgens:

- You were on an *androgen-suppressing* progestin such as drospirenone or cyproterone, so your body had to compensate by upregulating androgen production. (For a discussion of the "androgen-index" of birth control, see Chapter 2.)
- You had an underlying tendency to PCOS *before* you took birth control.
- You developed insulin resistance from hormonal birth control and so now tend to insulin-resistant PCOS.

We looked at the problem of a post-pill surge in androgens in both the Post-Pill Acne section in Chapter 2, and the Post-Pill PCOS section in Chapter 7.

What to do: If you're prone to acne and other androgen symptoms then, please start treatment at least one month *before* you stop the pill. For androgen-lowering and acne treatment ideas, see the Acne Treatment and Anti-Androgen Treatment sections in Chapter 7.

Real periods for the first time in years

If you want to know what to expect when going off hormonal birth control, here's one simple question: what were your periods like before you took birth control? I'm not talking about your pill-bleeds—because they are not periods. I'm talking about your real periods—the ones you had before you went on the pill ten or more years ago.

Were those real periods regular? Were they heavy or painful? Did your skin break out? Because those problems have not gone away. They have merely been masked by birth control, and they will most likely re-emerge.

What to do: Forget that you've just come off birth control and go back to the drawing board to treat the period problem that has *always been there*. For example, for PMS, see Chapter 8. For heavy or painful periods, see Chapter 9.

 If you have a history of endometriosis, I recommend you begin the natural treatment for endometriosis at least one month before you stop the pill.

Delay in establishing regular ovulation

If you're struggling with PCOS or amenorrhea after coming off birth control, you're not alone. It is sometimes called "post-pill syndrome," and as we saw with Christine in Chapter 1, it can take months, even years, to ovulate.

What to do: Try not to panic. It might take a long time to get your period and it's not a problem with you—but rather with the ovulation-suppressing drug you were given!

There are lots of things you can do to promote ovulation. For treatment ideas, see the Post-Pill PCOS and Hypothalamic Amenorrhea sections in Chapter 7.

How to Talk to Your Doctor

If you've ever come out of your doctor's office feeling frustrated and confused, then you know how important this section is. Your doctor did not mean to confuse you. She was trying to help, and she probably came away feeling pretty confused herself. It's because you were talking apples and oranges to each other.

For example, you wanted to talk about "estrogen dominance," but your doctor wasn't familiar with that term. All she knew is that you have heavy periods, and she wanted to treat you with a clinically proven treatment such as the Mirena® IUD. Your doctor doesn't know about the natural treatment options. Of course, she was perplexed as to why you hesitate or delay.

Going forward, it doesn't have to be like that. Your doctor wants to help you, and she *will* help you—if you just learn how to talk to each other.

Here is a list of questions and statements to keep the conversation on track.

No periods or irregular periods

- I'm not sure I'm eating enough. Could that be why I'm not getting periods?
- I feel quite anxious about food, and think I might have an eating disorder. Can you help me?
- Have I been screened for celiac disease? I've heard that can cause amenorrhea.
- Have I been tested for thyroid disease? What is my actual TSH reading? I've heard it should ideally be less than 3.
- Have I been tested for high prolactin?
- Could one of my medications be stopping my period?
- I'm vegetarian. Can you check my levels of iron, zinc, and vitamin B12?
- Is there any chance I'm in menopause? Have you checked my FSH?
- What is my actual diagnosis? Is it PCOS? Is it hypothalamic amenorrhea?

You're told you have PCOS

- Was this diagnosis based solely on my ultrasound? I understand that PCOS cannot be diagnosed that way.

- My symptoms are only since I came off the pill. I never had this problem before. Is it possible it's just a post-pill adjustment and might get better on its own?
- Have you ruled out a condition called adrenal hyperplasia?
- Do I have insulin resistance? I understand it cannot be diagnosed by a glucose test. Can you please test me for "fasting insulin" or a "glucose tolerance test with insulin"?
- Do I have elevated testosterone or another androgen such as androstenedione or DHEAS?
- Do I have elevated LH?
- Can you check me for deficiency of zinc and vitamin D?
- Can you please test my progesterone? I want to see if I ovulated. (Remember, a progesterone test must be timed to be about one week *after* ovulation or one week *before* your next expected period.)
- I know I used to have PCOS, but everything is fine now. My periods are coming regularly, and I have no symptoms. I don't think I meet the diagnostic criteria anymore.

Hair loss

- Have I been tested for thyroid? What is my actual TSH reading? I've heard it should be less than 3.
- Have I been tested for iron? What is my actual ferritin reading? I've heard it should ideally be greater than 50 ng/mL.
- Have I been tested for celiac disease?
- Could my hormonal birth control be causing my hair loss? (Your doctor may mistakenly say "no" to this one. Ask her to look it up.)
- My hair loss started a few months after _____. Could that be the cause?

You're being pressured to take hormonal birth control

- I want to try another method of birth control such as fertility awareness method, Daysy®, copper IUD, condoms, cervical cap, or diaphragm.

- I want the copper IUD. I understand it's safe and suitable for young women, even before children.
- I want the copper IUD. I understand it makes periods heavier, but only by 20 to 50 percent.
- Why exactly do I need the pill?
- I've heard that pill bleeds are not real bleeds. Could going on the pill now make it more difficult to get my real period later? (The answer is yes.)
- Are you saying I need the pill for my bone health? I understand that the new research says the pill doesn't actually help with bones.
- My periods were fine before I went on the pill. I understand it might take time to get my periods back. I'd like to give it a few more months.
- I've heard that hormonal birth control pill worsens insulin resistance and PCOS. Is it really the right choice for me?
- I am going to change my diet and take nutritional supplements to improve my insulin resistance and PCOS. I would like some time to do that.

Your doctor is skeptical of the fertility awareness method (FAM)

- You might be thinking of the rhythm method, which does not have a high efficacy. I'm doing something different. I'm using the symptothermal method of birth control where I track my morning temperature. Research shows that when done properly, it can be as effective as the pill.
- I'm using the Daysy Fertility Monitor®, which is a certified medical device with an efficacy of 99.4 percent.

You discover you're not ovulating

- I'm having periods, but I don't think I'm ovulating. I think they're called anovulatory cycles.
- Could you check this by testing my progesterone? (Remember, a progesterone test must be timed to be about one week *after* ovulation or one week *before* your

next expected period.)
- Do you think I could have PCOS? Can you test my insulin and testosterone?
- Can you please test my thyroid?

Heavy periods

- I lose__ mL of menstrual fluid per cycle, which is more than the acceptable upper limit of 80 mL.
- Have I been tested for thyroid? I understand it's a common reason for heavy periods.
- What is my actual TSH reading? I've heard it should be less than 3.
- My mother and sister have autoimmune thyroid disease. Can you check me for thyroid antibodies?
- My thyroid seems a little borderline. Could I please try some thyroid medication for a few months to see if it lightens my periods?
- Could I have a coagulation disorder like von Willebrand disease? I understand it's the reason for one in five cases of heavy periods.
- Have I been tested for iron? What is my actual ferritin reading? I've heard it should ideally be greater than 50 ng/mL.
- Do I have insulin resistance? Can you please test me for "fasting insulin" or a "glucose tolerance test with insulin?"
- Do I have fibroids? Are they contributing to my bleeding? I've heard that most fibroids do NOT cause heavy bleeding.
- Could I have endometriosis? Should I have a referral to a gynecologist to discuss this possibility?
- Could I have adenomyosis? Should I have a referral to a gynecologist to discuss this possibility?
- Can you consider prescribing Prometrium®? I understand it works as well as Primolut® to reduce heavy bleeding, but without the side effects.

Pelvic pain

- My pain is so bad I take ____ painkillers per month.
- My pain is so bad that I miss school or work.
- I experience pain between periods.
- I experience a deep, stabbing pain with sex.
- Could I have endometriosis? Should I have a referral to a gynecologist to discuss this possibility?
- Could I have adenomyosis? Should I have a referral to a gynecologist to discuss this possibility?
- Do you think a pelvic ultrasound would be helpful?
- A normal ultrasound doesn't mean I don't have endometriosis, correct? Should I have a referral to a gynecologist to discuss the possibility of endometriosis?

You're going to have surgery for endometriosis

- What type of surgical method will you use?
- I've heard there is a better long-term outcome with something called "excision surgery."
- Will you remove all the lesions?
- Will the tissue be sent to pathology for identification?
- Do you have experience removing endometriosis from the bladder or bowel?

Perimenopausal mood symptoms

- My premenstrual symptoms are getting worse. I understand it's because I'm perimenopausal and I don't make as much progesterone as I used to.
- Can you consider prescribing Prometrium®? According to this Canadian endocrinologist, it can relieve symptoms. (And then show her Dr Prior's document "Progesterone Therapy for Symptomatic Perimenopause" listed in the Resources section.)
- Have you tested my thyroid?
- What is my actual TSH reading? I've heard it should be less than 3.

You're being pressured to have a hysterectomy

- Is the Mirena® IUD an option for me?
- Is endometrial ablation an option for me?
- Is uterine artery embolization an option for me?
- Would you recommend this procedure for yourself, your wife, or your daughter?
- I understand that fibroids and bleeding often resolve with menopause. Can I try to hold on until then?
- Have you tested my FSH? If it is high, does that suggest I might enter menopause soon? Can I try to hold on until then?
- My mother went through menopause at 45 (for example). Does that suggest I might enter menopause soon? Can I try to hold on until then?
- Can you consider prescribing Prometrium®? I understand it works as well as Primolut® to reduce heavy bleeding, but without the side effects.

If you previously had a hysterectomy and want to know if you have reached menopause

- Have I reached menopause? Can you please test my FSH so we can find out?

How Long Will It Take to See Results?

I hope you are excited about all the new treatments to try! If you're like my patients, then your very next question is: "How long until I see results?"

It's a good question, and the answer depends on which symptoms you're trying to treat. Let's have a look.

Days or weeks

PMS can improve in just hours as soon as you boost GABA with magnesium and vitamin B6. It should then steadily improve over a few months as you avoid inflammatory foods and enhance progesterone.

Normal period pain should improve within the very first month of treatment as soon as you remove dairy and take zinc. It should then completely resolve after a few months.

There are two parts to the improvement of both PMS and period pain. The first part is to reduce estrogen and inflammation. That happens quickly over days or weeks. The next part is to enhance progesterone. That takes 100 days for your ovarian follicles to complete their journey to ovulation.

One to two months

Endometriosis can also start to improve fairly quickly. You can expect some results as inflammation goes down in the first one to two months. After that, improvement should be slow but steady over six months or more.

If you're a teenager, your **heavy periods** should improve from the second month after you remove dairy and take iron.

If you're in perimenopause, your **heavy periods** can also improve reasonably quickly with dairy-free diet, iron, turmeric, and progesterone capsules unless there's an underlying problem with thyroid or insulin resistance. Then your improvement will take longer (see below).

Fibroids should stop growing within the first couple of months. Then you will need to maintain the treatment until the fibroids shrink with menopause. Fibroids usually will not shrink with natural treatment.

Three to six months

If your **heavy periods of perimenopause** are due to a problem with thyroid or insulin resistance (or both), then you'll need at least three months to address those underlying conditions before you see improvement with your periods.

Irregular periods (due to PCOS or hypothalamic amenorrhea) take a minimum of three months because that's how long it takes your ovarian follicles to journey all the way to ovulation. Of all the conditions discussed in Chapter 7, hidden-driver PCOS is the fastest to improve. Once you get the right treatment, you can expect a period within three months. Insulin-resistant PCOS takes longer because you must first correct insulin resistance, and that can take a few months. Only *then* can your follicles begin their 100-day journey to ovulation.

Acne will improve somewhat in the first month or two as you reduce inflammation. After that, you will have to wait at least six months because that's how long it takes to expel the sebum plugs that are blocking your pores. Post-pill acne will usually reach its worst point about six months off the pill. You can then expect full improvement about six months after that.

Six months to a year or more

Hair loss is slow to change. At the bare minimum, you'll have to wait three months because that's how long your hair stays in its telogen or resting phase. But that's once you get everything just right. If you have underlying hormonal problems, you'll need a few months to fix that, and then still have to wait another three months to see improvement in your hair.

Hirsutism is the slowest symptom to change. The life cycle of facial hair follicles is even longer than scalp hair follicles, so you cannot expect hirsutism to improve for at least twelve months. In the meantime, you can use hair removal methods such as tweezing, waxing, laser, and electrolysis.

A Final Message: Trust Your Body

Your body wants to be healthy. It wants to have healthy periods.

Treat the cause, and play the long game.

Stick with your treatment. Trust your body.

Appendix A

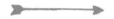

Resources

Author's Blog

- Lara Briden—The Period Revolutionary
  http://www.larabriden.com/

Period Apps and Body Literacy

- Clue: http://www.helloclue.com/
- Groove: http://www.readytogroove.com/
- Selene: http://daringplan.com/
- Daysy: https://daysy.me/
- Ovia: https://www.ovuline.com/

Menstrual Supplies

- Diva Cup: http://divacup.com/
- Lunette: http://www.lunette.com/
- Luna Pads: https://lunapads.com/

Contraception Resources

Fertility Awareness Method (FAM):

- Daysy fertility monitor: https://daysy.me/
- *Taking Charge of Your Fertility* by Toni Weschler
- http://sympto.org
- NaProTECHNOLOGY: http://www.naprotechnology.com/
- Fertility Friday: https://fertilityfriday.com/
- Kindara: https://www.kindara.com/home
- Justisse: https://www.justisse.ca/
- FACTS: http://www.factsaboutfertility.org/
- Natural Womanhood: https://naturalwomanhood.org/
- Tempdrop: https://tempdrop.xyz/

Other contraceptive methods

- Femcap cervical cap: https://femcap.com/
- Caya diaphragm: http://caya.us.com/
- Hex condoms: https://www.lelo.com/hex-condoms-original
- myONE Perfect Fit from ONE Condoms: https://myonecondoms.com/
- Gynefix frameless IUD: http://www.wildemeersch.com/products/gynefix/

PCOS Resources

- *8 Steps to Reverse Your PCOS* by Dr. Fiona McCulloch
- PCOS Diva: http://pcosdiva.com/
- The Centre for Menstrual Cycle and Ovulation Research (CeMCOR) *Cyclic progesterone therapy*: http://www.cemcor.ca/resources/topics/cyclic-progesterone-therapy

Endometriosis Resources

- *Endo-what* film: https://endowhat.com/
- *Citizen Endo* research project and app:

http://citizenendo.org/
- Nancy's Nook Endometriosis Education and Discussion Group: https://www.facebook.com/groups/418136991574617/

Perimenopause Resources

- The Centre for Menstrual Cycle and Ovulation Research (CeMCOR) *Daily Perimenopause Diary*: http://www.cemcor.ubc.ca/resources/daily-perimenopause-diary
- *Estrogen's Storm Season—stories of perimenopause* (second edition, 2017) by Dr. Jerilynn Prior
- Progesterone Therapy for Symptomatic Perimenopause: http://www.cemcor.ubc.ca/files/uploads/Progesterone_for_Symptomatic_Perimenopause.pdf
- Julva DHEA vaginal cream: https://order.julva.com/the-dream-cream

Menstruation Activism

- 5th Vital Sign: http://www.5thvitalsign.com/
- *Sweetening the Pill* by Holly Grigg-Spall http://www.sweeteningthepill.com/
- *Sweetening the Pill* documentary: https://vimeo.com/129738582
- The Centre for Menstrual Cycle and Ovulation Research (CeMCOR): http://www.cemcor.ubc.ca/
- Society of Menstrual Cycle Research: http://www.menstruationresearch.org/
- Hormones Matter: https://www.hormonesmatter.com/
- The Cup Effect: http://www.thecupeffect.org/
- Menstrual Hygiene Day: http://menstrualhygieneday.org/
- Nicole Jardim, The Period Girl: http://nicolejardim.com/

How to Locate a Naturopathic Doctor

In the US:

- The American Association of Naturopathic Physicians
  http://www.naturopathic.org/

In Canada:

- Canadian Association of Naturopathic Doctors
  http://www.cand.ca/

Help for Eating Disorders

In the US:

- Office on Women's Health—Eating Disorders
  https://www.womenshealth.gov/body-image/eating-disorders/

In Canada:

- National Eating Disorder Information Centre (NEDIC)
  http://nedic.ca/

In the UK:

- NHS—Eating Disorders
  http://www.nhs.uk/conditions/eating-disorders/

Information About Endocrine-Disrupting Chemicals

- Environmental Working Group (EWG):
  http://www.ewg.org/

Supplements

I've provided some suggested brands as a *starting point,* and not an exhaustive list. Please choose a supplement that is available to you and not too expensive.

Alpha lipoic acid

- **Useful for:** PCOS, insulin resistance, detoxification
- **Daily dose:** 100-600 mg
- **Suggested brand(s):** Douglas Laboratories Alpha-Lipoic Acid, Thorne Research Alpha-Lipoic Acid

Ashwagandha (Withania)

- **Useful for:** Functional hypothalamic amenorrhea, fatigue, perimenopause, thyroid disease
- **Daily dose:** As directed
- **Suggested brand(s):** Douglas Laboratories Ayur-Ashwagandha capsules, Douglas Laboratories AdrenoMend, Pure Encapsulations Phyto-ADR

B-complex

- **Useful for:** HPA axis dysfunction, anxiety, fatigue
- **Daily dose:** As directed
- **Suggested brand(s):** Thorne Research Stress B-Complex, Integrative Therapeutics Active B-Complex

Betaine HCl

- **Useful for:** Digestive problems, SIBO
- **Daily dose:** As directed
- **Suggested brand(s):** Thorne Research Betaine HCL & Pepsin

Berberine

- **Useful for:** PCOS, acne, digestive problems, SIBO
- **Daily dose:** As directed
- **Suggested brand(s):** Thorne Research Berberine 500 capsules, Metagenics CandiBactin-BR

Calcium d-glucarate

- **Useful for:** PMS, uterine fibroids, detoxification, perimenopause
- **Daily dose:** 1000-1500 mg

- **Suggested brand(s):** Thorne Research Calcium D-Glucarate

Coenzyme Q10
- **Useful for:** Perimenopause
- **Daily dose:** 100 mg
- **Suggested brand(s):** Thorne Research Q-Best, Douglas Laboratories Ubiquinol-QH

Diindolylmethane (DIM)
- **Useful for:** Hirsutism, acne, perimenopause
- **Daily dose:** 200 mg
- **Suggested brand(s):** Source Naturals DIM (Diindolylmethane)

Fish oil
- **Useful for:** Period pain
- **Daily dose:** 1000 mg
- **Suggested brand(s):** Thorne Research Super EPA, Nordic Naturals Omega-3

Glutathione
- **Useful for:** Detoxification and immune support
- **Daily dose:** 100-400 mg
- **Suggested brand(s):** LypriCel Liposomal GSH, Researched Nutritionals Tri-Fortify Liposomal Glutathione

Iodine
- **Useful for:** PMS, breast pain, uterine fibroids, heavy periods, ovarian cysts, thyroid disease, perimenopause
- **Daily dose:** 200-3000 mcg (0.2-3 mg)
- **Suggested brand(s):** Violet Daily

Iron
- **Useful for:** PMS, heavy periods

- **Daily dose:** 15-50 mg
- **Suggested brand(s):** Thorne Research Iron Bisglycinate

Magnesium

- **Useful for:** PCOS, insulin resistance, functional hypothalamic amenorrhea, PMS, migraines, fatigue, sleep, period pain, detoxification, perimenopause
- **Daily dose:** 300 mg
- **Suggested brand(s):** Designs for Health Magnesium Glycinate Chelate, Pure Encapsulations Magnesium Glycinate, Natural Factors WomenSense MagSense powder, Metagenics Australia CardioX, Orthoplex MagTaur Xcell

Melatonin

- **Useful for:** Sleep, PCOS, hair loss, migraines
- **Daily dose:** 0.5 to 3 mg

Milk thistle

- **Useful for:** Detoxification, SIBO
- **Daily dose:** As directed
- **Suggested brand(s):** Designs for Health LV-GB, Thorne Research S.A.T, Flordis Legalon

Mushroom extract

- **Useful for:** Immune support
- **Daily dose:** As directed
- **Suggested brand(s):** Thorne Research Myco-Immune liquid

Myo-inositol

- **Useful for:** PCOS
- **Daily dose:** 2000-3000 mg
- **Suggested brand(s):** Ovasitol Inositol Powder

N-acetyl cysteine

- **Useful for:** PCOS, endometriosis, detoxification
- **Daily dose:** 500-2000 mg
- **Suggested brand(s):** Pure Encapsulations NAC, Douglas Laboratories N-Acetyl-L-Cysteine

Peony and licorice

- **Useful for:** PCOS, hirsutism
- **Daily dose:** As directed
- **Suggested brand(s):** Kan Herbs Peony and Licorice Formula, Metagenics Australia T-Clear, Mediherb PCOS support tablets

Probiotics

- **Useful for:** Estrogen excess, PMS, endometriosis, digestive problems, yeast infections and bacterial vaginosis
- **Daily dose:** As directed
- **Suggested brand(s):** Please read the How to Choose a Probiotic section in Chapter 11

Progesterone (Micronized or Natural)

- **Useful for:** PCOS, hirsutism, PMS, migraines, heavy periods, endometriosis, perimenopause
- **Daily dose:** 10-100 mg
- **Suggested brand(s):** Metabolic Maintenance Progeste Cream, Now Foods Natural Progesterone, Prometrium capsules

Resveratrol

- **Useful for:** PCOS, endometriosis
- **Daily dose:** 40-200 mg
- **Suggested brand(s):** Pure Encapsulations Resveratrol

Rhodiola

- **Useful for:** PMS, fatigue

- **Daily dose:** 150-300 mg of a standardized preparation
- **Suggested brand(s):** Thorne Research Rhodiola, Metagenics Australia Adrenotone

S-adenosylmethionine (SAMe)

- **Useful for:** PMS, detoxification
- **Daily dose:** 200 mg
- **Suggested brand(s):** Pure Encapsulations SAMe (S-Adenosylmethionine)

Selenium

- **Useful for:** PMS, endometriosis, ovarian cysts, detoxification, thyroid disease
- **Daily dose:** 100-150 mcg
- **Suggested brand(s):** Thorne Research Selenomethionine

St John's wort

- **Useful for:** PMS
- **Daily dose:** 300 mg twice daily
- **Suggested brand(s):** Flordis Remotiv

Taurine

- **Useful for:** Insulin-resistant PCOS, perimenopause
- **Daily dose:** 1000-3000 mg
- **Suggested brand(s):** Natural Factors WomenSense MagSense powder, Metagenics Australia CardioX, Orthoplex MagTaur Xcell

Turmeric or Curcumin

- **Useful for:** Heavy periods, period pain, endometriosis, adenomyosis, detoxification
- **Daily dose:** As directed
- **Suggested brand(s):** Thorne Research Meriva 500-SF, Pure Encapsulations Curcumin 500 with Bioperine

Vitamin B2 (riboflavin)

- **Useful for:** Migraines
- **Daily dose:** Up to 200 mg twice daily
- **Suggested brand(s):** Thorne Research Riboflavin 5' Phosphate, Now Foods B-2,

Vitamin B6 (P5P)

- **Useful for:** PMS, histamine intolerance, heavy periods, perimenopause
- **Daily dose:** 10-150 mg
- **Suggested brand(s):** Thorne Research Pyridoxal 5'-Phosphate, Douglas Laboratories B-6,

Vitamin B12 (methylcobalamin)

- **Useful for:** PMS, heavy periods
- **Daily dose:** 1000 mcg
- **Suggested brand(s):** Douglas Laboratories Methyl B12 Plus

Vitex

- **Useful for:** Hirsutism, hypothalamic amenorrhea, high prolactin, PMS, breast pain
- **Daily dose:** 200-2000 mg
- **Suggested brand(s):** Flordis Premular

Zinc

- **Useful for:** HPA axis dysfunction, PCOS, acne, PMS, endometriosis, period pain
- **Daily dose:** 20-50 mg
- **Suggested brand(s):** Thorne Research Zinc Picolinate

Ziziphus

- **Useful for:** Sleep, perimenopause
- **Daily dose:** 20-30 mg
- **Suggested brand(s):** Douglas Laboratories Seditol Plus

Appendix B

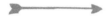

GLOSSARY

A1 dairy

Dairy products from Holstein cows, which contains a potentially inflammatory casein.

adaptogen

In herbal medicine, an adaptogen is a plant extract which helps the body adapt to stress. The term is not recognized by the scientific community.

adenomyosis

Adenomyosis is a gynecological condition in which uterine lining grows within the muscle of the uterine wall. It can cause pain and heavy periods.

adhesions

Adhesions are bands of connective tissue or scar tissue that bind together pelvic structures and cause pain. They are the result of both the disease process of endometriosis and the surgery used to treat it.

allopregnanolone (ALLO)

Allopregnanolone is a calming neurosteroid that acts like GABA in your brain.

alopecia

Alopecia means hair loss.

amenorrhea

Amenorrhea simply means no menstruation or no periods.

androgen

An androgen is a male hormone that promotes male characteristics.

androgenetic alopecia

Androgenetic alopecia is also called androgenic alopecia or female pattern hair loss. It's caused by androgen excess or androgen sensitivity.

anovulatory cycle

An anovulatory cycle is a menstrual cycle in which ovulation did not occur, and progesterone was not made.

anti-androgen

Anti-androgens (also known as androgen antagonists, androgen blockers, or testosterone blockers) are drugs or supplements that reduce androgens or block their effects.

anti-Müllerian hormone (AMH)

Anti-Müllerian hormone is made by your ovarian follicles.

autoimmune disease

Autoimmune disease occurs when immune system attacks healthy tissue.

bacterial vaginosis

Vaginosis is an overgrowth of one or more species of normal vaginal bacteria.

bioidentical hormone

A bioidentical or "body identical" hormone is a hormone that is structurally identical to your own human hormone.

blood count

Blood count is a blood test to determine the number of blood cells and hemoglobin.

body mass index (BMI)

Your BMI is your weight in kilograms divided by the square of your height in meters. A normal BMI is between 18.5 and 24.9.

congenital adrenal hyperplasia

Congenital adrenal hyperplasia is a genetic disorder that causes the adrenal glands to make too many androgens.

contraception failure rate

Contraception failure rate is the percentage of couples who experience an accidental pregnancy during one year of use. It is expressed as *perfect use* and *typical use*.

corpus luteum

The corpus luteum is a temporary endocrine gland that forms from the emptied ovarian follicle after ovulation.

cytokines

Inflammatory cytokines are chemical messengers that your body uses to fight infection. They are part of your body's inflammatory response.

DHEAS

DHEAS (dehydroepiandrosterone sulfate) is a steroid hormone made by the adrenal glands. It's often high with PCOS and low with HPA axis dysfunction. DHEAS naturally declines with age.

dysmenorrhea

Dysmenorrhea is the medical term for painful menstruation.

endocrine disrupting chemicals

Endocrine disrupting chemicals (EDCs) are substances that cause adverse health effects by altering the function of the endocrine or hormonal system. They include pesticides, metals, industrial pollutants, solvents, food additives, and personal care products.

estradiol

Estradiol is the type of estrogen made by the ovarian follicles.

ferritin

Serum ferritin is the blood test for stored iron.

FODMAPs

Fermentable, Oligo-, Di-, Mono-saccharides And Polyols. FODMAPs are a type of carbohydrate found in many foods, such as bread and fruit.

follicle

see ovarian follicle.

food allergy

Food allergy is an immediate reaction to food. It is mediated by a part of the immune system called IgE antibodies and causes symptoms such as hives or swollen airways.

food sensitivity

Food sensitivity is a broad category of adverse reactions to food. It is often a delayed reaction that involves inflammatory cytokines. Food sensitivity is different from a true food allergy.

FSH

FSH or follicle-stimulating hormone is a pituitary hormone that stimulates ovarian follicles to grow.

functional hypothalamic amenorrhea (FHA)

Functional hypothalamic amenorrhea is the absence of menstruation when no medical diagnosis can be found.

gamma-Aminobutyric acid (GABA)

GABA is a neurotransmitter that promotes relaxation and enhances sleep.

glutathione

Glutathione is a natural antioxidant made by your body.

gluten

Gluten is a protein found in grains such as wheat, rye, and barley.

hemoglobin

Hemoglobin is the iron-containing protein found in red blood cells.

hirsutism

Hirsutism is excessive growth of hair on the face and body.

histamine intolerance

Histamine intolerance is the temporary state of having too much histamine, which is the part of the immune system that causes allergies and swelling. In addition to its role in immune function, histamine also regulates stomach acid, stimulates the brain, boosts libido, and plays a key role in ovulation and female reproduction.

hormonal birth control

Hormonal birth control is the general term for all tablets, patches, and injections that deliver steroid drugs to suppress ovarian function. The combined pill (estrogen plus a progestin) is the most popular type.

hormone receptor

A hormone receptor is a docking station for hormones such as estrogen or progesterone. They exist in every type of cell and transmit hormonal messages deep into the cell.

HPA axis dysfunction

HPA axis dysfunction refers to a pattern of chronic stress that results in abnormal levels of cortisol.

hypothalamus

The hypothalamus is the part of the brain that sends messages to the pituitary gland.

hysterectomy

Hysterectomy is the surgical removal of the uterus. Surgical removal of both the uterus and the cervix and possibly the ovaries is called *total hysterectomy*. Surgical removal of the uterus, but not the cervix or the ovaries, is called *partial hysterectomy*.

insulin

Insulin is a hormone made by your pancreas. It stimulates your liver and muscles to take up sugar and convert it to energy.

insulin resistance

Insulin resistance is a metabolic disorder that results in high levels of the hormone insulin.

interstitial cystitis

Interstitial cystitis is also called painful bladder syndrome. It is the constant sensation of pressure or pain in the bladder and pelvis.

intestinal permeability

Intestinal permeability is a condition in which tiny microscopic leaks form between the cells of your intestinal wall.

luteal phase

The luteal phase of a menstrual cycle is the 10 to 16 days between ovulation and the bleed, and is determined by the lifespan of the corpus luteum.

luteinizing hormone (LH)

Luteinizing hormone is the pituitary hormone that signals your ovary to release an egg.

menopause

Menopause is the cessation of menstruation. It's the life phase that begins one year after your last period.[5]

microbiome

The genetic material of the microorganisms in a particular environment such as the body or part of the body.

micronized progesterone

Micronized progesterone is a form of replacement hormone. It is natural or bioidentical progesterone rather than a synthetic progestin. It can be taken as a topical cream or a capsule such as the brand Prometrium®.

MTHFR

MTHFR (methylenetetrahydrofolate reductase) is an enzyme that transforms folate (folic acid) to its active form. About one in three people have a variant of the gene that makes the enzyme. The MTHFR gene mutation can be assessed with a simple blood test. If you have the variant gene, then you may need a higher dose of B vitamins.

ovarian follicle

Ovarian follicle is the sac that contains one egg or oocyte.

perimenopause

Perimenopause means "around menopause," and refers to the hormonal changes (such as increased estrogen and decreased progesterone) that occur during the two to twelve years before menopause. The final part of perimenopause is called the menopause transition.

phytoestrogen

Phytoestrogens are a special group of phytonutrients that exert a weak estrogen-like effect.

phytonutrient

Phytonutrients are naturally occurring plant chemicals.

pituitary gland

The pituitary gland is a small endocrine gland attached to the base of the brain.

platelets

Platelets are blood cells whose function is to stop bleeding.

PMDD

Premenstrual dysphoric disorder is a condition of severe premenstrual depression, irritability, or anxiety. It affects about one in twenty women.

polycystic ovary syndrome (PCOS)

A common hormonal condition characterized by excess male hormones in women, covered in Chapter 7.

progesterone

Progesterone is a steroid hormone made by the ovary after ovulation.

progestin

Progestin is a general term for a group of molecules that are similar to the hormone progesterone.

prolactin

Prolactin is a pituitary hormone that stimulates breast development and breast milk. It suppresses normal cycling and ovulation.

prolactinoma

Prolactinoma is a benign pituitary tumor that releases prolactin.

prostaglandins

Prostaglandins are hormone-like compounds that have a variety of physiological effects, such as the constriction and dilation of blood vessels.

small intestinal bacterial overgrowth (SIBO)

Small intestinal bacterial overgrowth (SIBO) is the overgrowth of normal gut bacteria in your small intestine.

standard drink

In the US, a standard drink contains 0.6 ounces (18 mL) of alcohol which equates to a 12 ounce (350 mL) glass of beer or a 5 ounce (150 mL) glass of wine.

telogen phase

Hairs in the telogen phase are dormant or resting before they fall out. The telogen phase has a fixed duration of one to four months. In contrast, hairs in the anagen phase are actively growing. The anagen phase has a variable duration of years.

thyroid antibodies

Thyroid antibodies are autoimmune antibodies that your immune system makes against your thyroid.

TSH

TSH (thyroid stimulating hormone) is the pituitary hormone that stimulates the thyroid gland. It's the standard test for thyroid dysfunction and should be between 0.5 and 4 mIU/L.

ultrasound

A pelvic ultrasound is an imaging study to view your ovaries and uterus. It uses sound waves (not radiation) and is safe, noninvasive, and painless.

uterine polyps

Uterine polyps or endometrial polyps are outgrowths from the uterine lining (endometrium). They are usually benign or non-cancerous.

REFERENCES

1: . ACOG Committee Opinion No. 651: Menstruation in Girls and Adolescents: Using the Menstrual Cycle as a Vital Sign. Obstet Gynecol. 2015 Dec;126(6):e143-6. PubMed PMID: 26595586

2: https://www.psoriasis.org/advance/do-gluten-free-diets-improve-psoriasis

3: Pellicano R, Astegiano M, Bruno M, Fagoonee S, Rizzetto M. Women and celiac disease: association with unexplained infertility. Minerva Med. 2007 Jun;98(3):217-9. PubMed PMID: 17592443

4: Vollman RF. The menstrual cycle. In: Friedman EA, editor. Major Problems in Obstetrics and Gynecology, Vol 7. 1 ed. Toronto: W.B. Saunders Company; 1977 11-193

5: Personal communication with Dr Jerilynn Prior

6: https://www.ncbi.nlm.nih.gov/pmc/articles/PMC3520685/

7: Henderson VW, St John JA, Hodis HN, McCleary CA, Stanczyk FZ, Karim R, et al. Cognition, mood, and physiological concentrations of sex hormones in the early and late postmenopause. Proc Natl Acad Sci U S A. 2013 Dec 10;110(50):20290-5. PubMed PMID: 24277815

8: Skovlund CW, Mørch LS, Kessing LV, Lidegaard Ø. Association of Hormonal Contraception With Depression. JAMA Psychiatry. 2016 Nov 1;73(11):1154-1162. PubMed PMID: 27680324

9: Birch Petersen K, Hvidman HW, Forman JL, Pinborg A, Larsen EC, Macklon KT, et al. Ovarian reserve assessment in users of oral contraception seeking fertility advice on their reproductive lifespan. Hum Reprod. 2015 Oct;30(10):2364-75. PubMed PMID: 26311148

10: Cole JA, Norman H, Doherty M, Walker AM. Venous thromboembolism, myocardial infarction, and stroke among transdermal contraceptive system users. Obstet Gynecol. 2007 Feb;109(2 Pt 1):339-46. PubMed PMID: 17267834

11: Pattman, Richard; Sankar, K. Nathan; Elewad, Babiker; Handy, Pauline; Price, David Ashley, eds. (November 19, 2010). "Chapter 33. Contraception including contraception in HIV infection and infection reduction". Oxford Handbook of Genitourinary Medicine, HIV, and Sexual Health (2nd ed.). Oxford: Oxford University Press. p. 360.

12: GARCIA CR, PINCUS G, ROCK J. Effects of certain 19-nor steroids on the normal human menstrual cycle. Science. 1956 Nov 2;124(3227):891-3. PubMed PMID: 13380401

13: Lange HL, Belury MA, Secic M, Thomas A, Bonny AE. Dietary Intake and Weight Gain Among Adolescents on Depot Medroxyprogesterone Acetate. J Pediatr Adolesc Gynecol. 2015 Jun;28(3):139-43. PubMed PMID: 26046602

14: http://www.cemcor.ubc.ca/resources/depo-provera-use-and-bone-health

15: Li CI, Beaber EF, Tang MT, Porter PL, Daling JR, Malone KE. Effect of depo-medroxyprogesterone acetate on breast cancer risk among women 20 to 44 years of age. Cancer Res. 2012 Apr 15;72(8):2028-35. PubMed PMID: 22369929

16: Kailasam C, Cahill D. Review of the safety, efficacy and patient acceptability of the levonorgestrel-releasing intrauterine system. Patient Prefer Adherence. 2008 Feb 2;2:293-302. PubMed PMID: 19920976

17: Skovlund CW, Mørch LS, Kessing LV, Lidegaard Ø. Association of Hormonal Contraception With Depression. JAMA Psychiatry. 2016 Nov 1;73(11):1154-1162. PubMed PMID: 27680324

18: Aleknaviciute J, Tulen JHM, De Rijke YB, Bouwkamp CG, van der Kroeg M, Timmermans M, et al. The levonorgestrel-releasing intrauterine device potentiates stress reactivity. Psychoneuroendocrinology. 2017 Jun;80:39-45. PubMed PMID: 28315609

19: Mørch LS, Skovlund CW, Hannaford PC, Iversen L, Fielding S, Lidegaard Ø. Contemporary Hormonal Contraception and the Risk of Breast Cancer. N Engl J Med. 2017 Dec 7;377(23):2228-2239. PubMed PMID: 29211679

20: Seaman, Barbara. 1995. The Doctor's Case Against the Pill. Hunter House (CA); 25 Anv. Edition (July 1995). ISBN: 978-0-89793-181-6

21: Lidegaard O, Nielsen LH, Skovlund CW, Løkkegaard E. Venous thrombosis in users of non-oral hormonal contraception: follow-up study, Denmark 2001-10. BMJ. 2012 May 10;344:e2990. PubMed PMID: 22577198

22: Skovlund CW, Mørch LS, Kessing LV, Lidegaard Ø. Association of Hormonal Contraception With Depression. JAMA Psychiatry. 2016 Nov 1;73(11):1154-1162. PubMed PMID: 27680324

23: http://www.reuters.com/article/us-health-depression-hormones-idUSKCN11Z33J

24: Skovlund CW, Mørch LS, Kessing LV, Lange T, Lidegaard Ø. Association of Hormonal Contraception With Suicide Attempts and Suicides. Am J Psychiatry. 2018 Apr 1;175(4):336-342. PubMed PMID: 29145752

25: Aleknaviciute J, Tulen JHM, De Rijke YB, Bouwkamp CG, van der Kroeg M, Timmermans M, et al. The levonorgestrel-releasing intrauterine device potentiates stress reactivity. Psychoneuroendocrinology. 2017 Jun;80:39-45. PubMed PMID: 28315609

26: Macut D, Božić Antić I, Nestorov J, Topalović V, Bjekić Macut J, Panidis D, et al. The influence of combined oral contraceptives containing drospirenone on hypothalamic-pituitary-adrenocortical axis activity and glucocorticoid receptor expression and function in women with polycystic ovary syndrome. Hormones (Athens). 2015 Jan-Mar;14(1):109-17. PubMed PMID: 25402380

27: Petersen N, Touroutoglou A, Andreano JM, Cahill L. Oral contraceptive pill use is associated with localized decreases in cortical thickness. Hum Brain Mapp. 2015 Jul;36(7):2644-54. PubMed PMID: 25832993

28: https://www.marieclaire.com.au/article/news/yasmin-side-effects

29: https://kinseyconfidential.org/hormonal-birth-control-sexual-functioningwhats-deal/

30: Panzer C, Wise S, Fantini G, Kang D, Munarriz R, Guay A, et al. Impact of oral contraceptives on sex hormone-binding globulin and androgen levels: a retrospective study in women with sexual dysfunction. J Sex Med. 2006 Jan;3(1):104-13. PubMed PMID: 16409223

31: http://www.americanhairloss.org/women_hair_loss/oral_contraceptives.asp

32: http://www.sciencedaily.com/releases/2009/04/090417084014.htm

33: Scholes D, Ichikawa L, LaCroix AZ, Spangler L, Beasley JM, Reed S, et al. Oral contraceptive use and bone density in adolescent and young adult women. Contraception. 2010 Jan;81(1):35-40. PubMed PMID: 20004271

34: Scholes D, Hubbard RA, Ichikawa LE, LaCroix AZ, Spangler L, Beasley JM, et al. Oral contraceptive use and bone density change in adolescent and young adult women: a prospective study of age, hormone dose, and discontinuation. J Clin Endocrinol Metab. 2011 Sep;96(9):E1380-7. PubMed PMID: 21752879

35: Stewart ME, Greenwood R, Cunliffe WJ, Strauss JS, Downing DT. Effect of cyproterone acetate-ethinyl estradiol treatment on the proportions of linoleic and sebaleic acids in various skin surface lipid classes. Arch Dermatol Res. 1986;278(6):481-5. PubMed PMID: 2947544

36: Turner JV. Fertility-awareness practice and education in general practice. Aust J Prim Health. 2016 Sep 27;. PubMed PMID: 27671339

37: http://www.acog.org/Patients/FAQs/Fertility-Awareness-Based-Methods-of-Family-Planning

38: Frank-Herrmann P, Heil J, Gnoth C, Toledo E, Baur S, Pyper C, et al. The effectiveness of a fertility awareness based method to avoid pregnancy in relation to a couple's sexual behaviour during the fertile time: a prospective longitudinal study. Hum Reprod. 2007 May;22(5):1310-9. PubMed PMID: 17314078

39: Frank-Herrmann P, Heil J, Gnoth C, Toledo E, Baur S, Pyper C, et al. The effectiveness of a fertility awareness based method to avoid pregnancy in relation to a couple's sexual behaviour during the fertile time: a prospective longitudinal study. Hum Reprod. 2007 May;22(5):1310-9. PubMed PMID: 17314078

40: https://www.cdc.gov/reproductivehealth/contraception/index.htm

41: https://daysy.me/accuracy/

42: Personal communication with Dr Jerilynn Prior.

43: https://www.cdc.gov/reproductivehealth/contraception/index.htm

44: https://www.cdc.gov/reproductivehealth/contraception/index.htm

45: https://www.cdc.gov/reproductivehealth/contraception/index.htm

46: https://en.wikipedia.org/wiki/FemCap

47: http://www.independent.co.uk/life-style/health-and-families/features/the-best-contraception-is-an-iud-why-i-love-having-a-coil-9578198.html

48: Hurd, TM. 2007. Clinical reproductive medicine and surgery. Philadelphia: Mosby. p. 409. ISBN 978-0-32303-309-1

49: Mohllajee AP, Curtis KM, Peterson HB. Does insertion and use of an intrauterine device increase the risk of pelvic inflammatory disease among women with sexually transmitted infection? A systematic review. Contraception. 2006 Feb;73(2):145-53. PubMed PMID: 16413845

50: https://www.bustle.com/articles/100406-more-sexually-active-women-are-satisfied-with-iuds-than-with-birth-control-pills-new-research-shows

51: Hubacher D, Chen PL, Park S. Side effects from the copper IUD: do they decrease over time?. Contraception. 2009 May;79(5):356-62. PubMed PMID: 19341847

52: Andrade AT, Pizarro E, Shaw ST Jr, Souza JP, Belsey EM, Rowe PJ. Consequences of uterine blood loss caused by various intrauterine contraceptive devices in South American women. World Health Organization Special Programme of Research, Development and Research Training in Human Reproduction. Contraception. 1988 Jul;38(1):1-18. PubMed PMID: 3048870

53: Wu S, Hu J, Wildemeersch D. Performance of the frameless GyneFix and the TCu380A IUDs in a 3-year multicenter, randomized, comparative trial in parous women. Contraception. 2000 Feb;61(2):91-8. PubMed PMID: 10802273

54: Mohllajee AP, Curtis KM, Peterson HB. Does insertion and use of an intrauterine device increase the risk of pelvic inflammatory disease among women with sexually transmitted infection? A systematic review. Contraception. 2006 Feb;73(2):145-53. PubMed PMID: 16413845

55: Achilles SL, Austin MN, Meyn LA, Mhlanga F, Chirenje ZM, Hillier SL. Impact of contraceptive initiation on vaginal microbiota. Am J Obstet Gynecol. 2018 Jun;218(6):622.e1-622.e10. PubMed PMID: 29505773

56: De la Cruz D, Cruz A, Arteaga M, Castillo L, Tovalin H. Blood copper levels in Mexican users of the T380A IUD. Contraception. 2005 Aug;72(2):122-5. PubMed PMID: 16022851

57: Elizabeth G. Raymond, Pai Lien Chen, Joanne Luoto, for the Spermicide Trial Group. "Contraceptive Effectiveness and Safety of Five Nonoxynol-9 Spermicides: A Randomized Trial" Obstetrics & Gynecology. 2004; 103:430-439

58: Falconer H, Yin L, Grönberg H, Altman D. Ovarian cancer risk after salpingectomy: a nationwide population-based study. J Natl Cancer Inst. 2015 Feb;107(2). PubMed PMID: 25628372

59: Sadatmahalleh SJ, Ziaei S, Kazemnejad A, Mohamadi E. Menstrual Pattern following Tubal Ligation: A Historical Cohort Study. Int J Fertil Steril. 2016 Jan-Mar;9(4):477-82. PubMed PMID: 26985334

60: Morley C, Rogers A, Zaslau S. Post-vasectomy pain syndrome: clinical features and treatment options. Can J Urol. 2012 Apr;19(2):6160-4. PubMed PMID: 22512957

61: http://www.parsemusfoundation.org/vasalgel-faqs/

62: Mauvais-Jarvis F, Clegg DJ, Hevener AL. The role of estrogens in control of energy balance and glucose homeostasis. Endocr Rev. 2013 Jun;34(3):309-38. PubMed PMID: 23460719

63: http://www.abc.net.au/science/articles/2013/07/09/3798293.htm

64: Care AS, Diener KR, Jasper MJ, Brown HM, Ingman WV, Robertson SA. Macrophages regulate corpus luteum development during embryo implantation in mice. J Clin Invest. 2013 Aug;123(8):3472-87. PubMed PMID: 23867505

65: Mohammed H, Russell IA, Stark R, Rueda OM, Hickey TE, Tarulli GA, et al. Progesterone receptor modulates ERα action in breast cancer. Nature. 2015 Jul 16;523(7560):313-7. PubMed PMID: 26153859

66: Sathi P, Kalyan S, Hitchcock CL, Pudek M, Prior JC. Progesterone therapy increases free thyroxine levels--data from a randomized placebo-controlled 12-week hot flush trial. Clin Endocrinol (Oxf). 2013 Aug;79(2):282-7. PubMed PMID: 23252963

67: Melcangi RC, Giatti S, Calabrese D, Pesaresi M, Cermenati G, Mitro N, et al. Levels and actions of progesterone and its metabolites in the nervous system during physiological and pathological conditions. Prog Neurobiol. 2014 Feb;113:56-69. PubMed PMID: 23958466

68: Smith GI, Yoshino J, Reeds DN, Bradley D, Burrows RE, Heisey HD, et al. Testosterone and progesterone, but not estradiol, stimulate muscle protein synthesis in postmenopausal women. J Clin Endocrinol Metab. 2014 Jan;99(1):256-65. PubMed PMID: 24203065

69: Schüssler P, Kluge M, Yassouridis A, Dresler M, Held K, Zihl J, et al. Progesterone reduces wakefulness in sleep EEG and has no effect on cognition in healthy postmenopausal women. Psychoneuroendocrinology. 2008 Sep;33(8):1124-31. PubMed PMID: 18676087

70: Mong JA, Baker FC, Mahoney MM, Paul KN, Schwartz MD, Semba K, et al. Sleep, rhythms, and the endocrine brain: influence of sex and gonadal hormones. J Neurosci. 2011 Nov 9;31(45):16107-16. PubMed PMID: 22072663

71: Prior JC (2014) Progesterone within ovulatory menstrual cycles needed for cardiovascular protection- an evidence-based hypothesis. Journal of Restorative Medicine 3: 85–103.

72: Gordon JL, Girdler SS, Meltzer-Brody SE, Stika CS, Thurston RC, Clark CT, et al. Ovarian hormone fluctuation, neurosteroids, and HPA axis dysregulation in perimenopausal depression: a novel heuristic model. Am J Psychiatry. 2015 Mar 1;172(3):227-36. PubMed PMID: 25585035

73: Petersen N, Touroutoglou A, Andreano JM, Cahill L. Oral contraceptive pill use is associated with localized decreases in cortical thickness. Hum Brain Mapp. 2015 Jul;36(7):2644-54. PubMed PMID: 25832993

74: Prior JC, Naess M, Langhammer A, Forsmo S. Ovulation Prevalence in Women with Spontaneous Normal-Length Menstrual Cycles - A Population-Based Cohort from HUNT3, Norway. PLoS One. 2015;10(8):e0134473. PubMed PMID: 26291617

75: Prior JC, Naess M, Langhammer A, Forsmo S. Ovulation Prevalence in Women with Spontaneous Normal-Length Menstrual Cycles - A Population-Based Cohort from HUNT3, Norway. PLoS One. 2015;10(8):e0134473. PubMed PMID: 26291617

76: Mountjoy M, Sundgot-Borgen J, Burke L, Carter S, Constantini N, Lebrun C, et al. The IOC consensus statement: beyond the Female Athlete Triad--Relative Energy Deficiency in Sport (RED-S). Br J Sports Med. 2014 Apr;48(7):491-7. PubMed PMID: 24620037

77: Loucks AB, Thuma JR. Luteinizing hormone pulsatility is disrupted at a threshold of energy availability in regularly menstruating women. J Clin Endocrinol Metab. 2003 Jan;88(1):297-311. PubMed PMID: 12519869

78: http://www.pcosfoundation.org/what-is-pcos

79: Personal communication with Dr Jerilynn Prior.

80: Shepard MK, Senturia YD. Comparison of serum progesterone and endometrial biopsy for confirmation of ovulation and evaluation of luteal function. Fertil Steril. 1977 May;28(5):541-8. PubMed PMID: 856637

81: Stoddard FR 2nd, Brooks AD, Eskin BA, Johannes GJ. Iodine alters gene expression in the MCF7 breast cancer cell line: evidence for an anti-estrogen effect of iodine. Int J Med Sci. 2008 Jul 8;5(4):189-96. PubMed PMID: 18645607

82: Eldering J, Nay M, Hoberg L, Longcope C, McCracken J. Hormonal regulation of prostaglandin production by rhesus monkey endometrium. J Clin Endocrinol Metab 1990; 71(3):596-604.

83: García-Velasco JA, Menabrito M, Catalán IB. What fertility specialists should know about the vaginal microbiome: a review. Reprod Biomed Online. 2017 Jul;35(1):103-112. PubMed PMID: 28479120

84: Whirledge S, Cidlowski JA. Glucocorticoids, stress, and fertility. Minerva Endocrinol. 2010 Jun;35(2):109-25. PubMed PMID: 20595939

85: Aleknaviciute J, Tulen JHM, De Rijke YB, Bouwkamp CG, van der Kroeg M, Timmermans M, et al. The levonorgestrel-releasing intrauterine device potentiates stress reactivity. Psychoneuroendocrinology. 2017 Jun;80:39-45. PubMed PMID: 28315609

86: Cadegiani FA, Kater CE. Adrenal fatigue does not exist: a systematic review. BMC Endocr Disord. 2016 Aug 24;16(1):48. PubMed PMID: 27557747

87: Sjörs A, Ljung T, Jonsdottir IH. Long-term follow-up of cortisol awakening response in patients treated for stress-related exhaustion. BMJ Open. 2012;2(4). PubMed PMID: 22786949

88: Schumacher S, Kirschbaum C, Fydrich T, Ströhle A. Is salivary alpha-amylase an indicator of autonomic nervous system dysregulations in mental disorders?--a review of preliminary findings and the interactions with cortisol. Psychoneuroendocrinology. 2013 Jun;38(6):729-43. PubMed PMID: 23481259

89: Swardfager W, Herrmann N, McIntyre RS, Mazereeuw G, Goldberger K, Cha DS, et al. Potential roles of zinc in the pathophysiology and treatment of major depressive disorder. Neurosci Biobehav Rev. 2013 Jun;37(5):911-29. PubMed PMID: 23567517

90: Long SJ, Benton D. Effects of vitamin and mineral supplementation on stress, mild psychiatric symptoms, and mood in nonclinical samples: a meta-analysis. Psychosom Med. 2013 Feb;75(2):144-53. PubMed PMID: 23362497

91: Mikkelsen K, Stojanovska L, Prakash M, Apostolopoulos V. The effects of vitamin B on the immune/cytokine network and their involvement in depression. Maturitas. 2017 Feb;96:58-71. PubMed PMID: 28041597

92: Hung SK, Perry R, Ernst E. The effectiveness and efficacy of Rhodiola rosea L.: a systematic review of randomized clinical trials. Phytomedicine. 2011 Feb 15;18(4):235-44. PubMed PMID: 21036578

93: Olsson EM, von Schéele B, Panossian AG. A randomised, double-blind, placebo-controlled, parallel-group study of the standardised extract shr-5 of the roots of Rhodiola rosea in the treatment of subjects with stress-related fatigue. Planta Med. 2009 Feb;75(2):105-12. PubMed PMID: 19016404

94: Darbinyan V, Aslanyan G, Amroyan E, Gabrielyan E, Malmström C, Panossian A. Clinical trial of Rhodiola rosea L. extract SHR-5 in the treatment of mild to moderate depression. Nord J Psychiatry. 2007;61(5):343-8. PubMed PMID: 17990195

95: Jiang JG, Huang XJ, Chen J, Lin QS. Comparison of the sedative and hypnotic effects of flavonoids, saponins, and polysaccharides extracted from Semen Ziziphus jujube. Nat Prod Res. 2007 Apr;21(4):310-20. PubMed PMID: 17479419

96: Koetter U, Barrett M, Lacher S, Abdelrahman A, Dolnick D. Interactions of Magnolia and Ziziphus extracts with selected central nervous system receptors. J Ethnopharmacol. 2009 Jul 30;124(3):421-5. PubMed PMID: 19505549

97: Pedersen BK. Anti-inflammatory effects of exercise: role in diabetes and cardiovascular disease. Eur J Clin Invest. 2017 Aug;47(8):600-611. PubMed PMID: 28722106

98: Mountjoy M, Sundgot-Borgen J, Burke L, Carter S, Constantini N, Lebrun C, et al. The IOC consensus statement: beyond the Female Athlete Triad--Relative Energy Deficiency in Sport (RED-S). Br J Sports Med. 2014 Apr;48(7):491-7. PubMed PMID: 24620037

99: Zhang DM, Jiao RQ, Kong LD. High Dietary Fructose: Direct or Indirect Dangerous Factors Disturbing Tissue and Organ Functions. Nutrients. 2017 Mar 29;9(4). PubMed PMID: 28353649

100: Stanhope KL, Schwarz JM, Keim NL, Griffen SC, Bremer AA, Graham JL, et al. Consuming fructose-sweetened, not glucose-sweetened, beverages increases visceral adiposity and lipids and decreases insulin sensitivity in overweight/obese humans. J Clin Invest. 2009 May;119(5):1322-34. PubMed PMID: 19381015

101: Page KA, Chan O, Arora J, Belfort-Deaguiar R, Dzuira J, Roehmholdt B, et al. Effects of fructose vs glucose on regional cerebral blood flow in brain regions involved with appetite and reward pathways. JAMA. 2013 Jan 2;309(1):63-70. PubMed PMID: 23280226

102: Sugiyama M, Tang AC, Wakaki Y, Koyama W. Glycemic index of single and mixed meal foods among common Japanese foods with white rice as a reference food. Eur J Clin Nutr. 2003 Jun;57(6):743-52. PubMed PMID: 12792658

103: http://www.sciencedaily.com/releases/2007/12/071212201311.htm

104: http://www.bmj.com/content/357/bmj.j2353

105: Topiwala A, Allan CL, Valkanova V, Zsoldos E, Filippini N, Sexton C, et al. Moderate alcohol consumption as risk factor for adverse brain outcomes and cognitive decline: longitudinal cohort study. BMJ. 2017 Jun 6;357:j2353. PubMed PMID: 28588063

106: Zhang SM, Lee IM, Manson JE, Cook NR, Willett WC, Buring JE. Alcohol consumption and breast cancer risk in the Women's Health Study. Am J Epidemiol. 2007 Mar 15;165(6):667-76. PubMed PMID: 17204515

107: Sun K, Ren M, Liu D, Wang C, Yang C, Yan L. Alcohol consumption and risk of metabolic syndrome: a meta-analysis of prospective studies. Clin Nutr. 2014 Aug;33(4):596-602. PubMed PMID: 24315622

108: Lowe PP, Gyongyosi B, Satishchandran A, Iracheta-Vellve A, Ambade A, Kodys K, et al. Alcohol-related changes in the intestinal microbiome influence neutrophil infiltration, inflammation and steatosis in early alcoholic hepatitis in mice. PLoS One. 2017;12(3):e0174544. PubMed PMID: 28350851

109: Fasano A. Zonulin and its regulation of intestinal barrier function: the biological door to inflammation, autoimmunity, and cancer. Physiol Rev. 2011 Jan;91(1):151-75. PubMed PMID: 21248165

110: Aziz I, Hadjivassiliou M, Sanders DS. The spectrum of noncoeliac gluten sensitivity. Nat Rev Gastroenterol Hepatol. 2015 Sep;12(9):516-26. PubMed PMID:

26122473

111: Elli L, Roncoroni L, Bardella MT. Non-celiac gluten sensitivity: Time for sifting the grain. World J Gastroenterol. 2015 Jul 21;21(27):8221-6. PubMed PMID: 26217073

112: Vazquez-Roque M, Oxentenko AS. Nonceliac Gluten Sensitivity. Mayo Clin Proc. 2015 Sep;90(9):1272-7. PubMed PMID: 26355401

113: Peters SL, Biesiekierski JR, Yelland GW, Muir JG, Gibson PR. Randomised clinical trial: gluten may cause depression in subjects with non-coeliac gluten sensitivity - an exploratory clinical study. Aliment Pharmacol Ther. 2014 May;39(10):1104-12. PubMed PMID: 24689456

114: Peters SL, Biesiekierski JR, Yelland GW, Muir JG, Gibson PR. Randomised clinical trial: gluten may cause depression in subjects with non-coeliac gluten sensitivity - an exploratory clinical study. Aliment Pharmacol Ther. 2014 May;39(10):1104-12. PubMed PMID: 24689456

115: Woodford, Keith. 2009. Devil in the Milk: Illness, Health and the Politics of A1 and A2 Milk. Chelsea Green Publishing. ISBN: 978-1603581028

116: Ul Haq MR, Kapila R, Sharma R, Saliganti V, Kapila S. Comparative evaluation of cow β-casein variants (A1/A2) consumption on Th2-mediated inflammatory response in mouse gut. Eur J Nutr. 2014 Jun;53(4):1039-49. PubMed PMID: 24166511

117: Deth R, Clarke A, Ni J, Trivedi M. Clinical evaluation of glutathione concentrations after consumption of milk containing different subtypes of β-casein: results from a randomized, cross-over clinical trial. Nutr J. 2016 Sep 29;15(1):82. PubMed PMID: 27680716

118: Zierau O, Zenclussen AC, Jensen F. Role of female sex hormones, estradiol and progesterone, in mast cell behavior. Front Immunol. 2012;3:169. PubMed PMID: 22723800

119: Fogel WA. Diamine oxidase (DAO) and female sex hormones. Agents Actions. 1986 Apr;18(1-2):44-5. PubMed PMID: 3088928

120: Bódis J, Tinneberg HR, Schwarz H, Papenfuss F, Török A, Hanf V. The effect of histamine on progesterone and estradiol secretion of human granulosa cells in serum-free culture. Gynecol Endocrinol. 1993 Dec;7(4):235-9. PubMed PMID: 8147232

121: Martner-Hewes PM, Hunt IF, Murphy NJ, Swendseid ME, Settlage RH. Vitamin B-6 nutriture and plasma diamine oxidase activity in pregnant Hispanic teenagers. Am J Clin Nutr. 1986 Dec;44(6):907-13. PubMed PMID: 3098085

122: Ludwig DS, Willett WC. Three daily servings of reduced-fat milk: an evidence-based recommendation?. JAMA Pediatr. 2013 Sep;167(9):788-9. PubMed PMID: 23818041

123: Silvio Buscemi et al. Coffee and metabolic impairment: An updated review of epidemiological studies. NFS Journal, Volume 3, August 2016, Pages 1-7

124: Ding M, Bhupathiraju SN, Chen M, van Dam RM, Hu FB. Caffeinated and decaffeinated coffee consumption and risk of type 2 diabetes: a systematic review and a dose-response meta-analysis. Diabetes Care. 2014 Feb;37(2):569-86. PubMed PMID: 24459154

125: Schliep KC, Schisterman EF, Mumford SL, Pollack AZ, Zhang C, Ye A, et al. Caffeinated beverage intake and reproductive hormones among premenopausal women in the BioCycle Study. Am J Clin Nutr. 2012 Feb;95(2):488-97. PubMed PMID: 22237060

126: Ganmaa D, Willett WC, Li TY, Feskanich D, van Dam RM, Lopez-Garcia E, et al. Coffee, tea, caffeine and risk of breast cancer: a 22-year follow-up. Int J Cancer. 2008 May 1;122(9):2071-6. PubMed PMID: 18183588

127: Hahn KA, Wise LA, Riis AH, Mikkelsen EM, Rothman KJ, Banholzer K, et al. Correlates of menstrual cycle characteristics among nulliparous Danish women. Clin Epidemiol. 2013;5:311-9. PubMed PMID: 23983490

128: Patwardhan RV, Desmond PV, Johnson RF, Schenker S. Impaired elimination of caffeine by oral contraceptive steroids. J Lab Clin Med. 1980 Apr;95(4):603-8. PubMed PMID: 7359014

129: Patisaul HB, Jefferson W. The pros and cons of phytoestrogens. Front Neuroendocrinol. 2010 Oct;31(4):400-19. PubMed PMID: 20347861

130: Patisaul HB, Jefferson W. The pros and cons of phytoestrogens. Front Neuroendocrinol. 2010 Oct;31(4):400-19. PubMed PMID: 20347861

131: Hampl R, Ostatnikova D, Celec P, Putz Z, Lapcík O, Matucha P. Short-term effect of soy consumption on thyroid hormone levels and correlation with phytoestrogen level in healthy subjects. Endocr Regul. 2008 Jun;42(2-3):53-61. PubMed PMID: 18624607

132: Feinman RD, Pogozelski WK, Astrup A, Bernstein RK, Fine EJ, Westman EC, et al. Dietary carbohydrate restriction as the first approach in diabetes management: critical review and evidence base. Nutrition. 2015 Jan;31(1):1-13. PubMed PMID: 25287761

133: Spaulding SW, Chopra IJ, Sherwin RS, Lyall SS. Effect of caloric restriction and dietary composition of serum T3 and reverse T3 in man. J Clin Endocrinol Metab. 1976 Jan;42(1):197-200. PubMed PMID: 1249190

134: Loucks AB, Thuma JR. Luteinizing hormone pulsatility is disrupted at a threshold of energy availability in regularly menstruating women. J Clin Endocrinol Metab. 2003 Jan;88(1):297-311. PubMed PMID: 12519869

135: Sparta M, Alexandrova AN. How metal substitution affects the enzymatic activity of catechol-o-methyltransferase. PLoS One. 2012;7(10):e47172. PubMed PMID: 23056605

136: Wong CP, Rinaldi NA, Ho E. Zinc deficiency enhanced inflammatory response by increasing immune cell activation and inducing IL6 promoter demethylation. Mol Nutr Food Res. 2015 May;59(5):991-9. PubMed PMID: 25656040

137: Swardfager W, Herrmann N, McIntyre RS, Mazereeuw G, Goldberger K, Cha

DS, et al. Potential roles of zinc in the pathophysiology and treatment of major depressive disorder. Neurosci Biobehav Rev. 2013 Jun;37(5):911-29. PubMed PMID: 23567517

138: Jamilian M, Foroozanfard F, Bahmani F, Talaee R, Monavari M, Asemi Z. Effects of Zinc Supplementation on Endocrine Outcomes in Women with Polycystic Ovary Syndrome: a Randomized, Double-Blind, Placebo-Controlled Trial. Biol Trace Elem Res. 2016 Apr;170(2):271-8. PubMed PMID: 26315303

139: Stoddard FR 2nd, Brooks AD, Eskin BA, Johannes GJ. Iodine alters gene expression in the MCF7 breast cancer cell line: evidence for an anti-estrogen effect of iodine. Int J Med Sci. 2008 Jul 8;5(4):189-96. PubMed PMID: 18645607

140: Slebodziński AB. Ovarian iodide uptake and triiodothyronine generation in follicular fluid. The enigma of the thyroid ovary interaction. Domest Anim Endocrinol. 2005 Jul;29(1):97-103. PubMed PMID: 15927769

141: Medici M, Ghassabian A, Visser W, de Muinck Keizer-Schrama SM, Jaddoe VW, Visser WE, et al. Women with high early pregnancy urinary iodine levels have an increased risk of hyperthyroid newborns: the population-based Generation R Study. Clin Endocrinol (Oxf). 2014 Apr;80(4):598-606. PubMed PMID: 23992400

142: Luo Y, Kawashima A, Ishido Y, Yoshihara A, Oda K, Hiroi N, et al. Iodine excess as an environmental risk factor for autoimmune thyroid disease. Int J Mol Sci. 2014 Jul 21;15(7):12895-912. PubMed PMID: 25050783

143: Kessler JH. The effect of supraphysiologic levels of iodine on patients with cyclic mastalgia. Breast J. 2004 Jul-Aug;10(4):328-36. PubMed PMID: 15239792

144: Faris MA, Kacimi S, Al-Kurd RA, Fararjeh MA, Bustanji YK, Mohammad MK, et al. Intermittent fasting during Ramadan attenuates proinflammatory cytokines and immune cells in healthy subjects. Nutr Res. 2012 Dec;32(12):947-55. PubMed PMID: 23244540

145: Arnason TG, Bowen MW, Mansell KD. Effects of intermittent fasting on health markers in those with type 2 diabetes: A pilot study. World J Diabetes. 2017 Apr 15;8(4):154-164. PubMed PMID: 28465792

146: Marinac CR, Nelson SH, Breen CI, Hartman SJ, Natarajan L, Pierce JP, et al. Prolonged Nightly Fasting and Breast Cancer Prognosis. JAMA Oncol. 2016 Aug 1;2(8):1049-55. PubMed PMID: 27032109

147: . ACOG Committee Opinion No. 651: Menstruation in Girls and Adolescents: Using the Menstrual Cycle as a Vital Sign. Obstet Gynecol. 2015 Dec;126(6):e143-6. PubMed PMID: 26595586

148: http://www.cemcor.ubc.ca/resources/contraceptive-choices_effective-convenient-safe

149: Lundsgaard AM, Kiens B. Gender differences in skeletal muscle substrate metabolism - molecular mechanisms and insulin sensitivity. Front Endocrinol (Lausanne). 2014;5:195. PubMed PMID: 25431568

150: Scholes D, Hubbard RA, Ichikawa LE, LaCroix AZ, Spangler L, Beasley JM, et al. Oral contraceptive use and bone density change in adolescent and young adult women: a prospective study of age, hormone dose, and discontinuation. J Clin Endocrinol Metab. 2011 Sep;96(9):E1380-7. PubMed PMID: 21752879

151: Prior JC, Naess M, Langhammer A, Forsmo S. Ovulation Prevalence in Women with Spontaneous Normal-Length Menstrual Cycles - A Population-Based Cohort from HUNT3, Norway. PLoS One. 2015;10(8):e0134473. PubMed PMID: 26291617

152: Polson DW, Adams J, Wadsworth J, Franks S. Polycystic ovaries--a common finding in normal women. Lancet. 1988 Apr 16;1(8590):870-2. PubMed PMID: 2895373

153: Dewailly D, Lujan ME, Carmina E, Cedars MI, Laven J, Norman RJ, et al. Definition and significance of polycystic ovarian morphology: a task force report from the Androgen Excess and Polycystic Ovary Syndrome Society. Hum Reprod Update. 2014 May-Jun;20(3):334-52. PubMed PMID: 24345633

154: Teede H, Deeks A, Moran L. Polycystic ovary syndrome: a complex condition with psychological, reproductive and metabolic manifestations that impacts on health across the lifespan. BMC Med. 2010 Jun 30;8;41. PubMed PMID: 20591140

155: Copp T, Jansen J, Doust J, Mol BW, Dokras A, McCaffery K. Are expanding disease definitions unnecessarily labelling women with polycystic ovary syndrome?. BMJ. 2017 Aug 16;358:j3694. PubMed PMID: 28814559

156: Dewailly D, Lujan ME, Carmina E, Cedars MI, Laven J, Norman RJ, et al. Definition and significance of polycystic ovarian morphology: a task force report from the Androgen Excess and Polycystic Ovary Syndrome Society. Hum Reprod Update. 2014 May-Jun;20(3):334-52. PubMed PMID: 24345633

157: Granger DA, Shirtcliff EA, Booth A, Kivlighan KT, Schwartz EB. The "trouble" with salivary testosterone. Psychoneuroendocrinology. 2004 Nov;29(10):1229-40. PubMed PMID: 15288702

158: Rosenfield RL. The Diagnosis of Polycystic Ovary Syndrome in Adolescents. Pediatrics. 2015 Dec;136(6):1154-65. PubMed PMID: 26598450

159: Witchel SF. Nonclassic congenital adrenal hyperplasia. Curr Opin Endocrinol Diabetes Obes. 2012 Jun;19(3):151-8. PubMed PMID: 22499220

160: Hudecova M, Holte J, Olovsson M, Sundström Poromaa I. Long-term follow-up of patients with polycystic ovary syndrome: reproductive outcome and ovarian reserve. Hum Reprod. 2009 May;24(5):1176-83. PubMed PMID: 19168874

161: Palioura E, Diamanti-Kandarakis E. Industrial endocrine disruptors and polycystic ovary syndrome. J Endocrinol Invest. 2013 Dec;36(11):1105-11. PubMed PMID: 24445124

162: Zhang DM, Jiao RQ, Kong LD. High Dietary Fructose: Direct or Indirect Dangerous Factors Disturbing Tissue and Organ Functions. Nutrients. 2017 Mar 29;9(4). PubMed PMID: 28353649

163: Pande AR, Guleria AK, Singh SD, Shukla M, Dabadghao P. β cell function and insulin resistance in lean cases with polycystic ovary syndrome. Gynecol Endocrinol.

2017 Jul 13;:1-5. PubMed PMID: 28704124

164: Arnason TG, Bowen MW, Mansell KD. Effects of intermittent fasting on health markers in those with type 2 diabetes: A pilot study. World J Diabetes. 2017 Apr 15;8(4):154-164. PubMed PMID: 28465792

165: Van Der Heijden GJ, Wang ZJ, Chu Z, Toffolo G, Manesso E, Sauer PJ, et al. Strength exercise improves muscle mass and hepatic insulin sensitivity in obese youth. Med Sci Sports Exerc. 2010 Nov;42(11):1973-80. PubMed PMID: 20351587

166: Diamanti-Kandarakis E, Baillargeon JP, Iuorno MJ, Jakubowicz DJ, Nestler JE. A modern medical quandary: polycystic ovary syndrome, insulin resistance, and oral contraceptive pills. J Clin Endocrinol Metab. 2003 May;88(5):1927-32. PubMed PMID: 12727935

167: http://www.sciencedaily.com/releases/2009/04/090417084014.htm

168: Adeniji AA, Essah PA, Nestler JE, Cheang KI. Metabolic Effects of a Commonly Used Combined Hormonal Oral Contraceptive in Women With and Without Polycystic Ovary Syndrome. J Womens Health (Larchmt). 2016 Jun;25(6):638-45. PubMed PMID: 26871978

169: Hruby A, Meigs JB, O'Donnell CJ, Jacques PF, McKeown NM. Higher magnesium intake reduces risk of impaired glucose and insulin metabolism and progression from prediabetes to diabetes in middle-aged americans. Diabetes Care. 2014 Feb;37(2):419-27. PubMed PMID: 24089547

170: Hata A, Doi Y, Ninomiya T, Mukai N, Hirakawa Y, Hata J, et al. Magnesium intake decreases Type 2 diabetes risk through the improvement of insulin resistance and inflammation: the Hisayama Study. Diabet Med. 2013 Dec;30(12):1487-94. PubMed PMID: 23758216

171: Guerrero-Romero F, Tamez-Perez HE, González-González G, Salinas-Martínez AM, Montes-Villarreal J, Treviño-Ortiz JH, et al. Oral magnesium supplementation improves insulin sensitivity in non-diabetic subjects with insulin resistance. A double-blind placebo-controlled randomized trial. Diabetes Metab. 2004 Jun;30(3):253-8. PubMed PMID: 15223977

172: McCarty MF, DiNicolantonio JJ. The cardiometabolic benefits of glycine: Is glycine an 'antidote' to dietary fructose?. Open Heart. 2014;1(1):e000103. PubMed PMID: 25332814

173: Masharani U, Gjerde C, Evans JL, Youngren JF, Goldfine ID. Effects of controlled-release alpha lipoic acid in lean, nondiabetic patients with polycystic ovary syndrome. J Diabetes Sci Technol. 2010 Mar 1;4(2):359-64. PubMed PMID: 20307398

174: De Cicco S, Immediata V, Romualdi D, Policola C, Tropea A, Di Florio C, et al. Myoinositol combined with alpha-lipoic acid may improve the clinical and endocrine features of polycystic ovary syndrome through an insulin-independent action. Gynecol Endocrinol. 2017 Apr 23;:1-4. PubMed PMID: 28434274

175: De Cicco S, Immediata V, Romualdi D, Policola C, Tropea A, Di Florio C, et al. Myoinositol combined with alpha-lipoic acid may improve the clinical and endocrine features of polycystic ovary syndrome through an insulin-independent action. Gynecol

Endocrinol. 2017 Apr 23;:1-4. PubMed PMID: 28434274

176: Monastra G, Unfer V, Harrath AH, Bizzarri M. Combining treatment with myo-inositol and D-chiro-inositol (40:1) is effective in restoring ovary function and metabolic balance in PCOS patients. Gynecol Endocrinol. 2017 Jan;33(1):1-9. PubMed PMID: 27898267

177: La Marca A, Grisendi V, Dondi G, Sighinolfi G, Cianci A. The menstrual cycle regularization following D-chiro-inositol treatment in PCOS women: a retrospective study. Gynecol Endocrinol. 2015 Jan;31(1):52-6. PubMed PMID: 25268566

178: Brzozowska M, Karowicz-Bilińska A. [The role of vitamin D deficiency in the etiology of polycystic ovary syndrome disorders]. Ginekol Pol. 2013 Jun;84(6):456-60. PubMed PMID: 24032264

179: Wei W, Zhao H, Wang A, Sui M, Liang K, Deng H, et al. A clinical study on the short-term effect of berberine in comparison to metformin on the metabolic characteristics of women with polycystic ovary syndrome. Eur J Endocrinol. 2012 Jan;166(1):99-105. PubMed PMID: 22019891

180: An Y, Sun Z, Zhang Y, Liu B, Guan Y, Lu M. The use of berberine for women with polycystic ovary syndrome undergoing IVF treatment. Clin Endocrinol (Oxf). 2014 Mar;80(3):425-31. PubMed PMID: 23869585

181: Peng WH, Wu CR, Chen CS, Chen CF, Leu ZC, Hsieh MT. Anxiolytic effect of berberine on exploratory activity of the mouse in two experimental anxiety models: interaction with drugs acting at 5-HT receptors. Life Sci. 2004 Oct 1;75(20):2451-62. PubMed PMID: 15350820

182: Zhang X, Zhao Y, Xu J, Xue Z, Zhang M, Pang X, et al. Modulation of gut microbiota by berberine and metformin during the treatment of high-fat diet-induced obesity in rats. Sci Rep. 2015 Sep 23;5:14405. PubMed PMID: 26396057

183: Han J, Lin H, Huang W. Modulating gut microbiota as an anti-diabetic mechanism of berberine. Med Sci Monit. 2011 Jul;17(7):RA164-7. PubMed PMID: 21709646

184: Li L, Li C, Pan P, Chen X, Wu X, Ng EH, et al. A Single Arm Pilot Study of Effects of Berberine on the Menstrual Pattern, Ovulation Rate, Hormonal and Metabolic Profiles in Anovulatory Chinese Women with Polycystic Ovary Syndrome. PLoS One. 2015;10(12):e0144072. PubMed PMID: 26645811

185: Zhao L, Li W, Han F, Hou L, Baillargeon JP, Kuang H, et al. Berberine reduces insulin resistance induced by dexamethasone in theca cells in vitro. Fertil Steril. 2011 Jan;95(1):461-3. PubMed PMID: 20840879

186: Gu L, Li N, Gong J, Li Q, Zhu W, Li J. Berberine ameliorates intestinal epithelial tight-junction damage and down-regulates myosin light chain kinase pathways in a mouse model of endotoxinemia. J Infect Dis. 2011 Jun 1;203(11):1602-12. PubMed PMID: 21592990

187: Guler I, Himmetoglu O, Turp A, Erdem A, Erdem M, Onan MA, et al. Zinc and homocysteine levels in polycystic ovarian syndrome patients with insulin resistance. Biol Trace Elem Res. 2014 Jun;158(3):297-304. PubMed PMID: 24664271

188: Jamilian M, Foroozanfard F, Bahmani F, Talaee R, Monavari M, Asemi Z. Effects of Zinc Supplementation on Endocrine Outcomes in Women with Polycystic Ovary Syndrome: a Randomized, Double-Blind, Placebo-Controlled Trial. Biol Trace Elem Res. 2016 Apr;170(2):271-8. PubMed PMID: 26315303

189: Takahashi K, Kitao M. Effect of TJ-68 (shakuyaku-kanzo-to) on polycystic ovarian disease. Int J Fertil Menopausal Stud. 1994 Mar-Apr;39(2):69-76. PubMed PMID: 8012442

190: Arentz S, Smith CA, Abbott J, Fahey P, Cheema BS, Bensoussan A. Combined Lifestyle and Herbal Medicine in Overweight Women with Polycystic Ovary Syndrome (PCOS): A Randomized Controlled Trial. Phytother Res. 2017 Sep;31(9):1330-1340. PubMed PMID: 28685911

191: Takeuchi T, Nishii O, Okamura T, Yaginuma T. Effect of paeoniflorin, glycyrrhizin and glycyrrhetic acid on ovarian androgen production. Am J Chin Med. 1991;19(1):73-8. PubMed PMID: 1897494

192: Armanini D, Mattarello MJ, Fiore C, Bonanni G, Scaroni C, Sartorato P, et al. Licorice reduces serum testosterone in healthy women. Steroids. 2004 Oct-Nov;69(11-12):763-6. PubMed PMID: 15579328

193: Somjen D, Knoll E, Vaya J, Stern N, Tamir S. Estrogen-like activity of licorice root constituents: glabridin and glabrene, in vascular tissues in vitro and in vivo. J Steroid Biochem Mol Biol. 2004 Jul;91(3):147-55. PubMed PMID: 15276622

194: Takahashi K, Kitao M. Effect of TJ-68 (shakuyaku-kanzo-to) on polycystic ovarian disease. Int J Fertil Menopausal Stud. 1994 Mar-Apr;39(2):69-76. PubMed PMID: 8012442

195: http://www.cemcor.ca/resources/topics/cyclic-progesterone-therapy

196: Diamanti-Kandarakis E, Baillargeon JP, Iuorno MJ, Jakubowicz DJ, Nestler JE. A modern medical quandary: polycystic ovary syndrome, insulin resistance, and oral contraceptive pills. J Clin Endocrinol Metab. 2003 May;88(5):1927-32. PubMed PMID: 12727935

197: Adeniji AA, Essah PA, Nestler JE, Cheang KI. Metabolic Effects of a Commonly Used Combined Hormonal Oral Contraceptive in Women With and Without Polycystic Ovary Syndrome. J Womens Health (Larchmt). 2016 Jun;25(6):638-45. PubMed PMID: 26871978

198: Wang JG, Lobo RA. The complex relationship between hypothalamic amenorrhea and polycystic ovary syndrome. J Clin Endocrinol Metab. 2008 Apr;93(4):1394-7. PubMed PMID: 18230664

199: Loucks AB, Thuma JR. Luteinizing hormone pulsatility is disrupted at a threshold of energy availability in regularly menstruating women. J Clin Endocrinol Metab. 2003 Jan;88(1):297-311. PubMed PMID: 12519869

200: Takahashi K, Kitao M. Effect of TJ-68 (shakuyaku-kanzo-to) on polycystic ovarian disease. Int J Fertil Menopausal Stud. 1994 Mar-Apr;39(2):69-76. PubMed PMID: 8012442

201: Long X, Li R, Yang Y, Qiao J. Overexpression of IL-18 in the Proliferative Phase Endometrium of Patients With Polycystic Ovary Syndrome. Reprod Sci. 2017 Feb;24(2):252-257. PubMed PMID: 27313119

202: González F. Inflammation in Polycystic Ovary Syndrome: underpinning of insulin resistance and ovarian dysfunction. Steroids. 2012 Mar 10;77(4):300-5. PubMed PMID: 22178787

203: Bisanz JE, Enos MK, Mwanga JR, Changalucha J, Burton JP, Gloor GB, et al. Randomized open-label pilot study of the influence of probiotics and the gut microbiome on toxic metal levels in Tanzanian pregnant women and school children. MBio. 2014 Oct 7;5(5):e01580-14. PubMed PMID: 25293764

204: Thakker D, Raval A, Patel I, Walia R. N-acetylcysteine for polycystic ovary syndrome: a systematic review and meta-analysis of randomized controlled clinical trials. Obstet Gynecol Int. 2015;2015:817849. PubMed PMID: 25653680

205: Tagliaferri V, Romualdi D, Scarinci E, Cicco S, Florio CD, Immediata V, et al. Melatonin Treatment May Be Able to Restore Menstrual Cyclicity in Women With PCOS: A Pilot Study. Reprod Sci. 2017 Jan 1;:1933719117711262. PubMed PMID: 28558523

206: Gourgari E, Lodish M, Keil M, Sinaii N, Turkbey E, Lyssikatos C, et al. Bilateral Adrenal Hyperplasia as a Possible Mechanism for Hyperandrogenism in Women With Polycystic Ovary Syndrome. J Clin Endocrinol Metab. 2016 Sep;101(9):3353-60. PubMed PMID: 27336356

207: Azziz R, Carmina E, Dewailly D, Diamanti-Kandarakis E, Escobar-Morreale HF, Futterweit W, et al. The Androgen Excess and PCOS Society criteria for the polycystic ovary syndrome: the complete task force report. Fertil Steril. 2009 Feb;91(2):456-88. PubMed PMID: 18950759

208: Barrett ES, Sobolewski M. Polycystic ovary syndrome: do endocrine-disrupting chemicals play a role?. Semin Reprod Med. 2014 May;32(3):166-76. PubMed PMID: 24715511

209: Rasmusson AM, Vasek J, Lipschitz DS, Vojvoda D, Mustone ME, Shi Q, et al. An increased capacity for adrenal DHEA release is associated with decreased avoidance and negative mood symptoms in women with PTSD. Neuropsychopharmacology. 2004 Aug;29(8):1546-57. PubMed PMID: 15199367

210: Lobo RA, Granger LR, Paul WL, Goebelsmann U, Mishell DR Jr. Psychological stress and increases in urinary norepinephrine metabolites, platelet serotonin, and adrenal androgens in women with polycystic ovary syndrome. Am J Obstet Gynecol. 1983 Feb 15;145(4):496-503. PubMed PMID: 6824043

211: JONES GE, HOWARD JE, LANGFORD H. The use of cortisone in follicular phase disturbances. Fertil Steril. 1953 Jan-Feb;4(1):49-62. PubMed PMID: 13021206

212: Lu YH, Xia ZL, Ma YY, Chen HJ, Yan LP, Xu HF. Subclinical hypothyroidism is associated with metabolic syndrome and clomiphene citrate resistance in women with polycystic ovary syndrome. Gynecol Endocrinol. 2016 Oct;32(10):852-855. PubMed PMID: 27172176

213: Kontaxakis VP, Skourides D, Ferentinos P, Havaki-Kontaxaki BJ, Papadimitriou GN. Isotretinoin and psychopathology: a review. Ann Gen Psychiatry. 2009 Jan 20;8:2. PubMed PMID: 19154613

214: Leachman SA, Insogna KL, Katz L, Ellison A, Milstone LM. Bone densities in patients receiving isotretinoin for cystic acne. Arch Dermatol. 1999 Aug;135(8):961-5. PubMed PMID: 10456346

215: Melnik BC. Diet in acne: further evidence for the role of nutrient signalling in acne pathogenesis. Acta Derm Venereol. 2012 May;92(3):228-31. PubMed PMID: 22419445

216: Adebamowo CA, Spiegelman D, Danby FW, Frazier AL, Willett WC, Holmes MD. High school dietary dairy intake and teenage acne. J Am Acad Dermatol. 2005 Feb;52(2):207-14. PubMed PMID: 15692464

217: Gupta M, Mahajan VK, Mehta KS, Chauhan PS. Zinc therapy in dermatology: a review. Dermatol Res Pract. 2014;2014:709152. PubMed PMID: 25120566

218: Fouladi RF. Aqueous extract of dried fruit of Berberis vulgaris L. in acne vulgaris, a clinical trial. J Diet Suppl. 2012 Dec;9(4):253-61. PubMed PMID: 23038982

219: Murata K, Noguchi K, Kondo M, Onishi M, Watanabe N, Okamura K, et al. Promotion of hair growth by Rosmarinus officinalis leaf extract. Phytother Res. 2013 Feb;27(2):212-7. PubMed PMID: 22517595

220: Fischer TW, Trueb RM, Hanggi G, et al. Topical melatonin for treatment of androgenetic alopecia. Int J Trichology. 2012;4(4):236-245

221: Jamilian M, Foroozanfard F, Bahmani F, Talaee R, Monavari M, Asemi Z. Effects of Zinc Supplementation on Endocrine Outcomes in Women with Polycystic Ovary Syndrome: a Randomized, Double-Blind, Placebo-Controlled Trial. Biol Trace Elem Res. 2016 Apr;170(2):271-8. PubMed PMID: 26315303

222: Hwang C, Sethi S, Heilbrun LK, Gupta NS, Chitale DA, Sakr WA, et al. Anti-androgenic activity of absorption-enhanced 3, 3'-diindolylmethane in prostatectomy patients. Am J Transl Res. 2016;8(1):166-76. PubMed PMID: 27069550

223: Fujita R, Liu J, Shimizu K, Konishi F, Noda K, Kumamoto S, et al. Anti-androgenic activities of Ganoderma lucidum. J Ethnopharmacol. 2005 Oct 31;102(1):107-12. PubMed PMID: 16029938

224: Nichols AJ, Hughes OB, Canazza A, Zaiac MN. An Open-Label Evaluator Blinded Study of the Efficacy and Safety of a New Nutritional Supplement in Androgenetic Alopecia: A Pilot Study. J Clin Aesthet Dermatol. 2017 Feb;10(2):52-56. PubMed PMID: 28367262

225: Cassidy A, Bingham S, Setchell KD. Biological effects of a diet of soy protein rich in isoflavones on the menstrual cycle of premenopausal women. Am J Clin Nutr. 1994 Sep;60(3):333-40. PubMed PMID: 8074062

226: Loucks AB, Thuma JR. Luteinizing hormone pulsatility is disrupted at a threshold of energy availability in regularly menstruating women. J Clin Endocrinol Metab. 2003 Jan;88(1):297-311. PubMed PMID: 12519869

227: Wiksten-Almströmer M, Hirschberg AL, Hagenfeldt K. Menstrual disorders and associated factors among adolescent girls visiting a youth clinic. Acta Obstet Gynecol Scand. 2007;86(1):65-72. PubMed PMID: 17230292

228: Vescovi JD, Jamal SA, De Souza MJ. Strategies to reverse bone loss in women with functional hypothalamic amenorrhea: a systematic review of the literature. Osteoporos Int. 2008 Apr;19(4):465-78. PubMed PMID: 18180975

229: Falsetti L, Gambera A, Barbetti L, Specchia C. Long-term follow-up of functional hypothalamic amenorrhea and prognostic factors. J Clin Endocrinol Metab. 2002 Feb;87(2):500-5. PubMed PMID: 11836275

230: Webster DE, Lu J, Chen SN, Farnsworth NR, Wang ZJ. Activation of the mu-opiate receptor by Vitex agnus-castus methanol extracts: implication for its use in PMS. J Ethnopharmacol. 2006 Jun 30;106(2):216-21. PubMed PMID: 16439081

231: Higuchi K, Nawata H, Maki T, Higashizima M, Kato K, Ibayashi H. Prolactin has a direct effect on adrenal androgen secretion. J Clin Endocrinol Metab. 1984 Oct;59(4):714-8. PubMed PMID: 6090494

232: Takeyama M, Nagareda T, Takatsuka D, Namiki M, Koizumi K, Aono T, et al. Stimulatory effect of prolactin on luteinizing hormone-induced testicular 5 alpha-reductase activity in hypophysectomized adult rats. Endocrinology. 1986 Jun;118(6):2268-75. PubMed PMID: 3486119

233: Hantsoo L, Epperson CN. Premenstrual Dysphoric Disorder: Epidemiology and Treatment. Curr Psychiatry Rep. 2015 Nov;17(11):87. PubMed PMID: 26377947

234: Timby E, Bäckström T, Nyberg S, Stenlund H, Wihlbäck AC, Bixo M. Women with premenstrual dysphoric disorder have altered sensitivity to allopregnanolone over the menstrual cycle compared to controls-a pilot study. Psychopharmacology (Berl). 2016 Jun;233(11):2109-17. PubMed PMID: 26960697

235: Epperson CN, Hantsoo LV. Making Strides to Simplify Diagnosis of Premenstrual Dysphoric Disorder. Am J Psychiatry. 2017 Jan 1;174(1):6-7. PubMed PMID: 28041003

236: Dubey N, Hoffman JF, Schuebel K, et al. The ESC/E(Z) complex, an effector of response to ovarian steroids, manifests an intrinsic difference in cells from women with premenstrual dysphoric disorder. Molecular Psychiatry. Published online January 3 2017.

237: Bertone-Johnson ER, Ronnenberg AG, Houghton SC, Nobles C, Zagarins SE, Takashima-Uebelhoer BB, et al. Association of inflammation markers with menstrual symptom severity and premenstrual syndrome in young women. Hum Reprod. 2014 Sep;29(9):1987-94. PubMed PMID: 25035435

238: Melcangi RC, Giatti S, Calabrese D, Pesaresi M, Cermenati G, Mitro N, et al. Levels and actions of progesterone and its metabolites in the nervous system during physiological and pathological conditions. Prog Neurobiol. 2014 Feb;113:56-69. PubMed PMID: 23958466

239: Hantsoo L, Epperson CN. Premenstrual Dysphoric Disorder: Epidemiology and Treatment. Curr Psychiatry Rep. 2015 Nov;17(11):87. PubMed PMID: 26377947

240: Zimatkin SM, Anichtchik OV. Alcohol-histamine interactions. Alcohol Alcohol. 1999 Mar-Apr;34(2):141-7. PubMed PMID: 10344773

241: Fogel WA. Diamine oxidase (DAO) and female sex hormones. Agents Actions. 1986 Apr;18(1-2):44-5. PubMed PMID: 3088928

242: Nyberg S, Andersson A, Zingmark E, Wahlström G, Bäckström T, Sundström-Poromaa I. The effect of a low dose of alcohol on allopregnanolone serum concentrations across the menstrual cycle in women with severe premenstrual syndrome and controls. Psychoneuroendocrinology. 2005 Oct;30(9):892-901. PubMed PMID: 15979810

243: Gollenberg AL, Hediger ML, Mumford SL, Whitcomb BW, Hovey KM, Wactawski-Wende J, et al. Perceived stress and severity of perimenstrual symptoms: the BioCycle Study. J Womens Health (Larchmt). 2010 May;19(5):959-67. PubMed PMID: 20384452

244: Gordon JL, Girdler SS, Meltzer-Brody SE, Stika CS, Thurston RC, Clark CT, et al. Ovarian hormone fluctuation, neurosteroids, and HPA axis dysregulation in perimenopausal depression: a novel heuristic model. Am J Psychiatry. 2015 Mar 1;172(3):227-36. PubMed PMID: 25585035

245: Prior JC, Vigna Y, Sciarretta D, Alojado N, Schulzer M. Conditioning exercise decreases premenstrual symptoms: a prospective, controlled 6-month trial. Fertil Steril. 1987 Mar;47(3):402-8. PubMed PMID: 3549364

246: Walker AF, De Souza MC, Vickers MF, Abeyasekera S, Collins ML, Trinca LA. Magnesium supplementation alleviates premenstrual symptoms of fluid retention. J Womens Health. 1998 Nov;7(9):1157-65. PubMed PMID: 9861593

247: Abraham GE, Lubran MM. Serum and red cell magnesium levels in patients with premenstrual tension. Am J Clin Nutr. 1981 Nov;34(11):2364-6. PubMed PMID: 7197877

248: M. Wyatt, P.W. Dimmock, M.S. O'Brien. Efficacy of vitamin B-6 in the treatment of premenstrual syndrome: systematic review. BMJ, 318 (1999), pp. 1375–1381.

249: Cerqueira RO, Frey BN, Leclerc E, Brietzke E. Vitex agnus castus for premenstrual syndrome and premenstrual dysphoric disorder: a systematic review. Arch Womens Ment Health. 2017 Dec;20(6):713-719. PubMed PMID: 29063202

250: Webster DE, Lu J, Chen SN, Farnsworth NR, Wang ZJ. Activation of the mu-opiate receptor by Vitex agnus-castus methanol extracts: implication for its use in PMS. J Ethnopharmacol. 2006 Jun 30;106(2):216-21. PubMed PMID: 16439081

251: Reichman ME, Judd JT, Longcope C, Schatzkin A, Clevidence BA, Nair PP, et al. Effects of alcohol consumption on plasma and urinary hormone concentrations in premenopausal women. J Natl Cancer Inst. 1993 May 5;85(9):722-7. PubMed PMID: 8478958

252: Morimoto Y, Conroy SM, Pagano IS, Isaki M, Franke AA, Nordt FJ, et al. Urinary estrogen metabolites during a randomized soy trial. Nutr Cancer. 2012;64(2):307-14. PubMed PMID: 22293063

253: Calcium-d-glucarate monograph. Altern Med Rev 2002;7(4):336-339

254: Siahbazi S, Behboudi-Gandevani S, Moghaddam-Banaem L, Montazeri A. Effect of zinc sulfate supplementation on premenstrual syndrome and health-related quality of life: Clinical randomized controlled trial. J Obstet Gynaecol Res. 2017 Feb 11;. PubMed PMID: 28188965

255: Posaci C, Erten O, Uren A, Acar B. Plasma copper, zinc and magnesium levels in patients with premenstrual tension syndrome. Acta Obstet Gynecol Scand. 1994 Jul;73(6):452-5. PubMed PMID: 8042455

256: Atmaca M, Kumru S, Tezcan E. Fluoxetine versus Vitex agnus castus extract in the treatment of premenstrual dysphoric disorder. Hum Psychopharmacol. 2003 Apr;18(3):191-5. PubMed PMID: 12672170

257: Canning S, Waterman M, Orsi N, Ayres J, Simpson N, Dye L. The efficacy of Hypericum perforatum (St John's wort) for the treatment of premenstrual syndrome: a randomized, double-blind, placebo-controlled trial. CNS Drugs. 2010 Mar;24(3):207-25. PubMed PMID: 20155996

258: Hall SD, Wang Z, Huang SM, Hamman MA, Vasavada N, Adigun AQ, et al. The interaction between St John's wort and an oral contraceptive. Clin Pharmacol Ther. 2003 Dec;74(6):525-35. PubMed PMID: 14663455

259: Kessler JH. The effect of supraphysiologic levels of iodine on patients with cyclic mastalgia. Breast J. 2004 Jul-Aug;10(4):328-36. PubMed PMID: 15239792

260: Aceves C, Anguiano B, Delgado G. Is iodine a gatekeeper of the integrity of the mammary gland?. J Mammary Gland Biol Neoplasia. 2005 Apr;10(2):189-96. PubMed PMID: 16025225

261: Kessler JH. The effect of supraphysiologic levels of iodine on patients with cyclic mastalgia. Breast J. 2004 Jul-Aug;10(4):328-36. PubMed PMID: 15239792

262: Carmichael AR. Can Vitex Agnus Castus be Used for the Treatment of Mastalgia? What is the Current Evidence?. Evid Based Complement Alternat Med. 2008 Sep;5(3):247-50. PubMed PMID: 18830450

263: Pavlović JM, Allshouse AA, Santoro NF, Crawford SL, Thurston RC, Neal-Perry GS, et al. Sex hormones in women with and without migraine: Evidence of migraine-specific hormone profiles. Neurology. 2016 Jul 5;87(1):49-56. PubMed PMID: 27251885

264: Peres MF. Melatonin, the pineal gland and their implications for headache disorders. Cephalalgia. 2005 Jun;25(6):403-11. PubMed PMID: 15910564

265: Champaloux SW, Tepper NK, Monsour M, Curtis KM, Whiteman MK, Marchbanks PA, et al. Use of combined hormonal contraceptives among women with migraines and risk of ischemic stroke. Am J Obstet Gynecol. 2017 May;216(5):489.e1-489.e7. PubMed PMID: 28034652

266: Egger J, Carter CM, Wilson J, Turner MW, Soothill JF. Is migraine food allergy? A double-blind controlled trial of oligoantigenic diet treatment. Lancet. 1983 Oct 15;2(8355):865-9. PubMed PMID: 6137694

267: Mauskop A, Varughese J. Why all migraine patients should be treated with magnesium. J Neural Transm (Vienna). 2012 May;119(5):575-9. PubMed PMID: 22426836

268: Chiu HY, Yeh TH, Huang YC, Chen PY. Effects of Intravenous and Oral Magnesium on Reducing Migraine: A Meta-analysis of Randomized Controlled Trials. Pain Physician. 2016 Jan;19(1):E97-112. PubMed PMID: 26752497

269: Gonçalves AL, Martini Ferreira A, Ribeiro RT, Zukerman E, Cipolla-Neto J, Peres MF. Randomised clinical trial comparing melatonin 3 mg, amitriptyline 25 mg and placebo for migraine prevention. J Neurol Neurosurg Psychiatry. 2016 Oct;87(10):1127-32. PubMed PMID: 27165014

270: Boehnke C, Reuter U, Flach U, Schuh-Hofer S, Einhäupl KM, Arnold G. High-dose riboflavin treatment is efficacious in migraine prophylaxis: an open study in a tertiary care centre. Eur J Neurol. 2004 Jul;11(7):475-7. PubMed PMID: 15257686

271: Calhoun AH, Gill N. Presenting a New, Non-Hormonally Mediated Cyclic Headache in Women: End-Menstrual Migraine. Headache. 2017 Jan;57(1):17-20. PubMed PMID: 27704538

272: Mong JA, Baker FC, Mahoney MM, Paul KN, Schwartz MD, Semba K, et al. Sleep, rhythms, and the endocrine brain: influence of sex and gonadal hormones. J Neurosci. 2011 Nov 9;31(45):16107-16. PubMed PMID: 22072663

273: Baker FC, Kahan TL, Trinder J, Colrain IM. Sleep quality and the sleep electroencephalogram in women with severe premenstrual syndrome. Sleep. 2007 Oct;30(10):1283-91. PubMed PMID: 17969462

274: Baker FC, Driver HS. Circadian rhythms, sleep, and the menstrual cycle. Sleep Med. 2007 Sep;8(6):613-22. PubMed PMID: 17383933

275: Canning S, Waterman M, Orsi N, Ayres J, Simpson N, Dye L. The efficacy of Hypericum perforatum (St John's wort) for the treatment of premenstrual syndrome: a randomized, double-blind, placebo-controlled trial. CNS Drugs. 2010 Mar;24(3):207-25. PubMed PMID: 20155996

276: Chocano-Bedoya PO, Manson JE, Hankinson SE, Johnson SR, Chasan-Taber L, Ronnenberg AG, et al. Intake of selected minerals and risk of premenstrual syndrome. Am J Epidemiol. 2013 May 15;177(10):1118-27. PubMed PMID: 23444100

277: James AH. Women and bleeding disorders. Haemophilia. 2010 Jul;16 Suppl 5:160-7. PubMed PMID: 20590876

278: Weeks AD. Menorrhagia and hypothyroidism. Evidence supports association between hypothyroidism and menorrhagia. BMJ. 2000 Mar 4;320(7235):649. PubMed PMID: 10698899

279: Poppe K, Velkeniers B, Glinoer D. Thyroid disease and female reproduction. Clin Endocrinol (Oxf). 2007 Mar;66(3):309-21. PubMed PMID: 17302862

280: Lethaby A, Duckitt K, Farquhar C. Non-steroidal anti-inflammatory drugs for heavy menstrual bleeding. Cochrane Database Syst Rev. 2013 Jan 31;(1):CD000400. PubMed PMID: 23440779

281: Kim K, Wactawski-Wende J, Michels KA, Plowden TC, Chaljub EN, Sjaarda LA, et al. Dairy Food Intake Is Associated with Reproductive Hormones and Sporadic Anovulation among Healthy Premenopausal Women. J Nutr. 2017 Feb;147(2):218-226. PubMed PMID: 27881593

282: TAYMOR ML, STURGIS SH, YAHIA C. THE ETIOLOGICAL ROLE OF CHRONIC IRON DEFICIENCY IN PRODUCTION OF MENORRHAGIA. JAMA. 1964 Feb 1;187:323-7. PubMed PMID: 14085026

283: Seltzer VL, Benjamin F, Deutsch S. Perimenopausal bleeding patterns and pathologic findings. J Am Med Womens Assoc (1972). 1990 Jul-Aug;45(4):132-4. PubMed PMID: 2398224

284: Marshall LM, Spiegelman D, Goldman MB, Manson JE, Colditz GA, Barbieri RL, et al. A prospective study of reproductive factors and oral contraceptive use in relation to the risk of uterine leiomyomata. Fertil Steril. 1998 Sep;70(3):432-9. PubMed PMID: 9757871

285: Hunt PA, Sathyanarayana S, Fowler PA, Trasande L. Female Reproductive Disorders, Diseases, and Costs of Exposure to Endocrine Disrupting Chemicals in the European Union. J Clin Endocrinol Metab. 2016 Apr;101(4):1562-70. PubMed PMID: 27003299

286: Medikare V, Kandukuri LR, Ananthapur V, Deenadayal M, Nallari P. The genetic bases of uterine fibroids; a review. J Reprod Infertil. 2011 Jul;12(3):181-91. PubMed PMID: 23926501

287: Templeman C, Marshall SF, Clarke CA, Henderson KD, Largent J, Neuhausen S, et al. Risk factors for surgically removed fibroids in a large cohort of teachers. Fertil Steril. 2009 Oct;92(4):1436-46. PubMed PMID: 19019355

288: Calcium-d-glucarate monograph. Altern Med Rev 2002;7(4):336-339

289: Sakamoto S, Yoshino H, Shirahata Y, Shimodairo K, Okamoto R. Pharmacotherapeutic effects of kuei-chih-fu-ling-wan (keishi-bukuryo-gan) on human uterine myomas. Am J Chin Med. 1992;20(3-4):313-7. PubMed PMID: 1471615

290: http://www.medscape.com/viewarticle/459772

291: Struble J, Reid S, Bedaiwy MA. Adenomyosis: A Clinical Review of a Challenging Gynecologic Condition. J Minim Invasive Gynecol. 2016 Feb 1;23(2):164-85. PubMed PMID: 26427702

292: Nozaki C, Vergnano AM, Filliol D, Ouagazzal AM, Le Goff A, Carvalho S, et al. Zinc alleviates pain through high-affinity binding to the NMDA receptor NR2A subunit. Nat Neurosci. 2011 Jul 3;14(8):1017-22. PubMed PMID: 21725314

293: Janssen EB, Rijkers AC, Hoppenbrouwers K, Meuleman C, D'Hooghe TM. Prevalence of endometriosis diagnosed by laparoscopy in adolescents with dysmenorrhea or chronic pelvic pain: a systematic review. Hum Reprod Update. 2013 Sep-Oct;19(5):570-82. PubMed PMID: 23727940

294: Králíčková M, Vetvicka V. Immunological aspects of endometriosis: a review. Ann Transl Med. 2015 Jul;3(11):153. PubMed PMID: 26244140

295: Kaur, K. and Allahbadia, G. (2016) An Update on Pathophysiology and Medical Management of Endometriosis. Advances in Reproductive Sciences, 4, 53-73

296: Matalliotakis IM, Arici A, Cakmak H, Goumenou AG, Koumantakis G, Mahutte NG. Familial aggregation of endometriosis in the Yale Series. Arch Gynecol Obstet. 2008 Dec;278(6):507-11. PubMed PMID: 18449556

297: Bruner-Tran KL, Gnecco J, Ding T, Glore DR, Pensabene V, Osteen KG. Exposure to the environmental endocrine disruptor TCDD and human reproductive dysfunction: Translating lessons from murine models. Reprod Toxicol. 2017 Mar;68:59-71. PubMed PMID: 27423904

298: Hunt PA, Sathyanarayana S, Fowler PA, Trasande L. Female Reproductive Disorders, Diseases, and Costs of Exposure to Endocrine Disrupting Chemicals in the European Union. J Clin Endocrinol Metab. 2016 Apr;101(4):1562-70. PubMed PMID: 27003299

299: Maroun P, Cooper MJ, Reid GD, Keirse MJ. Relevance of gastrointestinal symptoms in endometriosis. Aust N Z J Obstet Gynaecol. 2009 Aug;49(4):411-4. PubMed PMID: 19694698

300: Feehley T, Belda-Ferre P, Nagler CR. What's LPS Got to Do with It? A Role for Gut LPS Variants in Driving Autoimmune and Allergic Disease. Cell Host Microbe. 2016 May 11;19(5):572-4. PubMed PMID: 27173923

301: Iba Y, Harada T, Horie S, Deura I, Iwabe T, Terakawa N. Lipopolysaccharide-promoted proliferation of endometriotic stromal cells via induction of tumor necrosis factor alpha and interleukin-8 expression. Fertil Steril. 2004 Oct;82 Suppl 3:1036-42. PubMed PMID: 15474070

302: Khan KN, Kitajima M, Inoue T, Fujishita A, Nakashima M, Masuzaki H. 17β-estradiol and lipopolysaccharide additively promote pelvic inflammation and growth of endometriosis. Reprod Sci. 2015 May;22(5):585-94. PubMed PMID: 25355803

303: Khan KN, Fujishita A, Hiraki K, Kitajima M, Nakashima M, Fushiki S, et al. Bacterial contamination hypothesis: a new concept in endometriosis. Reprod Med Biol. 2018 Apr;17(2):125-133. PubMed PMID: 29692669

304: https://www.endometriosisaustralia.org/single-post/2016/09/03/Can-you-diagnose-Endometriosis-via-Ultrasound

305: Ahn SH, Singh V, Tayade C. Biomarkers in endometriosis: challenges and opportunities. Fertil Steril. 2017 Mar;107(3):523-532. PubMed PMID: 28189296

306: http://www.abc.net.au/triplej/programs/hack/blood-test-could-diagnose-endometriosis-within-a-day/8318016

307: Cosar E, Mamillapalli R, Ersoy GS, Cho S, Seifer B, Taylor HS. Serum microRNAs as diagnostic markers of endometriosis: a comprehensive array-based analysis. Fertil Steril. 2016 Aug;106(2):402-9. PubMed PMID: 27179784

308: Pundir J, Omanwa K, Kovoor E, Pundir V, Lancaster G, Barton-Smith P. Laparoscopic Excision Versus Ablation for Endometriosis-associated Pain: An Updated Systematic Review and Meta-analysis. J Minim Invasive Gynecol. 2017 Apr

26;. PubMed PMID: 28456617

309: http://endowhat.com/

310: Guo SW. Recurrence of endometriosis and its control. Hum Reprod Update. 2009 Jul-Aug;15(4):441-61. PubMed PMID: 19279046

311: Kaur, K. and Allahbadia, G. (2016) An Update on Pathophysiology and Medical Management of Endometriosis. Advances in Reproductive Sciences, 4, 53-73

312: Marziali M, Venza M, Lazzaro S, Lazzaro A, Micossi C, Stolfi VM. Gluten-free diet: a new strategy for management of painful endometriosis related symptoms?. Minerva Chir. 2012 Dec;67(6):499-504. PubMed PMID: 23334113

313: Moore JS, Gibson PR, Perry RE, Burgell RE. Endometriosis in patients with irritable bowel syndrome: Specific symptomatic and demographic profile, and response to the low FODMAP diet. Aust N Z J Obstet Gynaecol. 2017 Apr;57(2):201-205. PubMed PMID: 28303579

314: Jana S, Paul S, Swarnakar S. Curcumin as anti-endometriotic agent: implication of MMP-3 and intrinsic apoptotic pathway. Biochem Pharmacol. 2012 Mar 15;83(6):797-804. PubMed PMID: 22227273

315: Jana S, Paul S, Swarnakar S. Curcumin as anti-endometriotic agent: implication of MMP-3 and intrinsic apoptotic pathway. Biochem Pharmacol. 2012 Mar 15;83(6):797-804. PubMed PMID: 22227273

316: Zhang Y, Cao H, Yu Z, Peng HY, Zhang CJ. Curcumin inhibits endometriosis endometrial cells by reducing estradiol production. Iran J Reprod Med. 2013 May;11(5):415-22. PubMed PMID: 24639774

317: Kuttan G, Kumar KB, Guruvayoorappan C, Kuttan R. Antitumor, anti-invasion, and antimetastatic effects of curcumin. Adv Exp Med Biol. 2007;595:173-84. PubMed PMID: 17569210

318: Messalli EM, Schettino MT, Mainini G, Ercolano S, Fuschillo G, Falcone F, et al. The possible role of zinc in the etiopathogenesis of endometriosis. Clin Exp Obstet Gynecol. 2014;41(5):541-6. PubMed PMID: 25864256

319: Finamore A, Massimi M, Conti Devirgiliis L, Mengheri E. Zinc deficiency induces membrane barrier damage and increases neutrophil transmigration in Caco-2 cells. J Nutr. 2008 Sep;138(9):1664-70. PubMed PMID: 18716167

320: Wong CP, Rinaldi NA, Ho E. Zinc deficiency enhanced inflammatory response by increasing immune cell activation and inducing IL6 promoter demethylation. Mol Nutr Food Res. 2015 May;59(5):991-9. PubMed PMID: 25656040

321: Nozaki C, Vergnano AM, Filliol D, Ouagazzal AM, Le Goff A, Carvalho S, et al. Zinc alleviates pain through high-affinity binding to the NMDA receptor NR2A subunit. Nat Neurosci. 2011 Jul 3;14(8):1017-22. PubMed PMID: 21725314

322: Li H, Li XL, Zhang M, Xu H, Wang CC, Wang S, et al. Berberine ameliorates experimental autoimmune neuritis by suppressing both cellular and humoral immunity. Scand J Immunol. 2014 Jan;79(1):12-9. PubMed PMID: 24354407

323: Chu M, Ding R, Chu ZY, Zhang MB, Liu XY, Xie SH, et al. Role of berberine in anti-bacterial as a high-affinity LPS antagonist binding to TLR4/MD-2 receptor. BMC Complement Altern Med. 2014 Mar 6;14:89. PubMed PMID: 24602493

324: Gu L, Li N, Gong J, Li Q, Zhu W, Li J. Berberine ameliorates intestinal epithelial tight-junction damage and down-regulates myosin light chain kinase pathways in a mouse model of endotoxinemia. J Infect Dis. 2011 Jun 1;203(11):1602-12. PubMed PMID: 21592990

325: Jeong HW, Hsu KC, Lee JW, Ham M, Huh JY, Shin HJ, et al. Berberine suppresses proinflammatory responses through AMPK activation in macrophages. Am J Physiol Endocrinol Metab. 2009 Apr;296(4):E955-64. PubMed PMID: 19208854

326: Kaur, K. and Allahbadia, G. (2016) An Update on Pathophysiology and Medical Management of Endometriosis. Advances in Reproductive Sciences, 4, 53-73

327: Kolahdouz Mohammadi R, Arablou T. Resveratrol and endometriosis: In vitro and animal studies and underlying mechanisms (Review). Biomed Pharmacother. 2017 Apr 27;91:220-228. PubMed PMID: 28458160

328: Chottanapund S, Van Duursen MB, Navasumrit P, Hunsonti P, Timtavorn S, Ruchirawat M, et al. Anti-aromatase effect of resveratrol and melatonin on hormonal positive breast cancer cells co-cultured with breast adipose fibroblasts. Toxicol In Vitro. 2014 Oct;28(7):1215-21. PubMed PMID: 24929094

329: Porpora MG, Brunelli R, Costa G, Imperiale L, Krasnowska EK, Lundeberg T, et al. A promise in the treatment of endometriosis: an observational cohort study on ovarian endometrioma reduction by N-acetylcysteine. Evid Based Complement Alternat Med. 2013;2013:240702. PubMed PMID: 23737821

330: Hernández Guerrero CA, Bujalil Montenegro L, de la Jara Díaz J, Mier Cabrera J, Bouchán Valencia P. [Endometriosis and deficient intake of antioxidants molecules related to peripheral and peritoneal oxidative stress]. Ginecol Obstet Mex. 2006 Jan;74(1):20-8. PubMed PMID: 16634350

331: Li Y, Adur MK, Kannan A, Davila J, Zhao Y, Nowak RA, et al. Progesterone Alleviates Endometriosis via Inhibition of Uterine Cell Proliferation, Inflammation and Angiogenesis in an Immunocompetent Mouse Model. PLoS One. 2016;11(10):e0165347. PubMed PMID: 27776183

332: Seifert B, Wagler P, Dartsch S, Schmidt U, Nieder J. [Magnesium--a new therapeutic alternative in primary dysmenorrhea]. Zentralbl Gynakol. 1989;111(11):755-60. PubMed PMID: 2675496

333: Eby GA. Zinc treatment prevents dysmenorrhea. Med Hypotheses. 2007;69(2):297-301. PubMed PMID: 17289285

334: Zekavat OR, Karimi MY, Amanat A, Alipour F. A randomised controlled trial of oral zinc sulphate for primary dysmenorrhoea in adolescent females. Aust N Z J Obstet Gynaecol. 2015 Aug;55(4):369-73. PubMed PMID: 26132140

335: Harel Z, Biro FM, Kottenhahn RK, Rosenthal SL. Supplementation with omega-3 polyunsaturated fatty acids in the management of dysmenorrhea in adolescents. Am J Obstet Gynecol. 1996 Apr;174(4):1335-8. PubMed PMID: 8623866

336: Shu J, Xing L, Zhang L, Fang S, Huang H. Ignored adult primary hypothyroidism presenting chiefly with persistent ovarian cysts: a need for increased awareness. Reprod Biol Endocrinol. 2011 Aug 23;9:119. PubMed PMID: 21861901

337: http://www.aafp.org/afp/1998/0601/p2843.html

338: http://www.cochrane.org/CD006134/FERTILREG_oral-contraceptives-to-treat-cysts-of-the-ovary

339: Bahamondes L, Hidalgo M, Petta CA, Diaz J, Espejo-Arce X, Monteiro-Dantas C. Enlarged ovarian follicles in users of a levonorgestrel-releasing intrauterine system and contraceptive implant. J Reprod Med. 2003 Aug;48(8):637-40. PubMed PMID: 12971147

340: Szelag A, Merwid-Lad A, Trocha M. [Histamine receptors in the female reproductive system. Part I. Role of the mast cells and histamine in female reproductive system]. Ginekol Pol. 2002 Jul;73(7):627-35. PubMed PMID: 12369286

341: Personal communication with Dr. Jerilynn Prior

342: Prior JC. Progesterone for Symptomatic Perimenopause Treatment - Progesterone politics, physiology and potential for perimenopause. Facts Views Vis Obgyn. 2011;3(2):109-20. PubMed PMID: 24753856

343: http://www.cemcor.ubc.ca/resources/estrogen%E2%80%99s-storm-season

344: http://www.cemcor.ubc.ca/resources/perimenopause-time-%E2%80%9Cendogenous-ovarian-hyperstimulation%E2%80%9D

345: Santoro N, Crawford SL, Lasley WL, Luborsky JL, Matthews KA, McConnell D, et al. Factors related to declining luteal function in women during the menopausal transition. J Clin Endocrinol Metab. 2008 May;93(5):1711-21. PubMed PMID: 18285413

346: White YA, Woods DC, Takai Y, Ishihara O, Seki H, Tilly JL. Oocyte formation by mitotically active germ cells purified from ovaries of reproductive-age women. Nat Med. 2012 Feb 26;18(3):413-21. PubMed PMID: 22366948

347: http://news.nationalgeographic.com/news/2012/02/120229-women-health-ovaries-eggs-reproduction-science/

348: Carla Aimé, Jean-Baptiste André, Michel Raymond. Grandmothering and cognitive resources are required for the emergence of menopause and extensive post-reproductive lifespan. PLOS Computational Biology, 2017; 13 (7): e1005631

349: https://www.theatlantic.com/science/archive/2017/01/why-do-killer-whales-go-through-menopause/512783/

350: Gordon JL, Girdler SS, Meltzer-Brody SE, Stika CS, Thurston RC, Clark CT, et al. Ovarian hormone fluctuation, neurosteroids, and HPA axis dysregulation in perimenopausal depression: a novel heuristic model. Am J Psychiatry. 2015 Mar 1;172(3):227-36. PubMed PMID: 25585035

351: Gordon JL, Girdler SS, Meltzer-Brody SE, Stika CS, Thurston RC, Clark CT, et al. Ovarian hormone fluctuation, neurosteroids, and HPA axis dysregulation in perimenopausal depression: a novel heuristic model. Am J Psychiatry. 2015 Mar 1;172(3):227-36. PubMed PMID: 25585035

352: Campbell KE, Dennerstein L, Finch S, Szoeke CE. Impact of menopausal status on negative mood and depressive symptoms in a longitudinal sample spanning 20 years. Menopause. 2017 May;24(5):490-496. PubMed PMID: 27922940

353: JC Prior. Perimenopause lost - Reframing the end of menstruation. November 2006. Journal of Reproductive and Infant Psychology. Pages 323-335

354: Campbell KE, Dennerstein L, Tacey M, Szoeke CE. The trajectory of negative mood and depressive symptoms over two decades. Maturitas. 2017 Jan;95:36-41. PubMed PMID: 27889051

355: https://www.futurity.org/women-aging-mood-1525342-2/

356: Zierau O, Zenclussen AC, Jensen F. Role of female sex hormones, estradiol and progesterone, in mast cell behavior. Front Immunol. 2012;3:169. PubMed PMID: 22723800

357: Prior JC. Progesterone for Symptomatic Perimenopause Treatment - Progesterone politics, physiology and potential for perimenopause. Facts Views Vis Obgyn. 2011;3(2):109-20. PubMed PMID: 24753856

358: Gill J. The effects of moderate alcohol consumption on female hormone levels and reproductive function. Alcohol Alcohol. 2000 Sep-Oct;35(5):417-23. PubMed PMID: 11022013

359: Nyberg S, Andersson A, Zingmark E, Wahlström G, Bäckström T, Sundström-Poromaa I. The effect of a low dose of alcohol on allopregnanolone serum concentrations across the menstrual cycle in women with severe premenstrual syndrome and controls. Psychoneuroendocrinology. 2005 Oct;30(9):892-901. PubMed PMID: 15979810

360: Ritz MF, Schmidt P, Mendelowitsch A. 17beta-estradiol effect on the extracellular concentration of amino acids in the glutamate excitotoxicity model in the rat. Neurochem Res. 2002 Dec;27(12):1677-83. PubMed PMID: 12515322

361: Jiang JG, Huang XJ, Chen J, Lin QS. Comparison of the sedative and hypnotic effects of flavonoids, saponins, and polysaccharides extracted from Semen Ziziphus jujube. Nat Prod Res. 2007 Apr;21(4):310-20. PubMed PMID: 17479419

362: Koetter U, Barrett M, Lacher S, Abdelrahman A, Dolnick D. Interactions of Magnolia and Ziziphus extracts with selected central nervous system receptors. J Ethnopharmacol. 2009 Jul 30;124(3):421-5. PubMed PMID: 19505549

363: Personal communication with Dr. Jerilynn Prior

364: Friess E, Tagaya H, Trachsel L, Holsboer F, Rupprecht R. Progesterone-induced changes in sleep in male subjects. Am J Physiol. 1997 May;272(5 Pt 1):E885-91. PubMed PMID: 9176190

365: Schüssler P, Kluge M, Yassouridis A, Dresler M, Held K, Zihl J, et al. Progesterone reduces wakefulness in sleep EEG and has no effect on cognition in healthy postmenopausal women. Psychoneuroendocrinology. 2008 Sep;33(8):1124-31. PubMed PMID: 18676087

366: Prior JC. Progesterone for Symptomatic Perimenopause Treatment - Progesterone politics, physiology and potential for perimenopause. Facts Views Vis Obgyn. 2011;3(2):109-20. PubMed PMID: 24753856

367: Massoudi MS, Meilahn EN, Orchard TJ, Foley TP Jr, Kuller LH, Costantino JP, et al. Prevalence of thyroid antibodies among healthy middle-aged women. Findings from the thyroid study in healthy women. Ann Epidemiol. 1995 May;5(3):229-33. PubMed PMID: 7606312

368: Sathi P, Kalyan S, Hitchcock CL, Pudek M, Prior JC. Progesterone therapy increases free thyroxine levels--data from a randomized placebo-controlled 12-week hot flush trial. Clin Endocrinol (Oxf). 2013 Aug;79(2):282-7. PubMed PMID: 23252963

369: http://www.cemcor.ubc.ca/resources/healthcare-providers-managing-menorrhagia-without-surgery

370: Longinotti MK, Jacobson GF, Hung YY, Learman LA. Probability of hysterectomy after endometrial ablation. Obstet Gynecol. 2008 Dec;112(6):1214-20. PubMed PMID: 19037028

371: McCausland AM, McCausland VM. Frequency of symptomatic cornual hematometra and postablation tubal sterilization syndrome after total rollerball endometrial ablation: a 10-year follow-up. Am J Obstet Gynecol. 2002 Jun;186(6):1274-80; discussion 1280-3. PubMed PMID: 12066109

372: Altman D, Falconer C, Cnattingius S, Granath F. Pelvic organ prolapse surgery following hysterectomy on benign indications. Am J Obstet Gynecol. 2008 May;198(5):572.e1-6. PubMed PMID: 18355787

373: Calcium-d-glucarate monograph. Altern Med Rev 2002;7(4):336-339

374: Prior JC. Progesterone for Symptomatic Perimenopause Treatment - Progesterone politics, physiology and potential for perimenopause. Facts Views Vis Obgyn. 2011;3(2):109-20. PubMed PMID: 24753856

375: Labrie F. All sex steroids are made intracellularly in peripheral tissues by the mechanisms of intracrinology after menopause. J Steroid Biochem Mol Biol. 2015 Jan;145:133-8. PubMed PMID: 24923731

376: Beck-Peccoz P, Persani L. Premature ovarian failure. Orphanet J Rare Dis. 2006 Apr 6;1:9. PubMed PMID: 16722528

377: Komorowska B. Autoimmune premature ovarian failure. Prz Menopauzalny. 2016 Dec;15(4):210-214. PubMed PMID: 28250725

378: Rivera CM, Grossardt BR, Rhodes DJ, Brown RD Jr, Roger VL, Melton LJ 3rd, et al. Increased cardiovascular mortality after early bilateral oophorectomy. Menopause. 2009 Jan-Feb;16(1):15-23. PubMed PMID: 19034050

379: Rocca WA, Bower JH, Maraganore DM, Ahlskog JE, Grossardt BR, de Andrade

M, et al. Increased risk of cognitive impairment or dementia in women who underwent oophorectomy before menopause. Neurology. 2007 Sep 11;69(11):1074-83. PubMed PMID: 17761551

380: Hreshchyshyn MM, Hopkins A, Zylstra S, Anbar M. Effects of natural menopause, hysterectomy, and oophorectomy on lumbar spine and femoral neck bone densities. Obstet Gynecol. 1988 Oct;72(4):631-8. PubMed PMID: 3419740

381: Segelman J, Lindström L, Frisell J, Lu Y. Population-based analysis of colorectal cancer risk after oophorectomy. Br J Surg. 2016 Jun;103(7):908-15. PubMed PMID: 27115862

382: Castelo-Branco C, Palacios S, Combalia J, Ferrer M, Traveria G. Risk of hypoactive sexual desire disorder and associated factors in a cohort of oophorectomized women. Climacteric. 2009 Dec;12(6):525-32. PubMed PMID: 19905904

383: Shuster LT, Gostout BS, Grossardt BR, Rocca WA. Prophylactic oophorectomy in premenopausal women and long-term health. Menopause Int. 2008 Sep;14(3):111-6. PubMed PMID: 18714076

384: Avis NE, Crawford SL, Greendale G, Bromberger JT, Everson-Rose SA, Gold EB, et al. Duration of menopausal vasomotor symptoms over the menopause transition. JAMA Intern Med. 2015 Apr;175(4):531-9. PubMed PMID: 25686030

385: Hitchcock CL, Prior JC. Oral micronized progesterone for vasomotor symptoms--a placebo-controlled randomized trial in healthy postmenopausal women. Menopause. 2012 Aug;19(8):886-93. PubMed PMID: 22453200

386: Labrie F, Archer D, Bouchard C, Fortier M, Cusan L, Gomez JL, et al. Intravaginal dehydroepiandrosterone (Prasterone), a physiological and highly efficient treatment of vaginal atrophy. Menopause. 2009 Sep-Oct;16(5):907-22. PubMed PMID: 19436225

387: Larmo PS, Yang B, Hyssälä J, Kallio HP, Erkkola R. Effects of sea buckthorn oil intake on vaginal atrophy in postmenopausal women: a randomized, double-blind, placebo-controlled study. Maturitas. 2014 Nov;79(3):316-21. PubMed PMID: 25104582

388: Gupte AA, Pownall HJ, Hamilton DJ. Estrogen: an emerging regulator of insulin action and mitochondrial function. J Diabetes Res. 2015;2015:916585. PubMed PMID: 25883987

389: Finkelstein JS, Brockwell SE, Mehta V, Greendale GA, Sowers MR, Ettinger B, et al. Bone mineral density changes during the menopause transition in a multiethnic cohort of women. J Clin Endocrinol Metab. 2008 Mar;93(3):861-8. PubMed PMID: 18160467

390: Rizzoli R, Cooper C, Reginster JY, Abrahamsen B, Adachi JD, Brandi ML, et al. Antidepressant medications and osteoporosis. Bone. 2012 Sep;51(3):606-13. PubMed PMID: 22659406

391: http://www.npr.org/2009/12/21/121609815/how-a-bone-disease-grew-to-fit-the-prescription

392: Järvinen TL, Michaëlsson K, Jokihaara J, Collins GS, Perry TL, Mintzes B, et al. Overdiagnosis of bone fragility in the quest to prevent hip fracture. BMJ. 2015 May 26;350:h2088. PubMed PMID: 26013536

393: Seifert-Klauss, V., Prior, J.C. Progesterone and bone: actions promoting bone health in women. J Osteoporos. 2010;2010:845180

394: Mohammed H, Russell IA, Stark R, Rueda OM, Hickey TE, Tarulli GA, et al. Progesterone receptor modulates ERα action in breast cancer. Nature. 2015 Jul 16;523(7560):313-7. PubMed PMID: 26153859

395: Thomas P, Pang Y. Protective actions of progesterone in the cardiovascular system: potential role of membrane progesterone receptors (mPRs) in mediating rapid effects. Steroids. 2013 Jun;78(6):583-8. PubMed PMID: 23357432

396: Campbell KE, Dennerstein L, Finch S, Szoeke CE. Impact of menopausal status on negative mood and depressive symptoms in a longitudinal sample spanning 20 years. Menopause. 2017 May;24(5):490-496. PubMed PMID: 27922940

397: http://www.ewg.org/research/dirty-dozen-list-endocrine-disruptors

398: Bruner-Tran KL, Gnecco J, Ding T, Glore DR, Pensabene V, Osteen KG. Exposure to the environmental endocrine disruptor TCDD and human reproductive dysfunction: Translating lessons from murine models. Reprod Toxicol. 2017 Mar;68:59-71. PubMed PMID: 27423904

399: Morgenstern R, Whyatt RM, Insel BJ, Calafat AM, Liu X, Rauh VA, et al. Phthalates and thyroid function in preschool age children: Sex specific associations. Environ Int. 2017 May 26;106:11-18. PubMed PMID: 28554096

400: https://www.ncbi.nlm.nih.gov/pmc/articles/PMC3988285/

401: Takeuchi T, Tsutsumi O, Ikezuki Y, Takai Y, Taketani Y. Positive relationship between androgen and the endocrine disruptor, bisphenol A, in normal women and women with ovarian dysfunction. Endocr J. 2004 Apr;51(2):165-9. PubMed PMID: 15118266

402: Palioura E, Diamanti-Kandarakis E. Polycystic ovary syndrome (PCOS) and endocrine disrupting chemicals (EDCs). Rev Endocr Metab Disord. 2015 Dec;16(4):365-71. PubMed PMID: 26825073

403: Grindler NM, Allsworth JE, Macones GA, Kannan K, Roehl KA, Cooper AR. Persistent organic pollutants and early menopause in U.S. women. PLoS One. 2015;10(1):e0116057. PubMed PMID: 25629726

404: http://www.acog.org/About-ACOG/ACOG-Departments/Health-Care-for-Underserved-Women/Toxic-Environmental-Agents

405: Gore AC, Chappell VA, Fenton SE, Flaws JA, Nadal A, Prins GS, et al. Executive Summary to EDC-2: The Endocrine Society's Second Scientific Statement on Endocrine-Disrupting Chemicals. Endocr Rev. 2015 Dec;36(6):593-602. PubMed PMID: 26414233

406: Sinha R, Sinha I, Calcagnotto A, Trushin N, Haley JS, Schell TD, et al. Oral supplementation with liposomal glutathione elevates body stores of glutathione and markers of immune function. Eur J Clin Nutr. 2018 Jan;72(1):105-111. PubMed PMID: 28853742

407: El-Ashmawy IM, Ashry KM, El-Nahas AF, Salama OM. Protection by turmeric and myrrh against liver oxidative damage and genotoxicity induced by lead acetate in mice. Basic Clin Pharmacol Toxicol. 2006 Jan;98(1):32-7. PubMed PMID: 16433888

408: Berggren A, Lazou Ahrén I, Larsson N, Önning G. Randomised, double-blind and placebo-controlled study using new probiotic lactobacilli for strengthening the body immune defence against viral infections. Eur J Nutr. 2011 Apr;50(3):203-10. PubMed PMID: 20803023

409: Finamore A, Massimi M, Conti Devirgiliis L, Mengheri E. Zinc deficiency induces membrane barrier damage and increases neutrophil transmigration in Caco-2 cells. J Nutr. 2008 Sep;138(9):1664-70. PubMed PMID: 18716167

410: Orlando A, Linsalata M, Notarnicola M, Tutino V, Russo F. Lactobacillus GG restoration of the gliadin induced epithelial barrier disruption: the role of cellular polyamines. BMC Microbiol. 2014 Jan 31;14:19. PubMed PMID: 24483336

411: Patil AD. Link between hypothyroidism and small intestinal bacterial overgrowth. Indian J Endocrinol Metab. 2014 May;18(3):307-9. PubMed PMID: 24944923

412: Chedid V, Dhalla S, Clarke JO, Roland BC, Dunbar KB, Koh J, et al. Herbal therapy is equivalent to rifaximin for the treatment of small intestinal bacterial overgrowth. Glob Adv Health Med. 2014 May;3(3):16-24. PubMed PMID: 24891990

413: Gu L, Li N, Gong J, Li Q, Zhu W, Li J. Berberine ameliorates intestinal epithelial tight-junction damage and down-regulates myosin light chain kinase pathways in a mouse model of endotoxinemia. J Infect Dis. 2011 Jun 1;203(11):1602-12. PubMed PMID: 21592990

414: Anukam K, Osazuwa E, Ahonkhai I, Ngwu M, Osemene G, Bruce AW, et al. Augmentation of antimicrobial metronidazole therapy of bacterial vaginosis with oral probiotic Lactobacillus rhamnosus GR-1 and Lactobacillus reuteri RC-14: randomized, double-blind, placebo controlled trial. Microbes Infect. 2006 May;8(6):1450-4. PubMed PMID: 16697231

415: Achilles SL, Austin MN, Meyn LA, Mhlanga F, Chirenje ZM, Hillier SL. Impact of contraceptive initiation on vaginal microbiota. Am J Obstet Gynecol. 2018 Jun;218(6):622.e1-622.e10. PubMed PMID: 29505773

416: AACE Medical Guidelines for Clinical Practice for the Evaluation and Treatment of Hyperthyroidism and Hypothyroidism, Endocrine Practice, Vol. 8, No. 6, Nov/Dec 2002.

417: Chen S, Zhou X, Zhu H, Yang H, Gong F, Wang L, et al. Preconception TSH and pregnancy outcomes: a population-based cohort study in 184 611 women. Clin Endocrinol (Oxf). 2017 Jun;86(6):816-824. PubMed PMID: 28295470

418: Wiersinga WM. Paradigm shifts in thyroid hormone replacement therapies for hypothyroidism. Nat Rev Endocrinol. 2014 Mar;10(3):164-74. PubMed PMID: 24419358

419: Wartofsky L. Combination L-T3 and L-T4 therapy for hypothyroidism. Curr Opin Endocrinol Diabetes Obes. 2013 Oct;20(5):460-6. PubMed PMID: 23974776

420: Hoang TD, Olsen CH, Mai VQ, Clyde PW, Shakir MK. Desiccated thyroid extract compared with levothyroxine in the treatment of hypothyroidism: a randomized, double-blind, crossover study. J Clin Endocrinol Metab. 2013 May;98(5):1982-90. PubMed PMID: 23539727

421: Sategna-Guidetti C, Volta U, Ciacci C, Usai P, Carlino A, De Franceschi L, et al. Prevalence of thyroid disorders in untreated adult celiac disease patients and effect of gluten withdrawal: an Italian multicenter study. Am J Gastroenterol. 2001 Mar;96(3):751-7. PubMed PMID: 11280546

422: Janegova A, Janega P, Rychly B, Kuracinova K, Babal P. The role of Epstein-Barr virus infection in the development of autoimmune thyroid diseases. Endokrynol Pol. 2015;66(2):132-6. PubMed PMID: 25931043

423: Gannon JM, Forrest PE, Roy Chengappa KN. Subtle changes in thyroid indices during a placebo-controlled study of an extract of Withania somnifera in persons with bipolar disorder. J Ayurveda Integr Med. 2014 Oct-Dec;5(4):241-5. PubMed PMID: 25624699

424: Mazokopakis EE, Papadakis JA, Papadomanolaki MG, Batistakis AG, Giannakopoulos TG, Protopapadakis EE, et al. Effects of 12 months treatment with L-selenomethionine on serum anti-TPO Levels in Patients with Hashimoto's thyroiditis. Thyroid. 2007 Jul;17(7):609-12. PubMed PMID: 17696828

425: Pirola I, Gandossi E, Agosti B, Delbarba A, Cappelli C. Selenium supplementation could restore euthyroidism in subclinical hypothyroid patients with autoimmune thyroiditis. Endokrynol Pol. 2016;67(6):567-571. PubMed PMID: 28042649

426: http://www.americanhairloss.org/types_of_hair_loss/effluviums.asp

427: Murata K, Noguchi K, Kondo M, Onishi M, Watanabe N, Okamura K, et al. Promotion of hair growth by Rosmarinus officinalis leaf extract. Phytother Res. 2013 Feb;27(2):212-7. PubMed PMID: 22517595

428: Fischer TW, Burmeister G, Schmidt HW, Elsner P. Melatonin increases anagen hair rate in women with androgenetic alopecia or diffuse alopecia: results of a pilot randomized controlled trial. Br J Dermatol. 2004 Feb;150(2):341-5. PubMed PMID: 14996107

429: Personal communication with Dr. Jerilynn Prior.

INDEX

ACKNOWLEDGMENTS

Thanks again to all my patients who entrusted me with their period problems. You helped me to learn what works for period health and also to *trust in* what works.

Thanks to the readers of my blog and first book. Your comments and questions helped me to better understand and communicate the ideas and concepts I am putting forward.

Thanks to the faculty at the Canadian College of Naturopathic Medicine who set me on the road to this work more than twenty years ago.

A big thanks to Dr. Jerilynn Prior for your very helpful suggestions and also for your decades of brilliant work in women's health. I don't know where we'd be without you.

Thanks to Daynor Missingham for designing the cover.

Thanks to my mother, Ginny Grinevitch, for your tireless help with the manuscript.

And finally, thanks to my husband, Jonathan Briden, for *everything*. Thanks for your incredible behind the scenes work of turning a manuscript into a book. And thanks for your support and care of me while I toiled away at another book.

CPSIA information can be obtained
at www.ICGtesting.com
Printed in the USA
LVHW040953261020
669802LV00003B/547